Compendium
of
Podiatric
Medicine
and
Surgery
2001

Stephen J. Kominsky, D.P.M., F.A.C.F.A.S.

Editor-in-Chief

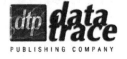

PUBLISHING COMPANY

**Published by
Data Trace Publishing Company
P.O. Box 1239
Brooklandville, Maryland 21022
410-494-4994 Fax: 410-494-0515**

ISBN 1-57400-062-4

Library of Congress Cataloging-in-Publication Data

Compendium of podiatric medicine and surgery 2000/Stephen J. Kominsky,
editor-in-chief.
  p.; cm.
  Reviews of published articles followed by a commentary by the chapter
  editor.
  Includes indexes.
  ISBN 1-57400-057-8
    1. Foot—Diseases—Surgery—Abstracts. 2. Podiatry—Abstracts.
    3. Surgery, Operative—Abstracts. I. Kominsky, Stephen J.
    [DNLM: 1. Foot Diseases. 2. Leg. 3. Skin Diseases. 4. Surgical
    Procedures, Operative. WE 880 C7362 2000]
  RD563. C6535 2000
  617.5'85—dc21
                                                            00-064537

Contents

Editors

Editor-in-Chief

Stephen J. Kominsky, D.P.M., F.A.C.F.A.S.
Diplomate, American Board of Foot and Ankle Surgery; Board Certified in
Foot and Ankle Surgery; Residency Director, Director of Podiatric Medical
Education, Washington Hospital Center, Washington, D.C.

Chapter Editors

Kenneth Bloom, D.P.M., A.A.C.F.A.S.
Private Practice, Huntersville, North Carolina
Thomas J. Chang, D.P.M.
Private Practice, Santa Rosa, and San Francisco, California; Clinical
Professor and Immediate Past Chairman, Department of Podiatric Surgery,
California College of Podiatric Medicine; Director of PSR-24, HealthSouth
Surgery Center, San Francisco; Faculty, The Podiatry Institute
Gary L. Dockery, D.P.M., F.A.C.F.A.S.
Founder and Scientific Chariman, Northwest Podiatric Foundation for
Education and Research, USA; Diplomate, American Board of Podiatric
Surgery; Diplomate, American Board of Podiatric Orthopedics and Primary
Podiatric Medicine; Fellow, American Society of Podiatric Dermatology;
Fellow, American College of Foot and Ankle Surgeons; Fellow, Amer-
ican College of Foot and Ankle Pediatrics; Fellow, American College of
Foot and Ankle Orthopedics and Medicine; Author: *Cutaneous Disorders of
the Lower Extremity*, W.B. Saunders Publishing Co., 1997; Author: *Color
Atlas of Foot & Ankle Dermatology*, Lippincott-Raven Publishing Co., 1999;
Private Practice, Seattle, Washington
John M. Giurini, D.P.M., F.A.C.F.A.S.
Assistant Professor in Surgery, Harvard Medical School, Boston; Chief,
Division of Podiatry, Beth Israel Deaconess Medical Center, Boston; Co-
Director, Joslin-BI Deaconess Diabetic Foot Center, Boston; Diplomate,
American Board of Podiatric Surgery; Fellow, American College of Foot
and Ankle Surgeons
Vincent J. Hetherington, D.P.M.
Vice President and Dean of Academic Affairs; Professor, Department of
Surgery, Ohio College of Podiatric Medicine
Richard M. Jay, D.P.M., F.A.C.F.A.S., F.A.C.F.A.O.
Director of Foot and Ankle Surgical Residency Program, The Graduate
Hospital, Philadelphia; Professor and Director, Pediatric Foot and Ankle

Orthopedics, Foot and Ankle Institute, Temple University School of Podiatric Medicine, Philadelphia, Pennsylvania

Gary Peter Jolly, D.P.M.
Chief of Podiatric Surgery and Director of PGY4 Fellowship in Reconstructive Foot Surgery, New Britain General Hospital, New Britain, Connecticut; Medical Director for the Center for Reconstructive Foot Surgery, P.C., Plainville, Connecticut; Clinical Professor of Surgery, California College of Podiatric Medicine; Clinical Professor of Surgery, College of Podiatric Medicine and Surgery, University of Des Moines

Stacey A. Paukovitz, D.P.M.
Private Practice, Washington, D.C.

Stephen M. Pribut, D.P.M., F.A.C.F.A.S., F.A.A.P.S.M., F.A.C.F.A.O.M.
Clinical Assistant Professor of Surgery, George Washington University Medical Center, Washington, D.C.; Diplomate, American Board of Podiatric Surgery; Diplomate, American Board of Podiatric Orthopedics and Primary Podiatric Medicine; Fellow, American College of Foot and Ankle Surgeons; Fellow, American Academy of Podiatric Sports Medicine; Fellow, American College of Foot and Ankle Orthopedics and Medicine; Member, American College of Sports Medicine; Member, American Association for the Advancement of Science; Member, New York Academy of Sciences; Private Practice, Washington, D.C.

Michael Rupp, D.P.M., M.D.
Vice Chairman, Department of Pathology, Chambersburg Hospital, Chambersburg, Pennsylvania

Barry Saffran, D.P.M., F.A.C.F.A.S.
Assistant Clinical Professor of Healthcare Sciences, George Washington University School of Medicine; Surgical Residency Training Committee, Northern Virginia Podiatric Residency Program; Private Practice, Fairfax, Virginia

G. Adam Shapiro, D.P.M., A.A.C.F.A.S.
Private Practice, Huntersville and Mooresville, North Carolina; Podiatric Advisor, Lake Norman Regional Medical Center

Stephen H. Silvani, D.P.M.
Past Chief of Podiatric Surgery, Kaiser Foundation Hospital, Walnut Creek, California; Diplomate, American Board of Podiatric Surgery; Fellow, American College of Foot Surgeons; Podiatric Advisor, Northwest Podiatric Foundation; President, American College of Foot and Ankle Pediatrics

Stuart Tessler, D.P.M., F.A.C.F.A.S.
Private Practice, Charleston, South Carolina

Ronald L. Valmassy, D.P.M.
Professor and Former Chairman, Division of Podiatric Biomechanics, California College of Podiatric Medicine; Staff Podiatrist, Center of

Sports Medicine, Saint Francis Hospital, San Francisco; Diplomate, American Board of Podiatric Orthopedics and Primary Podiatric Medicine; Editor: *Clinical Biomechanics of the Lower Extremities*, Mosby Yearbook, 1995

John H. Walter, Jr., D.P.M., M.S., F.A.C.F.A.S., F.A.C.F.A.O.M.

Diplomate, American Board of Podiatric Surgery; Diplomate, American Board of Podiatric Orthopedics and Podiatric Primary Care; Board of Directors, American College of Foot and Ankle Orthopedics and Medicine; Chairman and Professor, Department of Podiatric Orthopedics and Medicine; Course Director, Traumatology of Foot and Ankle; Faculty, Department of Surgery; Residency Director, TUSPM Podiatric Orthopedics Residency Program, Temple University School of Podiatric Medicine, Philadelphia, Pennsylvania

Ian Yu, D.P.M.

Private Practice, Vancouver, British Columbia; Courtesy Staff, Langley Memorial Hospital, Langley, British Columbia; Courtesy Staff, Richmond General Hospital, Richmond, British Columbia

Contributors

California College of Podiatric Medicine

Surgical Residents
Ali Ghamgosar, D.P.M.
Thomas C. Melillo, D.P.M.
David Tran, D.P.M.
Oliver Wang, D.P.M.

Students
David Carmack
Keenan Carriero
Ricky Childers
Dean Clement
David R. Collman (resident/student abstract coordinator)
John Michael Dawson
Amy Duckworth
Matt Garrison
Gregory Grant
Spencer B. Heninger
Brynn Hoffman
Ciaran Jacka
Gitanjali H. Jhala
Tyler Marshall
Farshid Nejad
Sandeep Patel
Quinton Solomon
Leslie T. Rowe
Kirsten E. Van Voris
Eugene Zarutsky

Journals Represented

Journals represented in this *Compendium* are listed below:

Acta Cytologica
American Journal of Clinical Oncology
American Journal of Dermatopathology
American Journal of Roentgenology
Annals of Plastic Surgery
Annals of Vascular Surgery
Archives of Dermatology
Archives of Family Medicine
Archives of Physical Medicine and Rehabilitation
Archives of Surgery
Arthritis Research
Biomaterials 21
British Journal of Dermatology
Canadian Journal of Surgery
Canadian Medical Association Journal
Cancer
Cleveland Clinic Journal of Medicine
Clinical Biomechanics (Bristol, Avon)
Clinical and Experimental Dermatology
Clinical Journal of Sports Medicine
Cinical Orthopaedics and Related Research
Clinics in Podiatric Medicine and Surgery
Connecticut Medicine
Dermatologic Surgery
Diabetes Care
Diabetes/Metabolism Research and Reviews
Diabetic Medicine
Drugs and Aging
Electromyography & Clinical Neurophysiology
Emergency Medical Services
European Journal of Dermatology

European Journal of Nuclear Medicine
European Journal of Surgical Oncology
European Journal of Vascular and Endovascular Surgery
Foot & Ankle International
Foot & Ankle Surgery
Gait & Posture
Hong Kong Medical Journal
Injury
International Angiology
International Journal of Dermatology
International Orthopaedics
Japanese Journal of Clinical Oncology
Journal of the American Academy of Dermatology
Journal of the American Academy of Orthopaedic Surgeons
Journal of the American Geriatrics Society
Journal of the American Podiatric Medical Association
Journal of Arthroscopic & Related Surgery
Journal of Biomechanics
Journal of Bone and Joint Surgery (American Volume)
Journal of Bone and Joint Surgery (British Volume)
Journal of Bone and Mineral Research
Journal of Cardiovascular Surgery (Torino)
Journal of Clinical Ultrasound
Journal of Computer Assisted Tomography
Journal of Emergency Medical Services
Journal of Family Practice
Journal of Foot & Ankle Surgery
Journal of the National Medical Association
Journal of Orthopaedic and Sports Physical Therapy
Journal of Pathology
Journal of Pediatric Orthopaedics
Journal of Vascular Surgery
Journal of Wound Care
Knee Surgery, Sports Traumatology, Arthroscopy
Medicine and Science in Sports and Exercise
Neurology

Nursing Clinics of North America
Orthopedic Clinics of North America
Ostomy/Wound Management
Pediatric Emergency Care
Pediatrics
Physical Medicine and Rehabilitation Clinics of North America
Plastic and Reconstructive Surgery
QJM
Radiographics
Rheumatology (Oxford)
Scandinavian Journal of Medicine and Science in Sports
Scandinavian Journal of Rehabilitation Medicine
Sports Medicine
Sportverletz Sportschaden
Strahlentherapie und Onkologie
Surgery
The Foot
Tissue Engineering
Transplantation
Ultrasound in Medicine & Biology
Wound Repair & Regeneration

Introduction

This edition of the *Compendium* marks a change in direction from last year's edition. The chapter editors have taken a more active role in the selection process of the articles chosen for this book. We have an outstanding collection of physicians with years of experience. Many of the chapter editors are well published on various topics and have established themselves as leaders in our profession. As such, I felt that it would be advantageous to the success of this book to afford them the opportunity to read and select the articles that would be appropriate for their respective chapters.

You, the subscriber of this series, have told us by your support for this book that you believe this format works for you and is providing you with an easy-to-read text. This book is filled with material and information that is pertinent to what you do every day in your practice.

We will continue to strive to be out front with what is new and current in our field. We will always provide this material to you in a format that you can easily access.

Stephen J. Kominsky, D.P.M., F.A.C.F.A.S.
Editor-in-Chief

1 Vascular Disorders Affecting the Lower Extremity

BARRY SAFFRAN, D.P.M.

Arrest of the Growth Plate After Arterial Cannulation in Infancy

Macnicol MF, Anagnostopoulos J (Princess Margaret Rose Orthopaedic Hospital and the Royal Hospital for Sick Children, Edinburgh, Scotland)
J Bone Joint Surg 82-B(2):172–175, 2000

Background—Newborns who suffer from cardiovascular abnormalities often have to undergo arterial cannulation. This procedure has recognized risks of thrombosis or stenosis of the vessel, compartment syndrome, skin breakdown due to the extravasation of infused fluids, infection, scarring, and impaired growth of bones due to ischemia of the limb. Ischemia of the limb and consequent limb shortening is reported to be present in 2–33% of patients who endured arterial cannulation in the neonatal period.

Cases—Seven cases of children who had arterial cannulation during the neonatal period were reviewed. The cannulation site was the femoral artery in four of the patients, the iliofemoral artery in one patient, the radial artery in one, and the brachial artery in one. The shortening that was observed in the femoral artery cannulation was seen in both the femur and tibia in three of the cases. A range 0.5–1.2 cm shortening of the femur and a range of 0.5–0.6 cm in the tibia was reported. One case only exhibited femur shortening of 1.2 cm. In the case in which the iliofemoral artery was used, the patient developed coxa valga. The radial artery affected the radius with 3.0 cm of shortening, and the brachial artery affected the humerus (1.2 cm), radius (8.0 cm), and ulna (5.0 cm).

Conclusion—Cannulation of the radial and brachial arteries should be avoided during the neonatal period. In the event of cannulation and limb ischemia, the child should be anticoagulated and carefully followed to

1

observe skeletal changes, in order to intervene before a limb discrepancy develops. — *T. Marshall*

◆ Pediatric patients who have undergone femoral arterial cannulation, secondary to cardiac abnormalities, should be carefully monitored for limb-length irregularities. Impaired growth due to the above has been well recognized for years. While this study clearly addresses growth cessation in the femur and tibia, it would be interesting to look for problems in the foot. Perhaps this is just a phenomenon of long bones. A high index of suspicion in children with congenital cardiac anomalies would prompt us to consider this cause of a developing limb-length problem or even an occult vascular problem presenting as a lower extremity pain in a young patient. — *B. Saffran, D.P.M.*

The Effects of Successful Intervention on Quality of Life in Patients with Varying Degrees of Lower-Limb Ischaemia

Klevsgård R, Hallberg IR, Risberg B, Thomsen MB (Lund University; Växjö University; Sahlgrenska University Hospital, Göteborg; County Hospital, Kristianstad, Sweden)
Eur J Vasc Endovasc Surg 19(3):238–245, 2000

Introduction—There are an increasing number of lower limb ischemia who undergo arterial reconstruction and percutaneous transluminal angioplasty (PTA) patients with primarily to provide symptomatic relief and help improve quality of life. It is unknown whether therapy impacts the patients' quality of life or if the effect is only related to the disease's severity. Other influential factors could be their sense of coherence (SOC), which if strong, can help manage life's stressors. Thus successful intervention should be based on lower limb perfusion, degree of ischemia, type of intervention, and the patient's SOC. This study assessed the quality of life 6 months after successful intervention (surgical or PTA) in patients with varying degrees of lower limb ischemia and compared them to healthy controls.

Materials and Methods—One hundred and twelve patients with varying degrees of ischemia were studied after 6 months status post successful revascularization (ankle-brachial pressure index, ABPI $\geq$ 0.15). Four treatments groups were utilized: PTA, surgical bypass graft, patch, and surgical thromboendarterectomy. A medical history and physical were done on admission and 6 months after intervention. The control group consisted of 102 healthy individuals with no diagnosed disease, no drug consumption, and normal clinical lab values, blood pressure, and weight. The Nottingham Health Profile (NHP) was utilized to measure quality of life and is designed to determine perceived health problems and their effects on daily activities. Subjects also completed a SOC questionnaire. All data were analyzed using several statistical tests.

Results—There are significant improvements in ABPI for both claudicants and critical ischemia patients and in walking distance for claudicants after intervention. There was no significant difference between the baseline SOC and the 6-month follow-up. The SOC significantly correlated with the total NPH for the entire group. The total NHP was significantly higher for patients than for controls, meaning a lower quality of life in the patients. All health problems improved dramatically for claudicants after either PTA or surgery, but not so for critical ischemia patients who improved significantly in only some of their health problems. There were no significant differences between the subgroups treated with PTA and surgery. After therapy, the NHP scores were similar to the control, but were still significantly higher. Logistic regression analysis yielded both a high sense of coherence and ABPI after therapy which significantly correlated with a low total NHP.

Discussion—The study showed that successful PTA or surgery can improve quality of life after 6 months in certain aspects of daily living within the claudicant group but not as successfully with the critical ischemia patients. The results also yielded that a high SOC and a high ABPI were associated with a high quality of life after intervention. Thus the successful treatment of chronic limb ischemia improved the quality of life significantly.—*F. Nejad*

◆ Most studies evaluate graft patency and mortality, while little attention is paid to the effect on the patient's daily life. As expected, the claudicants fared better than those with critical limb ischemia. The result may be a function of the study period representing only the first 6 months postop or the fact the patient with critical limb ischemia is more compromised secondary to underlying disease. Furthermore, a patient with a strong sense of coherence preop is expected to have an easier recovery and experience a better quality of life.—*B. Saffran, D.P.M.*

Combined Vascular Reconstruction and Free Flap Transfer in Diabetic Arterial Disease

Vermassen FEG, van Landuyt K (University Hospital, Ghent, Belgium)
Diabetes Metab Res Rev 16 (Suppl 1):S33–S36, 2000

Introduction—Diabetic patients with arterial disease may acquire gangrenous lesions of the foot or lower leg which may become so extensive as to expose bones or tendons. In such patients, major amputation is often the only possible treatment, even after attempts to revascularize the limb. However, an amputation is likely to compromise a patient's independence, rehabilitation, ambulation, and overall quality of life. One of the goals of this study was to determine if the proposed technique of combined vascular reconstruction and free tissue transfer could extend the possibility of limb salvage in this patient population.

Methods—The subject group consisted of 45 patients between the ages of 38 and 83 (63 years was the mean age) with peripheral vascular disease of diabetic origin. All patients had extensive gangrenous defects of the foot or lower leg with exposure of bones or tendons that could not be treated by simple wound closure or skin grafting without a more proximal amputation. Thirty-nine of the 45 patients were treated with the combined procedure. The combined procedure involved two teams working simultaneously to perform the arterial reconstruction and free tissue transfer, limiting the mean operating time to 6 hours. Donor muscles were cut to the size of the defect and were covered with a split-thickness skin graft. On average, patients wore a compressive stocking for 6 months to allow for remodeling of the muscle and ambulation began at the 3rd week.

Results—With a mean postoperative hospital stay of 40 days, a total of 39 (87%) patients left the hospital with a full-length limb. Three of the 45 patients died while in the hospital and another three had to undergo amputation as a result of free flap loss. Long-term follow-up ranged from 6 months to 72 months with a mean of 26 months. Combined survival and limb-salvage rate was 84% after 1 year, 77% after 2 years, and 65% after 3 years. Independent ambulation was achieved in 32 of the 39 patients who left the hospital with a full-length limb and these patients were able to resume their regular daily activities.

Conclusion—This combined technique offers several advantages:

1. It provides immediate soft-tissue coverage limiting amputation level and healing time, resulting in early ambulation.
2. The free flap transfer provides additional outflow to the bypass (decrease in peripheral resistance) and a positive effect on bypass patency.
3. The application of healthy, well vascularized tissue limits infection and enhances neovascularization.
4. A full-length limb is preserved.

The authors believe that this combined approach offers a valuable alternative to primary amputation in diabetic patients with extensive ischemic defects. Preservation of a full-length limb facilitates independent ambulation, thus helping to preserve patient independence and quality of life, as well as resulting in a lower overall socioeconomic cost.—*B. Hoffman*

♦ Gangrenous lesions in diabetics often present with concurrent infection. In those individuals, infection control often consists of wound drainage, as well as an ablative procedure before revascularization can be considered. It is essential that care is taken to consider and plan for future reconstruction both before and during resection of infected and necrotic tissue and bone.

Simultaneous revascularization and free flap transfers are best reserved for those cases of gangrene with no associated infection. The definition and discussion of a full-length versus a biomechanically functioning limb warrants further discussion. The hospital mortality (7%) and major medical complication (25%) rate was not low in this study, but the patient population had extensive risk factors. In addition, the mean hospital stay of 40 days raises significant cost concerns. All in all, consideration should be given to this procedure as an adjunctive approach to treating the diabetic dysvascular foot in a center where the appropriate peripheral vascular/plastic-reconstructive services are available and demonstrate interest in diabetic foot care.—*B. Saffran, D.P.M.*

Predictors of Health After Revascularization for Extremity Ischemia

Nackman GB, Horahan K, Banavage A, Ciocca RG, Graham AM (University of Medicine and Dentistry of New Jersey–Robert Wood Johnson Medical School and The Robert Wood Johnson University Hospital, New Brunswick, NJ)
Surgery 128(2):293–300, 2000

Objective—This study was performed to determine the functional health status impact of both inflow and outflow revascularization procedures for lower extremity ischemia.

Methods—The Medical Outcomes Study SF-36 Health Survey was given to 104 patients preoperatively and at intervals postoperatively to determine if outcomes are affected by age, gender, time since procedure, diabetes, indication, and inflow versus outflow procedures.

Results—Patients before an outflow procedure for either claudication or limb-threatening ischemia had decreased general health scores compared to patients with inflow disease. Gender distribution and mean patient age did not differ between inflow and outflow groups. There were no significant differences in the incidences of diabetes, end-stage renal failure, hypertension, smoking, chronic obstructed pulmonary disease, or coronary artery disease. There were no significant differences in survival rates between inflow and outflow procedures. The patency of the inflow procedures (100%) was superior to outflow procedures (70%) at 1 year. No noteworthy difference in limb salvage between inflow and outflow procedures was distinguished. Patients who had undergone outflow procedures were more likely to need a cane or walker postoperatively than those with inflow procedures. Patients after outflow procedures did not experience significant improvement in outcome scores. Only inflow procedures were related to improved functional health.

Conclusion—The functional outcome for patients after outflow revascularization procedures for lower extremity ischemia is worse than the outcome after those who go through the inflow procedures. Other factors such as diabetes and the indication for the procedure are also significant predictors of functional health. Insight into the patient's functional health may prove crucial in deciding among different therapeutic options.—*J.M. Dawson*

♦ This study looked at the differences between inflow (suprainguinal) and outflow (infrainguinal) lower extremity bypass. As expected, those individuals requiring outflow procedures for claudicating or limb-threatening ischemia had lower general health scores and did not demonstrate improved outcome scores postoperatively. We are well aware of the high incidence of associated cardiovascular and cerebrovascular disease in these patients. Diabetes also affected the functional outcome of these patients.—*B. Saffran, D.P.M.*

Improving Walking Ability and Ankle Brachial Pressure Indices in Symptomatic Peripheral Vascular Disease with Intermittent Pneumatic Foot Compression: A Prospective Controlled Study with One-Year Follow-up

Delis KT, Nicolaides AN, Wolfe JHN, Stansby G (Imperial College School of Medicine, St. Mary's Hospital, London, UK)
J Vasc Surg 31(4):650–651, 2000

Purpose—Using a mechanical pneumatic pump applied firmly to the foot facilitates artery leg inflow. It is suggested that the application of intermittent pneumatic foot compression (IPC_{foot}) 2–3 times a day by the patient while at home can alter and improve claudication caused by peripheral vascular disease (PVD), by improving collateral circulation. Delis et al. have set out to determine the effect of IPC_{foot} on the distance a patient can walk without discomfort (claudication distance) and arterial leg flow in patients with intermittent claudication.

Methods—Thirty-seven patients with stable intermittent claudication were admitted to the study. In group 1, 25 patients received the IPC_{foot} 2–3 periods a day with a total duration of >4 hours/day for 4.5 months. Group 2 was used as a control group with a total of 12 patients. IPC_{foot} was delivered with an A-V impulse system with settings of maximum inflation compression, 180 mm Hg; minimum deflation pressure, 0 mm Hg; inflation time, 3 seconds; deflation time, 17 seconds; and rise time <0.2 seconds. Both groups were advised to exercise unsupervised for a minimum of 1 hour/day and received aspirin (75 mg/d). After matching the groups for age, sex, risk factors, claudication distances, and ankle pressures at baseline, the following variables were then measured: the initial claudication distance, the absolute claudication distance, resting ankle index (r-ABI), ABI after exercise (p-eABI), and popliteal artery volume flow. Each measurement was taken at day 0, 2 weeks, and monthly for 5 months, followed by re-examination at 12 months, after which statistical analysis was performed. Results are expressed as median values in interquartile ranges.

Results—Over the 4.5 months, all those in group 1 showed improvement, with no relation to the severity of the baseline pathology. Delis et al. reported a median ICD in group 1 increased by 146% ($p < .001$), from 78 at baseline to 191.5 m; ICD did not significantly increase in group 2; median ACD in group 1 improved by 106% ($p < .001$), from 124 m to 255 m; no significant changes were documented in group 2; median r-ABI in group 1 rose by 18% ($p < .001$), from 0.57 to 0.67; no improvement was noted in group 2; median p-eABI in group 1 rose by 110% ($p < .001$), from 0.21 to 0.44; no changes were noted in group 2; and median popliteal artery volume flow in group 1 improved by 36% ($p < .001$), from 100 mL/min on day 0 to 136 mL/min at month 4.5; peak flows were between month 2 and 3 with no significant changes in artery flow of group 2.

Discussion—Delis et al. recognize a couple of mechanisms that may explain arterial calf inflow enhancement with the use of IPC_{foot}. In no particular order the first idea is that there is an increase of the arteriovenous pressure gradient as the result of the lower limb venous emptying. The second thought is that there may be a production of vasodilating factors such as nitric oxide and prostacyclin which form increased shear stress on the endothelial cells. A further causative factor that should be considered is the delay in the venoarteriolar (V/A) reflex with the decrease in venous pressure after pneumatic foot impulse. When there is a venous pressure increase, a local sympathetic reflex (V/A reflex) occurs, causing precapillary sphincters to contract and peripheral resistance to increase, thus decreasing arterial calf inflow.—*S.B. Heninger*

♦ Improved walking ability was clearly demonstrated in this study, in a patient population with stable intermittent claudication, secondary to the usage of intermittent pneumatic compression. It is interesting that the maximum results were achieved after 3 months of treatment and these results were maintained after 1 year, without any further treatment. Further studies are necessary to determine the ideal treatment time, as well as to evaluate results and consider further treatment beyond the 1-year time frame. In addition, some of the exclusion criteria (i.e., CAD, angina, and IDDM) encompass a large portion of a population that could very well benefit from this modality. If indeed it is shown that exercise is responsible for adverse inflammatory changes, then intermittent foot compression is worthy of significant further study and possible utilization in everyday practice.—*B. Saffran, D.P.M.*

Recombinant Human Platelet-Derived Growth Factor-BB (Becaplermin) for Healing Chronic Lower Extremity Diabetic Ulcers: An Open-Label Clinical Evaluation of Efficacy

Embil JM, Papp K, Sibbald G, Tousignant J, Smiell JM, Wong B, Lau CY, The Canadian Becaplermin Study Group (University of Manitoba, Winnipeg, Manitoba; Probity Medical Research, Waterloo, Ontario; Women's College Hospital, Toronto, Ontario; Hôpital Notre Dame, Montreal, Quebec, Canada; The R.W. Johnson Pharmaceutical Research Institute, Raritan, NJ; Janssen-Ortho Inc., Toronto, Ontario, Canada)

Wound Repair Regen 8(3):162–168, 2000

Introduction—Chronic, nonhealing ulcers are a major cause of the sequelae associated with diabetes mellitus. Approximately 20% of diabetics that develop lower extremity ulcers will require eventual amputation. Wound healing is comprised of inflammatory, proliferation and repair, and remodeling phases that are regulated by various growth factors. Platelet-derived growth factor (PDGF) is the predominant growth factor in this process and is released in all three stages. Becaplermin, a recombinant DNA product, closely mirrors the biological activity of endogenous PDGF-BB by inducing the chemotactic recruitment and proliferation of the cells involved in wound healing. This study was designed to evaluate the efficacy of becaplermin gel in closing and preventing the recurrence of chronic full-thickness lower extremity diabetic ulcers.

Methods—A total of 134 type I and type II diabetes patients with a maximum of two full-thickness lower extremity neuropathic ulcers were included. Palpable pedal pulses and normal noninvasive vascular studies were required. Patients with open lesions investing bone or affecting the plantar arch were excluded, as were those with concomitant diseases, certain medications, impaired renal function, or ulcers of an electrical, chemical, radiation burn, or venous origin. Wound care regimen consisted of sharp debridement, once-daily becaplermin gel application along with nonadherent and moist saline dressings, off-loading, and systemic infection control, if necessary. Biweekly visits were made until complete ulcer healing or 20 weeks, whichever occurred first. Patients were educated on application of the gel product and proper foot care. Efficacy was primarily defined by the number of patients who realized complete wound closure during the 20-week treatment period.

Results—Complete healing of ulcers was achieved in 57.5% of all patients treated with becaplermin gel (mean, 63 days). Significant evidence of wound healing was also evident in many patients who did not attain complete healing. In addition, 46% of the patients who showed ≥50% reduction in ulcer size realized complete closure by week 8. Ulcers recurred in 21% of the healed lesions during the 6-month follow-up period.

Discussion—As compared to previous studies, once-daily dressing changes combined with becaplermin use did not compromise wound healing. Factors associated with higher healing rates included patient compliance, small initial ulcer size, and low wound evaluation scores. The presence of infection, however, was negatively associated with wound healing. Application of becaplermin gel is a safe and effective method for the treatment of lower extremity diabetic neuropathic ulcers when accompanied by infection control, pressure off-loading, and a complete wound care regimen.—*E. Zarutsky*

♦ Becaplermin has been shown to aid in healing lower extremity diabetic ulcerations in several studies referenced in this paper. The study excluded individuals with several concomitant conditions including chronic renal insufficiency, uncontrolled hyperglycemia, and immunosuppressants. It also emphasized a good wound care regimen and proper off-weightbearing, all of which are basic tenants of good wound healing. Good results were achieved using becaplermin via a regimen of once-daily dressing changes. A controlled study is warranted to determine wound healing differences in a regimen of once- versus twice-daily dressing changes.—*B. Saffran, D.P.M.*

Vascular Imaging and Intervention in Peripheral Arteries in the Diabetic Patient

Dyet JF, Nicholson AA, Ettles DFE (Hull Royal Infirmary, Kingston upon Hull, UK)
Diabetes Metab Res Rev 16(Suppl 1):S16–S22, 2000

Introduction—Diabetic patients have a four-time higher chance of developing peripheral vascular disease than do nondiabetic patients. The vessels that are most often affected are the distal superficial femoral, the popliteal, and the proximal crural vessels. This pattern differs from the nondiabetic distribution of peripheral vascular disease, which also makes it harder to treat with current therapies. It is imperative in treating diabetic patients to determine if a patient is suffering from critical limb ischemia or neuropathic pain. The definition of critical limb ischemia is that it either has persistent recurring ischemic rest pain that requires analgesia for more than 2 weeks, with an ankle systolic pressure less than 50 mm Hg and/or a toe pressure of less than 30 mm Hg, or ulceration gangrene of the foot or toes with a ankle systolic pressure of less than 50 mmHg or a toe pressure of less than 30 mmHg. This definition is difficult to obtain in some diabetics because of Monkeberg's medial calcification in the intermediate-size vessels, which necessitate having a more definitive imaging to determine the true blood supply.

Imaging Techniques—

- *Duplex ultrasound*—This radiological imaging records velocity changes and is able to identify stenosis by combining cross-sectional imaging of vessels from the ultrasound and color flow and spectral information from the Doppler component. It has a high degree of sensitivity and specificity and is noninvasive. The assessment of the tibial vessels requires higher technical skill, but when done correctly the results can be superior to angiography. This is the first-line imaging technique in assessment of peripheral vascular disease in a diabetic patient.

- *Magnetic resonance imaging* (two types)—MRI is only capable of determine blood flowing in the vessel, it does not assess the vessel itself. In the event of an occluded vessel, there will be no signal at that point, but it will show flow further distally which could otherwise not be detected. Although MRI has this advantage, it is a time-consuming process.

  1. *2D time-of-flight sequences*—This technique visualizes blood in the arteries only. This technique has a presaturating of the venous inflow so no visualization of blood going to the heart is seen.
  2. *Gadolinium*—This is a rare earth compound that enhances the magnetic effect, thus provides a stronger signal.

- *Helical (spiral) computerized tomography* (CT)—CT can show artifact in a diabetic patient because of the presence of the calcification in the arteries.

- *Angiography*—A contrast agent is injected in the patient to visualize the arterial blood supply. The more recent contrast dyes have a much lower risk of complications and adverse reactions; however, there is still a risk of anaphylaxis and death. In addition, because diabetic patients often have concurrent kidney impairment, this can be a problem with using contrast agents. Patients who manage their diabetes with metformin have an added risk of developing lactic acidosis, especially if they suffer from kidney impairment. This is a second-line imaging technique despite all of its inherent risks and invasiveness.

Interventional Radiological Procedures—

- *Percutaneous transluminal angioplasty* (PTA)—PTA involves passing a guide wire across the stenotic or occluded area of the vessel and then a balloon is inflated to open the vessel. This causes disruption of the plaque and longitudinal splitting of the vessel endothelium, and disruption of the elastic media which all heals, but the patient must be heparinized during the procedure and is put on a lifetime of antiplatelet medication. The best results are found when this procedure is performed in the iliac arteries. Unfortunately, in the superficial femoral arteries there is a lower success rate. It does allow for some patency in critical limb ischemia.

- *Subintimal angioplasty*—Dissection of the arterial wall is achieved above the occlusion and then a balloon is inflated to form a new lumen. This has resulted in a smoother lumen than in those who had PCA, and has been more effective in the crural artery occlusions.

- *Thromobolysis*—Viability of the limb must be assessed for this procedure to be successful. After angiograpy has established the location of the occlusion, a catheter is inserted into the thrombus, then lytic agents are infused along with heparinization. Streptokinase and recombinant tissue plasminogen activator are used. Streptokinase is cheaper but has antigenic properties and a much longer half-life that can lead to side effects. Once serial angiograms have shown the clot to dissipate, balloon PTA or stent can be performed.

- *Endovascular stenting*—This reduces the reoccurrence that is inevitable when balloon PTA has been performed. Stents are also helpful in complications of angioplasty. Stenting is very efficient at the aorto-iliac level, but it has been less successful at the femoro-popliteal and tibial level. This is due in part to the smaller diameter and decreased blood flow volume, which allows for neointimal hyperplasia. Neointimal hyperplasia is formation of a pseudointima that has a large amount of intercellular matrix and on a few smooth muscles.

Conclusion—Although some of these techniques are not as successful in diabetic patients, it is imperative that they still be performed.—*T. Marshall*

♦ Studies dating back to the 1970s have shown that atheromatous disease is four times more common in the diabetic than in the general population. Duplex ultrasound remains the best noninvasive imaging method, as MRI continues to have limitations in its current state. Angiography remains the invasive treatment of choice, with some of the nonionic contrast agents decreasing the renal complications of the procedure. For those patients with renal concerns, it is important to stop metformin 48 hours in advance of an angiographic procedure. Subsequent percutaneous transluminal angioplasty works best in the proximal inflow vessels, despite more recent attempts at usage in the tibial vessels. Perhaps this is an area of promise in the future. Thrombolysis and stent placement function best when used on inflow vessels. Unfortunately, diabetic peripheral vascular disease affects the distal vessels, which precludes usage of some imaging and interventional modalities.—*B. Saffran, D.P.M.*

Reflex Sympathetic Dystrophy Syndrome of the Lower Limbs in a Renal Transplant Patient Treated with Tacrolimus

Mari JM, Martinez Miralles E, Perich X, Lloveras J, Mir M, Iñigo V, Barbosa F, Orfila A, Masramon J (Hospital del Mar, Barcelona, Spain)

Transplantation 70(1):210–211, 2000

Background—Reflex sympathetic dystrophy syndrome (RSDS) is an idiopathic disease that has been described in patients who have received major organ transplants in conjunction with cyclosporine (CsA) immunosuppression therapy. This disease typically affects the distal lower extremity joints causing periarticular bone pain with symmetrical vasomotor changes that may lead to patchy areas of osteoporosis. This article describes a new case of RSDS observed in a renal transplant patient treated with tacrolimus rather than CsA.

Methods and Results—A 49-year-old man received a renal transplant (RT) from a 58-year-old cadaver, with tacrolimus used as the immunosuppressive agent. Several months later, he complained of pain in both knees and ankles. Clinical exam revealed normal mobility with increased skin temperature and change in skin color. Edema was noted around the affected joints. Laboratory tests were relatively normal while bone scintography and MRI showed classic symptoms consistent with RSDS. Several months later the patient was asymptomatic even though there were no appreciable changes in the tacrolimus levels throughout the process.

Conclusion—The cause of RSDS is unknown, but injury to the central or peripheral neural tissue, specifically sympathetic efferent pathways, has been hypothesized. Tacrolimus and CsA are systemic immunosuppressive agents that have been reported to cause significant neurotoxicity. Therefore, these agents may be a risk factor for the development of RSDS in patients undergoing organ transplantation.—*D. Carmack*

♦ The development of reflex sympathetic dystrophy syndrome after solid organ transplantation is well recognized with symptoms primarily affecting the lower limbs. Cyclosporine has been raised as an etiologic agent on multiple occasions, but this is the first case described as a result of tacrolimus. While both agents have been associated with neurotoxicity, there is no known mechanism to induce RSDS. Fortunately, the RSDS symptoms seem to resolve independent of treatment. It would be interesting to study the effect of altering doses of cyclosporine, tacrolimus, and prednisone in an effort to reduce the intensity and duration of RSDS, once it has developed in transplant patients.—*B. Saffran, D.P.M.*

Long-Term Functional Status and Quality of Life After Lower Extremity Revascularization

Holtzman J, Caldwell M, Walvatne C, Kane R (University of Minnesota, Minneapolis, MN)

J Vasc Surg 29(3):395–402, 1999

Objective—The objective of this study was to examine the functional status outcomes and quality of life of patients for up to 7 years after undergoing revascularization at the University of Minnesota Hospital.

Methods—This study is a cross-sectional telephone survey and chart review of patients at the University of Minnesota Hospital. The subjects were patients who underwent their first lower extremity revascularization procedure or a primary amputation for vascular disease between January 1, 1989 and January 31, 1995. These patients had either granted consent or had died. The main outcomes measures were: ability to walk, SF-36 physical function, SF-12, subsequent amputation, and death.

Results—There were 329 subjects who qualified for the study; 166 were living and 163 were deceased. All living patients were surveyed.

Of the patients who qualified, 62.6% had undergone arterial bypass grafting, 36.8% had undergone angioplasty, and 0.6% had undergone atherectomy. The mean age at the time of the qualifying procedure was 63 years. At 7 years from the time of the qualifying procedure, 73% of the patients who were still alive still had the limb that was salvaged. Of those subjects, 63% of the subjects had died by the time the 7-year grace period had ended. All the 166 patients who were still living were surveyed by telephone. Overall, at the follow-up examination, 65% of the patients were walking independently, 43% reported few or no limitations in walking several blocks, and 71% of the patients reported the ability to walk one block with few or no limitations. In a multiple regression analysis of overall physical health, greater patient age and the presence of diabetes were the only factors that were significantly associated with overall physical health which gives a worse SF-36 and a lower physical health rating in the SF-12.

Conclusion—Patients who undergo limb revascularization are likely to keep the salvaged limb for many years and most are able to ambulate independently on it. Since there are underlying disease states present with almost all of these procedures, the overall time that a person will enjoy this benefit is unfortunately somewhat unknown.—*Q. Solomon*

♦ Limb preservation remains the prime goal, whether by angioplasty or bypass. While long-term patency rates are higher with bypass, limb salvage often remains viable after vessel occlusion. Unfortunately, the comorbidities found in these patients are responsible for the high mortality rates in the study period, despite successful limb salvage. This study as well as others presented in this chapter and throughout the literature show better functional outcome (i.e., independent ambulating) post bypass compared to amputation. It remains unclear if this is procedure dependent or rather the fact that the sick patient may not be a bypass candidate and will generally be subject to an amputation. As expected, these patients do not fare as well functionally.—*B. Saffran, D.P.M.*

Peripheral Arterial Disease: Insights from Population Studies of Older Adults

Newman AB (University of Pittsburgh, Pittsburgh, PA)
J Am Geriatr Soc 48(9):1157–1162, 2000

Prevalence of Peripheral Arterial Disease—Several studies have shown the incidence of peripheral arterial disease (PAD) to increase with age. Intermittent claudication (IC) prevalence ranged from 2% to 6% in older adults with greater incidence in men, as diagnosed by pulse palpation and questionnaire. Noninvasive testing, with use of a doppler probe, however, reveals a much higher incidence of the disease. Using an ankle-brachial systolic blood pressure index (ABI) of <0.9 as a cutoff, prevalence in adults aged 55 or older ranges from 12.4% to 24.6% with men being affected twice as much as women until age 85, when both sexes seem to be affected equally.

Symptoms and Disability—Signs and symptoms of PAD other than those classic for IC may mask ischemia of the limb. Signs include decreased lower limb strength, decrease in activity, and difficulty performing mobility tasks. People with diagnosed PAD show a decrease in endurance and gait abnormalities manifested by a slower cadence and smaller steps. Biopsy of the muscle reveals a decrease in the amount of type II fast twitch muscle with demyelination of the nerve.

Overlap Between Peripheral Arterial Disease and Cardiovascular Disease—The incidence of PAD increases with age, irrespective of cardiovascular disease (CVD). A majority (60%) of people with a history of PAD also had a history of myocardial infarction (MI), angina, or stroke. Thus a history absent of CVD does not rule out PAD. Populations with PAD show an increase in carotid wall thickness, carotid stenosis, ECG irregularities, and abnormalities in cardiac wall motion on echocardiography. Silent ischemia is also more prevalent in people with PAD. Due to the systemic nature of atherosclerosis, the presence PAD is strongly associated with CVD and all associated risk factors.

Natural History—Patients diagnosed with PAD show an increase risk and incidence of MI and stroke, in addition to total mortality. Less than 10% will require bypass revascularization and fewer than 5% will eventually have an amputation, whereas 20% will suffer from MI or stroke and total mortality is 30% in the 5 years post detection.

Treatment of PAD Patients—Medical treatment with aspirin, cholesterol-lowering agents, and newer drugs with various methods of action, along with regular exercise, is preferred to surgical treatment.

Reduction of Total CVD Risk—Due to risk factor similarities between CVD and PAD, prevention of CVD should decrease the incidence of PAD. Smoking and diabetes carry a particularly high risk, necessitating aggressive treatment. Treatment, as discussed previously for PAD, with antiplatelet medication, lipid-lowering agents, and aspirin should improve the prognosis.

Summary—Given the increased incidence of PAD, prevention and improved treatment of the disease could significantly improve lower extremity function and increase mobility and independence in the aging population. PAD can be easily detected with ABI measurements, allowing for timely treatment implementation.—*G. Grant*

♦ As podiatric physicians and surgeons, we routinely treat patients with peripheral arterial disease, some with and others without diabetes. Unfortunately, the disease is not localized to the extremities, as these patients are 2–4 times more likely to have associated cardiovascular or cerebrovascular disease. First-line treatment of these patients includes careful management of their smoking and diabetes. Exercise and antiplatelet drugs have a role in the early stages of treatment, while lipid-lowering drugs and ASA may modify cardiovascular disease. Based on the statistics, it is incumbent upon us to refer any patient with newly diagnosed PAD for cardiac evaluation and treatment.—*B. Saffran, D.P.M.*

Survival in Patients with Chronic Lower Extremity Ischemia: A Risk Factor Analysis

Cheng SWK, Ting ACW, Lau H, Wong J (The University of Hong Kong Medical Centre, Queen Mary Hospital, Hong Kong, China)
Ann Vasc Surg 14(2):158–165, 2000

Introduction—Peripheral arterial occlusive disease of the lower extremity (PAOD) is associated with decreased patient survival, as compared with the normal population. These patients typically have cardiovascular and cerebrovascular diseases, in particular, in addition to numerous multisystem disorders. The mortality rate for patients with PAOD is higher than for those with stable coronary heart disease, indicating the presence of risk factors inherent to PAOD.

Methods—A total of 665 consecutive patients presenting with PAOD symptoms were enrolled. Evaluation data consisted of demographic and biochemical risk factors, disease profiles, blood samples, and noninvasive vascular laboratory examination. Follow-up occurred on a regular basis at a dedicated vascular clinic.

Results—A mean age of 71.1 years was recorded for the 401 men (60.3%) and 264 women (39.7%) involved in the study. The follow-up period was between 6 and 90 months (mean, 27.0 months). During this time, 107 patients (16.1%) required a major amputation, and 181 patients (27.2%) died of various causes. Many patients (62.4%) were diagnosed with critical limb-threatening ischemia, a majority (52.9%) suffering from femoropopliteal occlusive disease, and 50.1% presenting with tissue loss. A total of 64 surgical procedures were performed to treat the primary ailment. Survival rates for patients at 1, 3, and 5 years were 86.1%, 71.2%, and 55.8%, respectively (median, 72.2 months). Statistical analysis revealed certain variables associated with a higher rate of mortality including female sex, advanced age (>70 years), smoking, heart disease, renal disease, respiratory disease, stroke, disease category (critical versus non-limb-threatening ischemia), and limb loss. Additionally, advanced age, disease category, ankle-brachial index (<0.5), vascular reconstruction, diabetes mellitus, and renal, cardiac, and respiratory diseases were identified as independent risk factors affecting patient survival.

Discussion—This study revealed that vascular reconstruction might be a worthwhile treatment modality for patients suffering from PAOD. The patients who underwent vascular reconstruction had a better survival rate than those who did not. Though vascular reconstruction leads to successful limb salvage and allows for the return to healthy life, patients are only selected for this procedure based upon their age and the extent of their disease. Those with severe multisystem or incapacitating symptoms are often treated with primary amputation and are not given the option of limb salvage surgery. With better patient education and subsequent early disease detection, timely vascular reconstruction can lead to an increased survival rate in patients with PAOD.—*E. Zarutsky*

♦ The patient population with peripheral arterial occlusive disease, studied from Hong Kong, showed a mortality rate of 32% from cardiovascular and cerebrovascular disease, compared to 70% typically seen from western studies. Respiratory disease accounted for an additional 9%, which is attributed to smoking in the Asian population. Diabetes, on average, was prevalent in 25% of the over-65-year-old population, providing a further significant risk factor.

The overall survival statistics must be carefully examined, as they are deceptive. The University of Hong Kong is the only full-time vascular surgery service on the island. As a result, early intervention is not possible in all cases which is reflected in the greater than 50% of patients presenting with tissue loss. Furthermore, one must realize that the sickest patients cannot tolerate extremity bypass and often undergo primary amputation. The higher mortality statistics are reflected by the greater degree of disease comorbidities in the patient undergoing a less complex surgical procedure.—*B. Saffran, D.P.M.*

The Diabetic Foot: A Global Review

Boulton AJM (Manchester Royal Infirmary, Manchester, UK)
Diabetes Metab Res Rev 16(Suppl 1):S2–S5, 2000

Introduction—There is currently an estimated 150 million people with diabetes mellitus in the world today with the majority of these patients having type 2 diabetes. Approximately 15% of diabetics will develop foot ulcers as a consequence of peripheral neuropathy and peripheral vascular diseases. Past studies suggest that 80% of these ulcers are preventable with proper screening, identification of high-risk patients, and patient education. For this to be accomplished, multidisciplinary foot clinics and podiatric services must be made available worldwide. This article gives a brief global review of the current situation regarding diabetes.

Discussion—Europe has provided the world with much of the research and clinical data regarding the management of diabetes. In the northern European countries, many diabetic foot clinics are being established along with podiatry services, while in the southern European countries, amputation rates still remain high. However, the need for diabetic health care has been recognized and foot clinics are being established in many countries such as Yugoslavia, Bosnia, Macedonia, Ukraine, Lithuania, Bulgaria, Czechoslovakia, Poland, and Hungary.

In China, over 15 million people currently have diabetes with an additional 18 million people with impaired glucose tolerance. Realizing the challenge of providing appropriate care for this many people, a national program for diabetes is underway. Meanwhile, amputation rates remain high.

In India, there are an estimated 30 million people with type 2 diabetes. The presence of full-blown foot infections is quite common because of the people's tendency to walk barefoot, attempt home surgery, and trust faith healers. It is not atypical to see rats eating at neuropathic feet, maggots pouring out of ulcers, and bandages covered with red ants.

Although the prevalence of type 2 diabetes is relatively high in the native Aborigines and Maoris of Australia and New Zealand, respectively, the health care system is well developed and a national diabetes foot care network is currently being established by the Australian government.

There is little current literature on diabetes in Africa. There have been recent reports of up to an 11% increase in foot ulcerations in some countries. The level of available health care varies tremendously across the continent because of the social inequalities and differences between urban and rural populations.

North America and the American Diabetes Association are responsible for a lot of the current publications and data on diabetic care. The importance of preventative care has long been acknowledged and the presence of diabetic health care is still ever-growing.

The prevalence of diabetes is high throughout South and Central America with a recent study reporting a prevalence of 6.5% in Hispanic populations and a further 11% with impaired glucose tolerance. Leprosy is also on the rise in the northern regions like Brazil and wound care clinics are currently being established.

Conclusion—Although diabetes varies worldwide, it is still an ever-growing pandemic. Many countries still lack the necessary health care services to manage this disease. Consequently, the morbidity and mortality from diabetes are devastating and the economic burden overwhelming. Fortunately, the importance of this disease has been recognized worldwide and most countries are establishing some form of diabetic health care.—*D. Carmack*

◆ The St Vincent's Declaration established the goal of reducing amputations by 50% in the European nations. The focus was based on screening, as well as the identification and education of the high-risk patient. A project of this type is worth pursuing on an international level in both developing and fully developed countries. Even in Europe where many foot care programs and multidisciplinary clinics exist, those countries, with available podiatric services seem to fare best. In many other countries, the treatment algorithm for diabetic foot problems flows from the primary care doctor, directly to the general surgeon, where a functionally and financially costly amputation is the next step. In addition, there is a scarcity of published literature on diabetic foot problems from the African and Asian continents. This publication void must be filled as there are unique social and cultural issues affecting the treatment of patients from these countries.—*B. Saffran, D.P.M.*

2 Dermatologic Conditions of the Lower Extremity

GARY L. DOCKERY, D.P.M.

Squamous Cell Carcinoma Arising from Lesions of Porokeratosis Palmaris et Plantaris Disseminata
Seishima M, Izumi T, Oyama Z, Maeda M (Ogaki Municipal Hospital, Ogaki, Japan; GiFu Prefectural GiFu Hospital, Japan)
Eur J Dermatol 10(6):478–480, 2000

Background—Porokeratosis palmaris et plantaris disseminata (PPPD) occurs sporadically or as an autosomal dominant trait; it is a rare form of porokeratosis. Lesions first appear on the palms and soles in the 3rd decade of life and gradually disseminate to the trunk. PPPD lesions have been associated with malignant epithelial tumors, i.e., squamous cell carcinoma (SCC). Oral retinoid treatment has thus far been successful.

Case Report—A Japanese man presented at the ages of 28 and 43 with 1- to 1.5-mm nonpruritic, nonpainful hyperkeratotic lesions on the palms and soles B/L. At the age of 49, the right middle finger was amputated due to possible squamous cell carcinoma; no specific information was obtained. At the age of 57, biopsies were taken making the diagnosis of PPPD. One year later, he began a discontinuous 14-year course of oral etretinate and topical 10% urea. No involvement of the trunk, face, mucous membranes, arms, or legs was ever noted. This school teacher denied family history of the disease, treatment for syphilis, and exposure to arsenic or irradiation.

Seven months after cessation of oral etretinate, the patient noted a singular change, erosion on the left heel over a hyperkeratotic lesion. Two months later, this same erosion had increased to 2 mm and was thus biopsied revealing atypical keratinocytes with mononuclear infiltration. Further biopsies were taken from different locations, revealing SCC at all sites. Human papilloma virus DNAs were not detected. Lab values were WNL including negative results for syphilis. Further testing did not reveal metastasis. Diagnosis of SCC from PPPD was made.

Discussion—Diagnosis of PPPD was made by histological findings of punch biopsies. Use of oral retinoids for treatment of PPPD has been controversial. Whereas there have been excellent results obtained in some patients with relapses after several weeks or months after cessation of retinoid treatment, there have also been exacerbations of the condition.

The literature points out that retinoids may decrease cytological atypia and inhibit dermal carcinogenesis in porokeratotic lesions. This case presents development of SCC 9 months post oral retinoid cessation, which suggests that retinoids have inhibitory effects on PPPD malignancy, although the complete dosage of etretinate was low, totaling 21 g over 14 years.—*G. Grant*

♦ As foot and ankle specialists, we have the potential of seeing many patients with different variations of the punctate keratodermas involving the soles. These chronic dermatoses have the potential for malignant conversion, most often to squamous cell carcinoma. In this case report, the authors describe the malignant conversion of several lesions of porokeratosis palmaris et plantaris disseminata (PPKD) to squamous cell carcinoma. If, at any time during treatment, similar lesions spontaneously ulcerate or fail to heal, the physician should be concerned about conversion of the condition of the neoplastic variants. This is where the understanding of developing good differential diagnoses and the adequate use of biopsy techniques provides the most accurate and fast diagnosis and allows for appropriate and early treatment. — *G.L. Dockery, D.P.M.*

Desmoid Tumors in a Woman with Idiopathic Multicentric Osteolysis: Result of Three Etiologic Factors or Coincidence?

Nuyttens JJ, Jenrette JM, Thomas CR Jr (Medical University of South Carolina, Charleston, SC)
Am J Clin Oncol 23(4):376–378, 2000

Background—Desmoid tumors, or aggressive fibromatosis, pose a challenge to the experienced surgeon and pathologist due to their general acellular, collagenized histologic appearance. These lesions lack a pseudocapsule and typically originate in muscle or fascia. Without respect for tissue planes, desmoid processes have been known to attach to or invade muscle and bone. Idiopathic multicentric osteolysis (IMO), or disappearing bone disease, occurs in early childhood and is of unknown etiology with both autosomal dominant and recessive forms. Multiple small joint effusions with pain and crepitation often mimic juvenile arthritis. Common deformities resulting from this disease process are ulnar-deviation of the hands, equinovarus of the feet, and cubitus varus of the elbows. Radiographic signs indicative of this disease process are juxta-articular osteolysis initially with resultant fibrofatty deposition in vacant bone. Progressive neuropathy usually appears in the 2 decade of life.

Case Report—A 21-year-old female diagnosed with IMO at 2.5 years and confined to a wheelchair was treated by the authors. At age 8, the patient developed a nodule on the posterior neck, which enlarged in 2 years to the size of 15 × 7 cm. Biopsy revealed a "keloid" and a wide local skin excision was performed twice. At age 14, the patient was treated for endometriosis with medroxyprogesterone acetate (MPA:Depo-Provera). At age 20, the patient had 10 total matrixectomies which resulted in the subsequent growth of small nodules within the scar tissue in 9 out of 10 digits. Biopsy of one nodule revealed desmoid tumor. All nine nodules were resected and postoperative radiotherapy was administered.

Discussion—Three theories exist to explain the growth of desmoid tumors: 1) autosomal inheritance, 2) trauma, and 3) hormonal induction. The authors believe that the aggressive fibromatosis seen in this patient can be linked to family members lending support to the autosomal pattern of inherited disease. In support of the second theory, the patient developed small tumors on 9 out of 10 digits violated during matrixectomies producing scar tissue. An abnormal response to healing in conjunction with excessive immature fibroblast formation may cause tumor formation and therefore the resection of the nails may have contributed to the tumor growth. In support of hormonal induction as a causative agent in desmoid tumor growth, studies have shown that the middle-aged women are at risk, suggesting that estrogens may stimulate growth. In addition, high-dose estrogen treatment in a man with prostate cancer induced an abdominal desmoid tumor, which was shown to regress upon cessation of hormonal therapy. In addition, estrogen and antiestrogen binding sites have been located in desmoid tumors.

Conclusion—At age 8, with increasing levels of estrogen, this patient induced the growth of the tumor on the posterior neck. Subsequently, she was protected from the further development of tumors by the MPA and when discontinued, the patient developed multiple tumors on her toes. As shown by this patient, trauma, estrogens, and genetic predisposition may all be factors that cause desmoid tumor growth.—*K. Van Voris*

♦ Desmoid tumors usually occur in young females and arise from the anterior abdominal wall but occasionally are extra-abdominal. The extra-abdominal lesions occur most frequently in the shoulder girdle and on the thighs. As a result, foot and ankle specialists rarely get to see these tumors on the lower extremities. When they do occur in this region, as in this case report of lesions on the digits, it may be difficult to make a clinical diagnosis based upon visual appearance alone, another good reason for making a differential diagnostic list of tumors and using excisional biopsy techniques for an accurate diagnosis.—*G.L. Dockery, D.P.M.*

Acral Cutaneous Melanoma in Caucasians: Clinical Features, Histopathology and Prognosis in 112 Patients

Kuchelmeister C, Schaumburg-Lever G, Garbe C (Eberhard-Karls-University, Tuebingen, Germany)
Br J Dermatol 143(2):275–280, 2000

Background—The four clinical subtypes of cutaneous melanoma are superficial spreading melanoma (SSM), lentigo maligna melanoma (LMM), nodular melanoma (NM), and acral lentiginous melanoma (ALM). ALM, unlike the other three, is still controversial regarding its histopathological diagnosis and prognosis. A distinct histological picture of ALM, a correlation with its anatomical location, and a prognostic impact of its diagnosis are sought.

Methods—A total of 2642 melanoma patients were identified from 1986 to 1997. Of these, 187 presented with acral melanomas; 112 were biopsied. Histological evaluation proceeded and diagnoses were made. Modified Reed criteria were used for ALM diagnosis. All 112 were invasive according to Clark's criteria (Clark level of invasion $\geq$ II). Patients were followed for an average of 32 months.

Results—

- *Stage and anatomical presentation*: 101 of 112 presented without metastasis. Four presented with satellite metastasis and seven with lymph node metastasis. Eighty-eight of 112 tumors occurred on feet. Histopathological exam of ALM yielded results similar to Reed in 1976. Tumors were histologically classified as 67 (60%) ALM, 34 (30%) SSM, 10 (9%) NM. No lesions were diagnosed as LMM. All ALM were palmoplantar or subungual. All SSM were dorsal. NM occurred at all acral sites.

- *Age classification by location and subtype*: Lesions on dorsum of hands and feet were mostly found among 21- to 30-year-olds, lesions on palmoplantar and subungual areas were mostly found among 61- to 70-year-olds. Median ages by subtype were as follows: 48 years for SSM, 55.5 years for NM, 51.5 years for ALM, and 68.7 years for LMM.

- *Prognosis*: Three-year survival for all acral melanomas without metastasis was 93%. Five-year survival was 82%. Five-year survival was 100% for SSM and 71% for ALM. There was a statistically significantly poorer prognosis for ALM compared with SSM or LMM, but not with ALM compared to NM.

Discussion—The present study was one of the largest ever undertaken on the subject. Epidemiological results were similar to other large studies of melanoma. This study confirmed the fact that most ALM occurs on plantar sites and fewer on palmar sites, and that subungual melanomas occur more commonly on hands than feet. Location is shown to be the single most reliable predictor of ALM. There is a distinctive age distribution of ALM and SSM, with most ALM (palmoplantar location) in 61- to 70-year-olds and most SSM (dorsal location) among 21- to 30-year olds. The etiology of ALM remains unknown, although there is a significantly lower finding of nevus remnants in ALM (10%) vs. other melanomas (20–30%).

It is proposed that the histology of ALM is characteristic but not distinct. Therefore, the characteristics outlined by Reed should be used—at least for the initial stages of ALM—although in the early stages it may resemble LMM. Tumor location takes on increased significance given these early-stage similarities and the poorer prognosis of ALM. Complete diagnosis of ALM is dependent upon histological exam together with the location of the tumor.—*D. Clement*

♦ This is a very large study of 112 patients with a complete review of acral melanomas including individual exams of the histology slides and long-term follow-up. The consequences of this neoplastic group of conditions are rather severe and the fact that tumors occurred on the feet in 88 patients, and of these lesions 58 were on the plantar sites, indicates the need for an accurate and early diagnosis. In comparison with the other types of melanoma, survival of acral lentiginous melanoma (ALM) patients was significantly worse than the survival of lentigo maligna melanoma (LMM) or superficial spreading melanoma (SSM), and unfortunately, this is often due to delayed diagnosis of plantar ALM cases.—*G.L. Dockery, D.P.M.*

Large Plantar Wart Caused by Human Papillomavirus-66 and Resolution by Topical Cidofovir Therapy

Davis MD, Gostout BS, McGovern RM, Persing DH, Schut RL, Pittelkow MR (Mayo Clinic and Mayo Foundation, Rochester, MN; Hennepin County Medical Center, Minneapolis, MN)
J Am Acad Dermatol 43(2):340–343, 2000

Background—Human papillomavirus (HPV) represents a heterogenous group of viruses. Currently, 77 different genotypes have been identified in humans. Certain HPV types have been linked with the development of some cancers. The virus infects the epithelial layers and leads to epithelial cell proliferation and acanthosis. This, in turn, leads to the development of epithelial tumors. HPV-66 is often found in verruca vulgaris and is genotypically related to HPV-30 and HPV-56, which are also linked with cervical dysplasia and squamous cell carcinoma (SCC) of the cervix.

Introduction—Cidofovir is an acyclic nucleotide analog of deoxycytidine monophosphate. It has broad-spectrum activity against viruses like cytomegalovirus, herpesvirus, adenovirus, human papillomavirus, and poly-omavirus. Cidofovir may work by inhibiting viral DNA synthesis. Cidofovir has many clinical uses including HPV-related anogenital warts in patients with AIDS, HSV in patients with AIDS, and molluscum contagiosum in patients with AIDS.

Case Report—A 37-year-old HIV-positive Kenyan female presents with a verrucous plaque on her right foot. The lesion first appeared in February 1997 on her lateral foot, and by October 1997, when she presented to the Department of Dermatology, the lesion had grown to include her right heel and medial foot. The clinical differential diagnosis included viral wart, deep fungal infection, SCC, and verrucous carcinoma. The lesion was resistant to antimicrobial and antifungal therapy. Special stains and cultures were negative for bacterial fungus. The biopsy showed minimal viral change and revealed papillomatosis, ancanthosis, hyperkeratosis, and superficial telangiectasia, and was thought to have verrucous characteristics. Polymerase chain reaction (PCR) from the biopsy of the foot lesion identified HPV-66. Since HPV-66 can also be found in the genital tract, a Papanicolaou smear was performed and showed a high-grade squamous intraepithelial lesion, which is in accordance with carcinoma-in-situ. A reverse line-blot HPV detection assay identified HPV types 11, 16, 53, and 66 in the foot lesion, and HPV types 11, 16, 52, 53, 66, and MM9 in the cervical lesions. The patient was told to apply cidofovir cream (3% in emollient cream) twice a day and by the 3rd day of therapy, she stated that the lesion had improved dramatically. By the 5th day, the wart was half of its original size and almost undetectable after a week. When the patient stopped using the drug, the verrucous lesion reappeared. However, when she reapplied the cream, the wart disappeared after 3–4 weeks.

Discussion—To recap, in February 1997, the patient noticed the lesion and had a CD4 count of 216. By August 1997, her CD4 count dropped to 108, her lesion had spread, and the patient changed her HIV drug regimen. In October 1997, the CD4 count increased to 234 and remained at this level throughout the cidofovir therapy. The disappearance of the patient's wart may have been due to her increased CD4 count following her changed HIV drug regimen. On the other hand, the patient had noticed the drastic decrease in size of her lesion following cidofovir application. The dramatic regression occurred while her CD4 count remained constant at 234. This supports the conclusion that the drug was responsible for the improvement of her lesion.—*G.H. Jhala*

◆ Patients who present with large verrucous lesions on the feet and positive test results for human immunodeficiency (HIV) represent a special problem for foot and ankle specialists. This case report outlines the association of a large foot wart secondary to human papillomavirus HPV-66, which is frequently associated with anogenital lesions and the use of topical 3% cidofovir cream (Vanicream®, Pharmaceutical Specialties, Inc. Rochester, MN). The use of these acyclic nucleotide analogs, with broad-spectrum antiviral activity against DNA viruses, and other drugs such as the immune response modifiers, 5% imiquimod (Aldara®, 3 M Pharmaceuticals, St. Paul,

MN), may totally change how we treat resistant and large foot warts in the very near future.—*G.L. Dockery, D.P.M.*

Plantar Hidradenitis in Children Induced by Exposure to Wet Footwear

Naimer SA, Zvulunov A, Ben-Amitai D, Landau M (Goosh Katif Health Center, Hof Gaza, Israel; Ben Gurion University, Beer-Sheva, Israel; Josephthal Hospital, Eilat, Israel; Tel Aviv University, Israel)

Pediatr Emerg Care 16(3):182–183, 2000

Introduction—When a physician is confronted with a relatively healthy pediatric patient who has painful erythematous papules and nodules on their palms and soles of the feet, they should be aware of palmoplantar hidradenitis as a possible differential. Although the pathogenesis of palmoplantar hidradenitis is unclear, it is histologically specific in that the eccrine gland is targeted by neutrophilic infiltrates.

Case Studies—Each of the four cases of palmoplantar hidradenitis discussed revealed healthy young (ages 6–11) pediatric patients who under cold wet conditions, and events of continuous impact such as walking, presented 1–3 days later with painful red-purple nodules on the soles of the feet. The treatment was conservative in nature, such as bed rest and observation, which ended in complete resolution. The similarities in clinical presentation between these individual cases contributes to the correlation of palmoplantar hidradenitis with physical activity and a wet environment. Furthermore, the evidence of cold dampness proceeding the abrupt onset of the characteristically painful red-purple lesions proposes a pathogenetic mechanism.

Discussion and Conclusions—In 1988 Metzker and Brodsky first brought this condition to light, naming it "traumatic plantar urticaria" due to its propensity to occur under conditions of physical activity, and other studies done by Stahr added the element of dampness to the pathogenesis. The role of an immunologic process and infection remains inconclusive, but it is clear that a child walking in wet shoes indeed triggers a process that leads to palmoplantar hidradnitis. It is reported that mechanical or thermal trauma may lead to eccrine glandular rupture, resulting in the expulsion of glandular secretions which activates a cytokine cascade encouraging neutrophils to infiltrate the area as is histologically evident. As noted in the case studies, the suggested current treatment is bed rest. The differential diagnosis of insect bites, chilblains, panniculitis or plantar erythema nodosum, thrombophlebitis, vasculitis, embolic phenomena, cellulitis, and migratory angioedema can generally be ruled out with a proper history and clinical findings.—*S.B. Heninger*

◆ This condition appears to be limited to children and is associated with the condition of hyperhidrosis and increased activities as well as with cold, wet exposure for extended amounts of time. These cases appear to present as exquisitely tender nodules and papules on the plantar soles of the feet. As in axillary and groin hidradenitis, there is probably some association with keratinous obstruction of the eccrine sweat duct resulting in ductal and tubular dilatation. In this case, plantar hidradenitis, the cause of obstruction is most likely the overmacerated plantar skin and the treatment with bedrest allows this tissue to dry and subsequently heal without the use of steroids or antibiotics. This may represent a severe form of miliaria that is seen as diaper rash with prolonged exposure to moisture and occlusion. This condition (plantar hidradenitis) should be in the differential diagnosis of painful plantar lesions in children. — *G.L. Dockery, D.P.M.*

The Prevalence and Management of Onychomycosis in Diabetic Patients

Gupta AK, Humke S (University of Toronto, Toronto, Canada; Universitats Kliniken Hautklinik, Moorenstrabe, Germany)
Eur J Dermatol 10(5):379–384,2000

Introduction—Diabetic patients are faced with a multitude of problems, including neuropathy, retinopathy, immunopathy, circulatory problems, and skin manifestations. The combined effects leave the diabetic prone to the development of onychomycosis. There is an increased incidence of onychomycosis in diabetics with potential morbidity and mortality resulting. Dystrophic, thickened fungal nails combined with neuropathy are a potential cause of soft-tissue injury and trauma. Mycotic nails may also serve as a reservoir for pathogenic organisms which can gain entry to circulation through a small abrasion.

Methods—Based on two studies, one conducted in North America and the Achilles prevalence study conducted in Europe, it is determined that the prevalence of onychomycosis is higher in diabetics than in non-diabetics. The studies showed that diabetics are about twice as likely to develop onychomycosis. The studies have the advantage of a large study population from which to base their results. It is also noted that onychomycosis and tinea pedis are often a concurrent finding. The most common causes of onychomycosis are dermatophytes (88.2%), nondermatophyte molds (9.1%), and candida species (2.7%).

Results—The possible sequelae of onychomycosis pose a great risk to diabetic patients. High-risk diabetics with neuropathy and impaired circulation are at increased risk of developing abrasions, ulcerations, paronychia, celluitis, bacterial infection, and osteomyelitis. The treatment of onychomycosis may improve quality of life and enhance the well-being of the patient. Itraconazole, fluconazole, and terbinafine are found to be effective in onychomycosis treatment. The dosing regimen for each has a high benefit–risk ratio with shorter treatment duration. The duration of treatment is in the range of 9–15 months. Of the three drugs, only fluconazole has drug interactions with the oral hypoglycemic drugs tolbutamide, glyburide, and glipizide. Clinical experience has shown that itraconazole and terbinafine are safe and effective in the treatment of onychomycosis.

Conclusion—It is of utmost importance to protect the diabetic foot through safe and effective treatment of mycotic nails. As diabetic patients age, they are more prone to develop onychomycosis and other systemic sequelae. Treatment with terbinafine and itraconazole may decrease the risk of ulceration, infection, and ultimately foot amputation. Proper foot care, as well as diabetic education, is a must to protect the diabetic foot.—*K. Carriero*

♦ As tired as we all are of papers and lectures on the treatment of fungal toenails, this paper takes an important look at the incidence of onychomycosis in diabetic patients and reviews two recent papers regarding this issue (see Tables 1–3) Since a significant portion of our patients with diabetes also have onychomycosis and because this group of patients can potentially have more severe complications with toenail infections, this is a meaningful topic.—*G.L. Dockery, D.P.M.*

TABLE 1. Clinical impression of the feet in individuals with or without diabetes

Clinical impression	Diabetes mellitus	
	Absent ($n = 15,940$)	Present ($n = 1,064$)
Foot not affected	6,447 (40.5%)	186 (17.5%)
Foot affected	9,493 (59.6%)	878 (82.2%)

TABLE 2. Clinical evidence of fungal infection in an affected foot in individuals with or without diabetes

Fungal infection	Diabetes mellitus	
	Absent ($n = 9,493$)	Present ($n = 878$)
No	3,175 (33.4%)	182 (20.7%)
Yes	6,318 (66.6%)	696 (79.3%)

TABLE 3. Location of the fungal infection in individuals with or without diabetes (data on 7,002 cases)

Location of fungal infection	Diabetes mellitus	
	Absent ($n = 6,307$)	Present ($n = 695$)
Only skin or nails	3,897 (61.8%)	182 (48.6%)
Skin and nails	2,410 (38.2%)	357 (51.4%)

Symmetrical Black Plaques on the Toes

Robinson C, Yee BYF, Kelly AP (King/Drew Medical Center, Los Angeles, CA)
Arch Dermatol 136(6):792, 795–796, 2000

Introduction—Acanthosis nigricans is described as a symmetrical, velvety, papillomatous, gray-brown to black thickening of the skin. It can be classified as being benign or malignant depending on the disease with which it is associated. The benign form is associated with certain disorders such as insulin-resistant diabetes, Addison's disease, polycystic ovarian disease, pituitary tumors, pinealoma, and hirsutism. It can also be associated with certain drugs, such as oral contraceptives, nicotinic acid, corticosteroids, and diethylstilbestrol.

The malignant form of acanthosis nigricans most commonly occurs with intra-abdominal adenocarcinoma, particularly gastric adenocarcinoma. The maliganant forms usually regress after the tumor is excised, and may recur with metastatic disease. Malignant acanthosis usually presents with a sudden onset, rapid progression, pruritis, and a diffuse keratoderma of the palms and soles. Peptide production by the carcinoma may be a factor in the pathogenesis of malignant acanthosis nigricans.

The most common sites of involvement are the base of the neck, axillae, groin, and the antecubital fossa. They have also been reported to affect the dorsum of the hands, elbow, periumbical skin, vermilion border of the lips, eyelids, and mucous membranes. Mucosal involvement is more common in the malignant form.

Microscopic findings show hyperkeratosis and papillomatosis with slight, irregular acanthosis and occasional hyperpigmentation. One may also see hypertrophy of the dermal papillae and increased melanin production in the stratum corneum.

Case Report—A 52-year-old African American female presents with a black rash that has progressively thickened over the past 3 years. Patient denies pruritis. Patient also has a 5-year history of tinea pedis. Five months prior to her initial visit, the patient underwent a total mastectomy for poorly differentiated infiltrating ductal breast carcinoma. Postsurgery, patient began a course of chemotherapy with methotrexate, cyclophosphamide, and fluorouracil. Patient also has a 10-year history of type II diabetes mellitus which is controlled with glipizide.

Physical Exam—There was a presence of bilateral, symmetrical hyperpigmented papillomatous plaques on the dorsum of the toes that extended from the metatarsal phalangeal joint to the proximal nail fold. There was a brown discoloration of all the nails. The hyponychium was normal. A 3-mm punch biopsy was taken. This revealed a hyperkeratosis, papillomatosis, and regular acanthosis with minimal basilar hyperpigmentation.

Conclusions—The patient in this article had an unusual presentation as far as location and association with breast cancer. The patient was diagnosed with the malignant form of acanthosis nigricans. Acanthosis nigricans is not commonly associated with breast cancer. A recent review showed that out of 247 cases of carcinoma associated with acanthosis nigricans, only 11 were breast cancers. The rest of the results showed 112 gastric, 20 lung, 18 liver, 18 uterine, and 9 ovarian cancers. Acanthosis nigricans may appear at any point in time of the malignancy.—*S. Patel*

♦ This short case report is presented in the quiz format in which the reader is given a very brief history of the patient and provided with two clinical photos of the feet and one 40-power close-up view of the histology slide from the biopsy specimen. Based upon the history and the findings of the biopsy, a diagnosis of malignant acanthosis nigricans associated with carcinoma of the breast is made. This is a relatively rare condition and one that makes another good point for the use of diagnostic biopsy techniques in clinical practice. It seems that this 52-year-old female patient could walk into any of our offices on any given day and ask us what was on her toes.—*G.L. Dockery, D.P.M.*

Necrolytic Acral Erythema Associated with Hepatitis C: Effective Treatment with Interferon Alfa and Zinc

Khanna VJ, Shieh S, Benjamin J, Somach S, Zaim, MT, Dorner WJ, Shill M, Wood GS (Case Western Reserve University, Cleveland, OH; General Medical Center, Akron, OH)
Arch Dermatol 136(6):755–757, 2000

Introduction—Necrolytic acral erythema has been described as part of a group of necrolytic erythemas, which are similar clinically and histologically but differ in etiology. Necrolytic acral erythema has been associated with hepatitis C infection. A case of necrolytic acral erythema effectively treated with interferon alfa-2b and oral zinc is presented.

Case Report—A 43-year-old African American woman was referred with a medical history of atopic dermatitis, asthma, and allergic rhinitis with a 4-year history of recurrent, pruritic, erythematous, papular eruptions on her feet and ankles. Previous biopsy specimens were diagnosed as lichen simplex chronicus and erythema multiforme with direct immunofluorescence yielding negative results. The patient was treated unsuccessfully with several conventional treatments. Physical exam showed large, painful, partially eroded violaceous patches on the proximal half of the dorsal aspect of the feet extending over the medial and lateral malleolus with 2+ to 3+ pedal edema. Laboratory studies were normal except for an elevated leukocyte count with left shift, decreased albumin level, and an elevated cholesterol, AST, ALT, and LDH. The patient was also hepatitis C positive. A current biopsy specimen yielded hyperkeratosis, parakeratosis, superficial necrosis, pallor, intercellular edema, and regenerative and/or inflammatory cytologic atypia in the epidermis. Examination of the dermis revealed telangiectasia, extravasation of red blood cells, and a perivascular sparse lymphocytic inflammatory cell infiltrate. Collectively, these findings are consistent with necrolytic erythema.

The patient began oral zinc sulfate with some clinical improvement after 5 weeks. Then subcutaneous interferon alfa-2b injections were begun 3 times weekly. Three weeks passed with marked improvement and at 6 months all the lesions had cleared with liver enzyme test results at normal values. The therapy was discontinued and the patient has been asymptomatic with normal liver function tests for 3½ years after treatment.

Summary—In comparison to an earlier report by El Darouti and El Ela of seven cases of necrolytic acral erythema, in five of their patients, oral zinc worked in varied degrees. Interferon alfa was extremely effective in two of their patients and in this case, with one of the former having complete resolve. In two other cases interferon alfa with oral zinc resulted in total clearance. This suggests that interferon alfa alone could be utilized for treatment or it could enhance the effect of oral zinc.

The association of necrolytic acral erythema and hepatitis C is important because its exclusive acral distribution of its lesions could precede the diagnosis of hepatitis C infection and can therefore be a marker of systemic disease.—*F. Nejad*

♦ This is thought to be a new entity and is considered to be rare in nature. This report is the first case in the United States and only seven other cases have been documented in the past 5 years. This unique dermatosis is exclusively located on the hands, lower legs, and feet and is strongly associated with hepatitis C. Recognition of this association is important since the skin lesions usually precede the diagnosis of hepatitis C and, therefore, are considered to be a prodrome or precursor.—*G.L. Dockery, D.P.M.*

An Unusual Case of Pemphigus Vulgaris Presenting as Bilateral Foot Ulcers

Tan HH, Tay YK (National Skin Centre, Singapore)
Clin Exp Dermatol 25(3):224–226, 2000

Background—Pemphigus vulgaris, an autoimmune mucocutaneous bullous disease caused by autoantibodies against desmosomal antigens, rarely presents in the feet. Commonly, it is characterized by lesions restricted to stratified squamous epithelia in the oral mucosa, followed by skin of the upper trunk, head and neck, and intertriginous areas. Previous studies have shown that the distribution of pemphigus antigens is regional, with higher expression in the buccal mucosa and scalp, and lower expression in the dorsum of the feet and soles. This may serve as a basis for the infrequency of pemphigus vulgaris presentation in the feet.

Case Report—A 60-year-old male with a 20-year history of type II diabetes presented with slowly enlarging ulcers on the dorsum of both feet that were unresponsive to previous amoxicillin and cloxacillin treatment. Lower extremity physical examination revealed ulcerated plaques on the dorsum of both feet, with slough over the ulcer base, along with surrounding cellulitis and macerated interdigital spaces. Additional vascular, neurological, and radiographic exams were unremarkable. Following a diagnosis of cellulitis complicating pyoderma of both feet, the lesions did not improve with 10-day courses of erythromycin or cephalexin. Swab cultures of the ulcers indicated presence of group B *Streptococcus*. On a follow-up visit 4 months later, the patient related the appearance of ulcers in his mouth, along with erosions on his neck and groin. Histological analysis of the neck lesions revealed eosinophilic infiltrate, acantholysis, and suprabasal clefts, while foot specimens showed red blood cells, acantholysis, and suprabasal clefts. Cellular deposits of IgG were noted within the epidermis upon direct immunofluorescence, while indirect serum immunofluorescence demonstrated intercellular antibody with a titer of 1:160. Noticeable improvement was attained with treatment of prednisone (45 mg/day) and dapsone (50 mg/day increased to 100 mg/day). Following 6 months of maintenance therapy with prednisolone (10 mg/day) and dapsone (100 mg/day), the patient's indirect immunofluorescence anti-intercellular IgG titer decreased to 1:20. All foot, oral, neck, and groin lesions healed well, with postinflammatory hyperpigmentation and no scarring.

Conclusion—The early recognition of pemphigus vulgaris lesions and subsequent prompt therapy are essential for a favorable prognosis. Possible differential diagnoses are of infectious origin and include lupus vulgaris, *Mycobacterium ulcerans*, deep fungal infections, and cutaneous leishmaniasis. Dapsone has been shown to be effective in the treatment of pemphigus vulgaris, and its steroid-sparing properties help to diminish the complications associated with concomitant steroid administration.—*E. Zarutsky*

♦ Another unusual and possibly rare presentation of a well-known condition, pemphigus vulgaris, is discussed in this case report. This report of chronic ulcerated plaques on both feet, in a 60-year-old male, that were slowly enlarging and presented with foul-smelling drainage represents a very important clinical lesson. That lesson is simple: when a condition does not respond as expected, then a new diagnosis should be considered. In this case, the patient was given a presumptive diagnosis of infection and treated by his family physician with 2 weeks of amoxicillin and cloxacillin. When there was no improvement, he was then placed on a 10-day course of erythromycin. When there was still no improvement, he was placed on a 10-day course of cephalexin. On a follow-up 4 months later, he still had the problem but now presented with erosions on the neck and groin area. Now, finally, a biopsy was performed and direct and indirect immunofluorescence studies combined to make a diagnosis of pemphigus vulgaris. Appropriate therapy was then started and the lesions healed and the patient went into remission. The message is: when something is not responding as it should, don't continue the same line of therapy simply by changing the name of the drug in the same category. It is time to do some investigative work.—*G.L. Dockery, D.P.M.*

Topical Corticosteroid Phobia in Patients with Atopic Eczema

Charman CR, Morris AD, Williams HC (Queen's Medical Centre, Nottingham, UK)
Br J Dermatol 142(5):931–936, 2000

Introduction—Topical corticosteroids are considered to be one of the most important treatments prescribed by dermatologists for patients with atopic dermatitis. This study was aimed at quantifying the prevalence of topical corticosteroid phobia in patients with atopic dermatitis and to examine the implication that these fears have on patient compliance. The study also aimed at discovering the patients' knowledge of the potencies of the medications they were using and where they were obtaining this information.

Methods—This was a questionnaire-based study of 200 dermatology patients (or a parent, if the subject was a child) whose ages ranged from 4 months to 67.8 years. The questionnaire was aimed at assessing the prevalence and source of topical corticosteroid phobia and the patients' knowledge of the potencies of various topical corticosteroids.

Results—Results showed that 72.5% of people worried about using topical corticosteroids on their own skin or their child's skin. There was no significant effect due to age, gender, or whether the subjects were new patients or follow-up patients. Of the total number of patients, 24% admitted to having been noncompliant with treatment because of these worries. This may be an underestimate because patients may be reluctant to admit noncompliance with treatment. The most common reasons for topical corticosteroid phobias in these patients were: skin thinning (34.5%), nonspecific long-term effects (24%), and systemic absorption leading to effects on growth and development (9.5%). While skin atrophy is a potential side effect of topical corticosteroid therapy, the concern about skin thinning is out of proportion to the evidence obtained from the article's literature review. In addition, the article discusses a few studies that show that neither adult height nor adrenal function are significantly affected by topical corticosteroids.

The study also pointed out the confusion among dermatology patients regarding the strengths of the topical corticosteroids prescribed to them. Hydrocortisone was the most commonly used topical corticosteroid and despite the fact that it has a relatively weak potency, 31% of those patients who have taken hydrocortisone thought it was either strong, very strong, or did not know the potency. Of the 48 patients who have used both Dermovate and hydrocortisone, only 62.5% of them classified Dermovate as being more potent than hydrocortisone. Thus, there is confusion among patients concerning the potencies of topical corticosteroid preparations. General practitioners were the most common source of patient education (33%) regarding the safety and side effects of topical corticosteroids, followed by magazines and newspapers (17.5%), friends (14.5%), and family (11.5%).

Conclusion/Discussion—General practitioners need access to accurate information regarding the safety, potency, and appropriate use of topical corticosteroids so that they may better educate their patients and ultimately reduce irrational fears and achieve better patient compliance.—*B. Hoffman*

◆ This is an interesting paper based upon the results of a detailed questionnaire checking steroid phobia in 200 patients with atopic eczema. The conclusions of this survey were not too surprising but were enlightening. More than 72% of those surveyed were concerned about the consequences of topical steroids and 24% were noncompliant in the use of these products due to their fears (see Table 1) What was surprising to me was the fact that the majority of patients relied upon information supplied by their general practitioner, indicating that these physicians may be providing less than optimal information to the patients regarding the use and side effects of topical steroids. Another interesting finding in this study was that patients relied upon information from magazines, friends, and family at a higher rate than they relied upon information from the pharmacist, medical books, and consultants. This may show the influence of these sources on our treatment programs.—*G.L. Dockery, D.P.M.*

TABLE 1. The reasons for patients' fears about using topical corticosteroids

Reasons for topical corticosteroid phobia	% of patients (n = 200)
Skin thinning	34.5
Nonspecific long-term effects	24.0
Absorption/effects on growth and development	9.5
Ageing/wrinkling	3.5
Changes in skin colour	3.0
Makes eczema worse	3.0
May become immune to effect	3.0
May become dependent	2.5
Scarring	2.0
Stretch marks	1.0
Pain/stinging	1.0
Reduced immunity to infections	0.5
Cataracts	0.5
Cancer	0.5
Sunburn	0.5
Bruising	0.5
Increased body hair	0.5

Lichenoid and Granulomatous Dermatitis

Magro CM, Crowson AN (Medical College of Thomas Jefferson University, Philadelphia, PA; Central Medical Laboratories, Winnipeg, Manitoba, Canada; Regional Medical Laboratories, St. John Medical Center, Tulsa, OK)
Int J Dermatol 39(2):126–133, 2000

Introduction—Lichenoid dermatitis is characterized by a microscopic pattern of superficial bandlike lymphocytic infiltrate accompanied by alterations that cause degeneration in the epithelial layers of the skin. The common causative agents are lichen planus (LP), lichenoid drug reactions, secondary syphilis, mixed connective tissue disease (MCTD), and subacute cutaneous lupus erythematosus (SCLE). All of the previously mentioned conditions have the characteristic microscopic pattern, but in addition have a distinguishing pattern to enable a better diagnosis. This article discusses the lichenoid dermatitis with a granulomatous component.

Methods—Forty patients with a lichenoid and granulomatous dermatitis were sequestered from two outpatient dermatopathology databases by a random computer selection over a 4-year period. Clinical impression and lesion distribution were obtained from the referring clinician, who was also contacted to review the patients' history and possible triggering factors. The impressions that the study group exhibited were lichenoid dermatitis, a linear eruption lichen striatus (LS), or a zosteriform process lichen nitidus (LN), drug eruption, erythroderma, necrobiosis lipoidica, granulomatous dermatitis, psoriasis, cutaneous T-cell lymphoma (CTCL) tinea capitis, pityriasis lichenoides, secondary syphilis, tuberculoid leprosy, and guttate psoriasis. The concurrent infections or medical illnesses that caused the eruptions were hepatitis C, human immunodeficiency when combined exposure to cytomegalovirus retinitis and nasal herpes, Epstein-Barr virus, syphilis, post varicella eruptions, rheumatoid arthritis (RA), hepatobiliary disease, Crohn's disease, hypercholesterolemias, hypertension, thyroiditis, diabetes, hypothyroidism, and streptococcal tonsillitis. Several cases had a drug-induced etiology. The drugs included antibiotics, lipid-lowering agents, anti-inflammatory drugs, antihistamines, hydroxychloroquine sulfate, and angiotensin-converting enzyme inhibitors. Skin biopsies were obtained from the 40 patients and were reviewed to determine if one could discriminate between the various diseases and triggers that cause these lichenoid eruptions. The biopsies were prepared into 5-μm sections of formalin-fixed, paraffin-embedded tissue stained with hematoxylin and eosin.

Results—A bandlike infiltrate of lymphocytes among histiocytes that obscured the dermoepidermal junction was found in all cases in addition to discriminating histopathology. The histiocytic component had one or more of five light microscopic patterns:

1. Superficially arranged loose histiocytic collection
2. cohesive granulomata within zones of bandlike lymphocytic infiltration with or without deeper dermal involvement
3. A diffuse interstitial pattern
4. Scattered singly arranged with giant cells
5. Granulomatous vasculitis

It was possible to break up the cases further into those representing LP, LN, LS, drug-associated cases, previous infection, hepatobiliary disease, CTCL, and RA.

1. *LP*—One case illustrated hypergranulosis and orthohyperkeratosis without mid or deep dermal perivascular extension with multicentric reticulohistiocytosis in the granular layer. Another case did not have the characteristic change in the granular cell layer and stratum corneum, but showed rare eosinophils, with the histiocytes arranged as poorly defined small aggregates within a superficially confined lymphoid infiltrate. One case of lichen planopilaris had a folliculocentric infiltrate with destruction of the outer root sheath epithelium and scattered plasma cells.

2. *LN*—This finding had a focal lichenoid infiltrate that could be selective with only two dermal papillae being affected to a much broader pattern with more dermal papillae being affected. In addition, the weakened epidermis had parakeratosis with slight suprabasilar exocytosis. The histiocytes and scattered giant cell made up the granulomatous component.

3. *LS*—A broad band of lymphocytes connected to a flattened epidermis with loose aggregates of varying histiocytes, focal suprabasilar lymphocytosis to necrotic keratinocytes, basilar vaculopathy, neutrophil saturated parakeratosis, and focal hemorrhage.

4. *Drug-associated*—Tissue eosinophilia and plasmacellular infiltrates with interface inflammation prominent in eccrine, acrosyringeal, and straight ducts, were evident. In addition a superficial vasculopathy consisting of endothelial swelling with hemorrhage was noted. The extravascular granulomatous had occasional giant cells or loose histiocytic aggregate among the lymphoid tissue.

5. *Previous infection*—Infiltration of hair follicles, perineurium, and eccrine structures. Some cases illustrated granulomatous vasculitis and/or focal cell-poor vacuolar interface dermatitis. Each infection had distinctive patterns.

6. *Hepatobiliary*—The findings were deep extension of the infiltrate, a lymphocytic eccrine hidradenitis, granulomatous vasculitis, and variable tissue eosinophilia. The granulomatous component was represented by two patterns, a diffuse interstitial granuloma anulare like pattern, and the other a superficially random disposed histiocytic aggregates.

7. *CTCL*—Lymphoid atypia with Sezary cells in the epidermis and dermis, with laminated papillary dermal sclerosis were present.

8. *RA*—These reactions were found to be due solely to RA. A vasculitic eruption showed pigmentary purpura-like lichenoid dermatitis with foci of superficial granulomatous vasculitis.

Conclusion—It is helpful to be able to recognize the characteristic microscopic patterns of the various manifestations of lichenoid and granulomatous dermatitis. It allows the clinician to distinguish the causative agents and medical conditions that may predispose a patient to these eruptions.—*T. Marshall*

♦ This important study looked at skin biopsies from 40 separate patients diagnosed with lichenoid or granulomatous dermatitis in an effort to correlate any underlying prodromes or medical conditions. This group of dermatoses includes lichen planus, lichenoid dermatitis, secondary syphilis, mixed connective tissue disease, and subacute cutaneous lupus erythematosus. The associated conditions included hepatobiliary disease, endocrinopathy, rheumatoid arthritis, Crohn's disease, infections, or drug reactions. It was interesting that 35% of the cases were secondary to the "anti-" agents, namely, the anti-inflammatory drugs, antibiotics, antihypertensive drugs, antihistamines, and anticholesterol drugs. Only seven cases were listed as idiopathic and therefore unclassified. Since we see many patients on the "anti-" drugs, it is important to understand the association with these types of reactions.—*G.L. Dockery, D.P.M.*

Pediatric Dermatology: That Itchy Scaly Rash

Boerio M, Brooker J, Freese L, Phares P, Yazvec S (Pediatric Associates of Fairfield/Hamilton, Fairfield, OH)
Nurs Clin North Am 35(1):147–157, 2000

Introduction—Skin problems have commonly driven parents to bring their children to the primary care physician for advice. Those skin disturbances that prove to be persistent, like seborrheic dermatitis and tinea infections, and those that itch, like contact and atopic dermatitis, tend to be the most frequently seen by the pediatrician.

Methods—Atopic dermatitis has a typical distribution and is characteristically pruritic. It presents symmetrically on the cheeks and extensor surfaces of children under 3, flexor surfaces of those over 3, and may be generalized. There is usually a family history of asthma and allergies, the etiology of which is increased levels of serum IgE and peripheral eosinophilia. Antigens in the environment or diet precipitate symptoms of pruritis and the child will commonly scratch areas even without rash which initiates an inflammatory response leading to erythema and possible skin breakdown. Treatment involves keeping the skin cool as sweaty skin itches the child; wearing cotton clothes helps whisk away moisture. Sedating oral antihistamines, such as hydroxyzine, before bedtime can help prevent scratching. Topical steroid creams also decrease inflammation. Avoiding the causative irritant is ideal and parents are advised to watch the skin's integrity as new foods are tried. Maintaining the integrity of the skin is essential, and the skin of atopic children is usually dry. Too much soaking, however, can dry even further. Parents are thus advised to keep baths under 10 minutes a day and to apply moisturizing ointment immediately after to trap the moisture next to the skin (ointment > cream > lotion).

Contact dermatitis is broken down to two types: irritant and allergic dermatitis, both of which can present at any age. Irritant dermatitis is more common and can be caused by such things as diapers, urine or stool, nickel, powders, or perfumes. The severity of the accompanying rash has been found to be a factor of the duration of exposure, the concentration of the irritant, and the integrity of the exposed skin. In contrast, allergic dermatitis is an immune response to an antigen, for instance poison oak or ivy. A careful history of exposure is key to a proper diagnosis. Initial contact establishes sensitization where white blood cells are primed with memory. The immune cells proliferate and secrete inflammatory cytokines upon reintroduction of the antigen, hence causing the clinically seen skin reaction. The typical rash is less demarcated and linear in distribution; the fine, erythematous, papular rash can erupt with vesicles. Treatment for both types of contact dermatitis includes patient education on the causative agent (for example, what the poisonous plant looks like); avoidance is ideal.. Mid to high potency topical steroids should be used for 1–2 weeks to help relieve the erythema and pruritis; cool compresses do the same. If the rash is generalized, oral corticosteroids can be used. Allergic dermatitis responds best to Prednisone dosed at 1–2 mg/kg per day, tapering off over 1–2 weeks. Patients are advised to avoid scratching and to keep the area clean as vesicles may weep and open if scratched; antibiotics may be necessary to combat any secondary infections.

Seborrheic dermatitis presents as mild erythema with flaky desquamation or as greasy plaques of yellow-red scales in the distribution of sebaceous glands. Young boys are affected more so than girls, and more so in either early infancy or postpuberty. The infantile type is seen diffusely on the scalp with discrete lesions on the face, trunk, and intertriginous areas and is noted to spontaneously resolve. With the adolescent type, the same red, greasy, scaly lesion with well defined borders is seen on the scalp, eyebrows, eyelids, forehead, nasolabial folds, and behind the ears. Both of the above forms are self-limiting so treatment should not be aggressive. Prolonged application of baby shampoo to the scalp, when scrubbed and rinsed, helps loosen the scales. One theory of etiology involves *Pitrosporum ovale*, so shampoos with ketoconazole can be used with recalcitrant cases. Infants with facial lesions respond well to low potency topical steroids; shampoos with salicylic acid should be avoided. Adolescents can use shampoos with salicylic acid or sulfur, progressing to those with zinc pyrithion or selenium sulfide; or they can try topical corticosteroids with or without 2–5% sulfur precipitate or salicylic acid twice a day. Steroids should be avoided on the eyelids; instead, use warm compresses and gentle cleansing to remove the scales, and topical application of sulfacetamide ointment. Compliance is stressed with adolescents as some untreated cases become chronic.

Tinea infections are diagnosed by clinical presentation, and definitively diagnosed by KOH microscopy. Tinea capitis produces inflammation of the scalp and damaged hair follicles, possibly leaving either "black dots" or boggy nodules with superficial pustules called kerion which can scar. Tinea corporis presents annular patches with papular scaly borders either with a clear center or red throughout with superficial pustules. With tinea pedis, the red scaly itchy lesions seen between the toes are exacerbated by the warm and moist environment inside a shoe and are common in adolescent athletes. Treatment

TABLE 1. Differential table of common pediatric dermatoses

Dermatoses	Onset	Presentation	Distribution	Diagnosis
Atopic dermatitis	Infancy	Dry, scaly Erythema Pruritis	Bilateral Cheeks Extensor Surfaces flexor surfaces	Family history Distribution Pruritis
	Childhood	Dry, scaly Erythema Pruritis		Family history Distribution Pruritis
Contact dermatitis	Any age	Fine papular Erythema Vesicular	Point of contact	History Appearance
Seborrheic dermatitis	Infancy	Scaly Mild erythema Greasy plaques Well defined borders	Parallels sebaceous glands Diffuse on scalp	Presentation Limited pruritis location
	Adolescence	Scaly Mild erythema Greasy plaques Well defined borders	Scalp Eyebrows Forehead Nasolabial folds Beard area	Presentation Limited pruritis Location
Tinea capitis	Any age	Inflammation Broken or lost hair follicles Kerions Pustules	Scalp	Location Black dot appearance Fungal culture KOH preparation
Tinea corporis	Any age	Annular Papular Scaly border with central clearing Erythema	Face, trunk, and extremities	Location Appearance Fungal culture KOH preparation
Tinea pedis	Adolescence	Scaly Erythema Pruritis	Between the toes	Location Appearance Fungal culture KOH preparation Pruritis

against tinea capitis involves oral antifungals because topicals do not reach the hair shaft. Griseofulvin at 10–20 mg/kg/day for 6 weeks works well; and selenium sulfide 2.5% shampoo can be added as a possible adjunct. Patients with tinea corporis and pedis need to keep the affected area clean and dry. Topical terbinafine, clotrimazole, ketoconazole, miconazole, or oxiconazole can be used twice a day for 3–6 weeks. The practitioner should follow-up each 2–4 weeks and should examine family members to avoid recurrence.

Discussion—By noting differences in the distribution and presentation of these common pediatric dermatoses, an appropriate diagnosis and plan can be constructed (Table 1).—*C. Jacka*

♦ This nursing presentation reviews the four most common pediatric skin conditions that present to the pediatrician office along with a brief description of the clinical presentation, the pathophysiology, and treatment of each group. These conditions are atopic dermatitis, contact dermatitis, seborrheic dermatitis, and the tinea infections (tinea capitis, tinea corporis, and tinea pedis). There is nothing new or advanced presented in this paper but, since foot and ankle specialists may encounter many of these cases in general practice, this is a good basic review.—*G.L. Dockery, D.P.M.*

3 Internal Medicine: Endocrinology and Rheumatology

IAN YU, D.P.M.

Impact of Genomics on Drug Discovery and Clinical Medicine

Emilien G, Ponchon M, Caldas C, Isacson O, Maloteaux J-M (Université Catholigue de Louvain, Brussels, Belgium; University of Cambridge, Addenbrookes's Hospital, Cambridge, UK; Harvard Medical School, Mclean & Massachusetts General Hospital, Belmont, MA)
Q J Med 93:391–423, 2000

Introduction—Genomics is opening the door for drug discovery and clinical medicine as it introduces new opportunities and efficiency to each area. However, it does not escape ethical concerns.

Discussion—Genomics is the scientific approach to mapping, sequencing, and analyzing an organism's compete set of genes and chromosomes. This discipline has opened the door for Pharmacogenomics which is the detection, monitoring, and treating of the molecular causes of a disease. It applies the genomic approach to drugs in development and in clinical trial by identifying genes' responses to drugs in trial. In turn, the efficacy and toxicity of a medication can be targeted. This effects drug development greatly since a patient's response to the medication can be more accurately analyzed and a subgroup of patients who showed higher efficacy and fewer side effects can be implemented to phases II and III of the drug's trial. Basically, we will be able to define populations that would benefit from the drug. Medications can work for one group of people, while being detrimental to another group of people. Genomics will allow the prediction of drug efficacy and medications will be customized for a beneficial population. However, this leads to very crucial ethical concerns. First, we do not know the unforeseen consequences of manipulating the human gene, and second, we will have to know which individuals carry the targeted gene. This will violate patient confidentiality unless a patient consents to the screening.—*R. Childers*

◆ Although this paper does not provide much information useful for clinical practice at this point and time, it is an excellent review of the potential impact of genomics on the future of drug discovery and clinical medicine. At first glance, one may not think that podiatric medicine would be greatly affected by genomics. However, with pharmacogenics, the study of the linkage between an individual's genotype and that individual's ability to metabolize a foreign compound, the development of drugs targeted towards specific problems will change. In addition, the major targets of research and development in this field are in the fields of diabetes, arthritis, and many neurological diseases which the podiatric physician participates in treating. It is important for the podiatric physician to understand the future of genomics and the potential implications on clinical practice.—*I. Yu, D.P.M.*

Meeting American Diabetes Association Guidelines in Endocrinologist Practice

Miller CD, Phillips LS, Tate MK, Porwoll JM, Rossman SD, Cronmiller N, Gebhart SSP (Emory University School of Medicine, Atlanta, GA)
Diabetes Care 23(4):444–448, 2000

Introduction—It has been shown that tight glycemic control, lower cholesterol, and lower blood pressure reduce complications in patients with type I and type II diabetes. This study was designed to see if patients could maintain the American Diabetes Association (ADA) guidelines for these factors while under the care of a specialist, more specifically an endocrinologist.

Research Design and Methods—Charts from 1998 were reviewed until 120 type II diabetes patients and 31 type I diabetes patients meeting select criteria were found. Information regarding the patient's control of risk factors was obtained from the charts and compared with ADA guidelines. Statistical analysis was conducted; value differences were deemed significant if p values were $<.05$.

Results—The most common complication of type II diabetes was hypertension (80%) followed closely by peripheral neuropathy (78%) and hyperlipidemia (64%). Types of screening studies that patients had received within the year were led by foot screenings (87%) and dilated eye exams (74%). Most (95%) patients were managed with pharmacological agents, over half (57%) used insulin either solely or in combination with oral hypoglycemics. HbA_{1c} was ≤ 7 in 61% and $\leq 8\%$ in 87% of type II diabetes patients. HbA_{1c} measured ≤ 7 in 57% of patients and ≤ 8 in 80% of patients with type I diabetes.

Conclusions—Based on the results given, specialists can help patients with type I and type II diabetes maintain lab values within ADA-approved limits. These data are not the first to reveal that specialists may be able to meet ADA guidelines better than primary care settings. New prospective studies should be conducted to evaluate concurrent management, outcomes, and costs for care of patients with diabetes in the generalist and specialist settings.—*G. Grant*

♦ This article is confirmation that the endocrinology community is becoming more aware of the potential complications associated with diabetic foot. In this review of clinical practice patterns of this particular group, it was nice to see that 87% of the diabetics had a foot examination at their previous visit with their endocrinologist. These findings were in contrast to previous studies which involve primary care physicians. However, one needs to keep in mind that the studies done on the primary care physicians were prior to the completion of the Diabetes Control and Complications Trials and the current practice standards may have changed. Future research should involve outcome studies to establish whether or not referrals made to podiatrists reduced the rate of diabetic foot complications.—*I. Yu, D.P.M.*

A Statement for Health Care Professionals on Type 2 Diabetes Mellitus in Hong Kong

Chan JCN (Hong Kong Society for Endocrinology, Metabolism, and Reproduction, Prince of Wales Hospital, Shatin, Hong Kong)
Hong Kong Med J 6(1):105–107, 2000

Introduction—One in 10 people in Hong Kong have diabetes mellitus (DM), 2% are less than 35 years old, and 20% are greater than 65 years old. Diabetes is on the rise due to obesity, physical inactivity, and aging. Diabetic patients often have hypertension, dyslipidemia, and albuminuria and have complications of kidney failure, leg amputations, heart disease, and stroke. DM is defined as fasting plasma glucose greater than 7 mmol/L or a random plasma glucose greater than 11.1 mmol/L. Patients with impaired glucose tolerance and impaired fasting glycemia are prone to develop diabetes and have increased cardiovascular risks. Diabetes risk factors include family history, obesity, dyslipidemia, hypertension, and age greater than 45 years. Control of blood glucose combined with patient education has been shown to reduce the complications associated with diabetes.

Physical/Lab Assessment—At least two visits a year should be made to the internist and at each visit, blood pressure and body weight should be measured. An annual foot exam should include pulses, sensation, skin changes, and deformities. An annual eye exam and lipid profile should also be performed. Glycosylated hemoglobin (HbA1c) levels should be measured biannually.

Urine samples should be checked for microalbuminuria. Electrocardiogram and chest radiograph should be performed when appropriate.

Discussion—Treatment should be directed at reducing glycosylated hemoglobin, blood pressure, weight, and an improvement in the lipid profile. Health care needs to be directed at the prevention of DM by educating the community about prevention and the severe complications it carries. Promote physical activity, and reduce obesity. Prevention and proper treatment are detrimental in preventing the morbity and mortality of diabetes.—*K. Carriero*

♦ Lifestyle factors, physical inactivity, and lack of patient education may be some of the factors resulting in the increasing prevalence of diabetes mellitus in the population. This is a very well put together statement for health professionals to follow, although some of the parameters may be different from those used in the United States. The inclusion of podiatrists and other health care professionals in the development of this statement has led to a very multidisciplinary approach.—*I. Yu, D.P.M.*

Prognostic Factors in Early Rheumatoid Arthritis

Scott DL (GKT School of Medicine, London, UK)
Rheumatology 39(Suppl 1):24–29, 2000

Introduction—Currently, the model for rheumatoid arthritis defines the disease as a persistent synovitis that leads to erosive damage and that progression of erosive damage itself results in functional disability. Prediction of disease progression is possible through the determination of prognostic factors such as joint involvement, high C-reactive protein (CRP), rheumatoid factor (RF) positivity, erythroctye sedimentation rate (ESR), and the presence of nodules.

Methods—Based upon evaluations of numerous studies published, rate and predictors of x-ray progression, rate and predictors of functional disability, factors predictive of x-ray progression, factors predictive of functional disability, and rheumatoid factor subtypes have been established.

Results—In a large 19-year study, radiographic damage occurred at a constant rate throughout the course of the disease. However, when progression was analyzed in two other studies, varying patterns of progression were observed. X-ray progression and RF positivity clearly correlated in all but one study. Similarly, the rate of progression of functional disability followed the disease duration. Several studies confirmed poor functional status at presentation as one of the best predictors of subsequent outcome. In addition, RF positivity and CRP correlated with progression of functional disability.

Erosion status in 79% of the patients was predicted using a combination of the following: positive RF, swelling of two or more large joints, and duration of at least 3 months. Compared with long-term x-ray progression, ESR levels significantly correlated. Patients who were seronegative showed a good prognosis, while 95% of seropositive individuals had a poor prognosis. Consequently, it was determined that RF positivity at presentation is one of the best predictors of disability. At present, an association has been found between IgA RF positivity and more increased joint damage and more active disease; however, other studies have failed to reproduce the association.

Conclusion—Identification of prognostic factors for patients who are at risk for a poor outcome could allow intervention at an early disease stage to prevent worsening of the disease and to limit joint damage. Prediction of joint damage and functional disability can be accomplished most consistently with the RF positivity prognostic factor.—*A. Duckworth*

◆ Given the complex and ever-changing nature of rheumatoid arthritis, the rheumatoid foot needs to be managed aggressively. We have all witnessed how dynamic the changes can be and wondered what the best prognostic factors are. This article does outline some of the prognostic predictors in the rheumatoid patient. However, other individual factors such as biomechanics can effect the therapeutic management within the foot. Therefore, the role of the podiatrist is extremely important. Our assessment and management should include serial x-rays and laboratory values. It is important to individualize treatment and routinely monitor the progression of changes in the rheumatoid foot in order to properly manage the patient both medically and surgically.—*I. Yu, D.P.M.*

Remitting Seronegative Symmetrical Synovitis with Pitting Edema (RS3PE) Syndrome: A Review of the Literature and a Report of Three Cases

Finnell JA, Cuesta IA (Madison, WI; Botsford General Hospital, Farmington Hills, MI)
J Foot Ankle Surg, 39(3):189–193, 2000

Introduction—Remitting seronegative symmetrical synovitis with pitting edema (RS3PE) syndrome is a disease that produces acute synovitis and tenosynovitis in the hands and feet and bilateral pitting edema. It lasts for about 18 months and has an older Caucasian male predominance. Serological tests tend to be negative, but there is a mild to moderate elevation of the erythrocyte sedimentation rate (ESR). The etiology is unknown but has been linked with *Campylobacter jejuni* infections, paraneoplastic syndrome, and seronegative arthropathies. RS3PE responds to low-dose corticosteroid therapy or hydroxychloroquine. Although the differential diagnosis for RS3PE syndrome includes polymyalgia rheumatica (PR), rheumatoid arthritis (RA), seronegative arthropathies, connective tissue diseases, calcium pyrophosphate dihydrate deposition disease, carpal/tarsal tunnel syndromes, amyloidosis, complex regional pain syndrome, and panarteritis nodosa, RS3PE most closely resembles rheumatoid arthritis and polymyalgia rheumatica.

Case Studies—

- *Case 1*—A 72-year-old Caucasian male presents with acute, bilateral hand swelling and symmetrical pitting edema in the legs that is worse in the morning and lasts throughout the day. He had a history of cancer, heart disease, and hypertension (HTN). He had no history of rheumatological disorders, although his sister had RA and systemic sclerosis. This patient responded well to low-dose prednisone and finished his treatment regimen in 25 weeks without complications.

- *Case 2*—A 78-year-old Caucasian male presents with an acute onset of bilateral stiffness, edema, and pain in his legs. He also has symmetrical pitting edema of his hands and feet. This patient has a history of HTN, left rotator cuff tendinitis, right knee replacement, and a benign lung biopsy. Neither he nor his family had a history of rheumatologic disorders. He had an elevated ESR. This patient's complaints improved with corticosteroid therapy, although he suffered a steroid-induced acne attack.

- *Case 3*—An 89-year-old Caucasian male presents with acute bilateral pitting edema of the hands and legs that was unsuccessfully treated with diuretics and anti-inflammatory medications. This stiffness was worse in the morning but persisted throughout the day. His past medical history included anemia. He had a slightly elevated ANA and ESR. This patient was successfully treated with low-dose prednisone therapy without complications.

Discussion—It is important for podiatric physicians to be aware of the signs and symptoms of RS3PE since patients often present with bilateral pitting edema. Bilateral edema may be attributed to systemic diseases (congestive heart failure, renal/liver failure, etc.) while unilateral edema may be caused by local factors (deep vein thrombosis, cellulitis, etc.) However, RS3PE will not respond to conventional therapy like elevation, compression, anti-inflammatories, or diuretics. It will, on the other hand, respond to low-dose corticosteroid therapy or hydroxycholoroquine. If a patient presents with these symptoms, it would be prudent to order a rheumatology workup. RS3PE remits within 18 months.—*G.H. Jhala*

♦ How many times has edema in the lower extremity been attributed to systemic diseases such as congestive heart failure, renal disease, nephrotic syndrome, etc. All too often it goes ignored and untreated and patients are simply told to elevate their feet. As podiatrists, we are often the first to hear the complaint that "my legs are swollen." This is a good article which reviews some of the causes of both unilateral and bilateral pitting edema. The presentation of RS3PE and the treatment are well presented. This is a clinical condition which should be added to the differential diagnosis in order to allow early detection and appropriate treatment.—*I. Yu, D.P.M.*

Frontiers in Transplantation of Insulin-Secreting Tissue for Diabetes Mellitus

Warnock GL (University of Alberta, Edmonton, Alberta, Canada)
Can J Surg 42(6):421–426, 1999

Introduction—Intensive insulin therapy has been shown to significantly reduce the risk of neurovascular complications. Transplantation of the pancreas provides an effective, physiologic treatment option where insulin delivery can be precisely regulated. Reports suggest that peripheral neuropathy is improved and retinopathy is stabilized after these procedures. However, most of the pancreas transplantations are done in conjunction with simultaneous kidney transplantation. This is associated with an increased risk of infection, rejection, hospitalization, and surgical complications. The morbidity of these procedures has prompted the investigation of islet cell transplant.

Method—Six insulin-dependent diabetic patients ranging from 23 to 36 years of age were selected for islet cell transplants. Each of the subjects had end-stage diabetic nephropathy and received simultaneous kidney transplantation. The results were compared to nine individuals who only received kidney transplants. In two of the subjects, 4000 islets/kg body weight from one donor were embolized to the liver through a mesenteric vein during the kidney transplant procedure. In the other four patients, islets from 3 to 10 additional donors were cryopreserved, thawed, and implanted at a dose of 10,000 islets/kg body weight. Immunosuppression was obtained with polyclonal antilymphocyte serum, cyclosporine, steroids, and azathioprine.

Results—The patients who received 4000 islets/kg achieved insulin production of 1–2 ng/mL during fasting and 3–4 ng/mL after eating a mixed meal. There was a decrease of their exogenous insulin requirements. However, the graft function decreased after 8 weeks. There were greater improvements observed in the patients who received 10,000 islets/kg. One of the patients was insulin independent for more than 2 years. Another patient had graft function for up to 5 years with repeated intervals of insulin independence. There was an 83% survival rate at 5 years, with one patient dying due to sepsis at 3 years.

Conclusions—Islet cell transplantation provides the potential for a low-risk invasive procedure with a reduction in the need for aggressive, toxic immunosuppression. This study showed that when combinations of multidonor fresh islet cells plus cryopreserved islets were implanted, better results were achieved. Other studies have shown that several factors improve the success of islet cell transplants. These characteristics include: 1) preservation of the pancreas for less than 8 hours before islet cell isolation, 2) an islet cell dose greater than 6000/kg, 3) embolization of islet cells into the liver through the portal vein, and 4) use of antilymphocyte globulin to induce immunosuppression.

There has been some progress made in regards to the supply of donor tissue, immune-mediated injury of the transplanted islets, and deterioration of transplanted islet function with time. This is promising for future research and clinical application of islet cell transplants.—*S. Patel*

◆ This is an exciting area of research in which medicine and surgery converge. As the search for the best method of "physiologically reversing diabetes mellitus" continues, it will be important for podiatric research to focus attention on the impact it has on the diabetic foot-related complications. Individual reports suggest that peripheral but not autonomic neuropathy is improved. As the number of successful transplantations become more widespread, there will be greater opportunity to study the outcomes. Multi-centered, controlled trials to examine the effects of these transplantations still need to be completed with attention on the impact on diabetic-related complications.—*I. Yu, D.P.M.*

Investigation and Treatment of Osteoporosis in Patients with Fragility Fractures

Hajcsar EE, Hawker G, Bogoch ER (McMaster University, Hamilton, Ontario, Canada; Sunnybrook & Women's College Health Sciences Centre; University of Toronto, Toronto, Ontario, Canada)
Can Med Assoc J 163(7):819–822, 2000

Introduction—Osteoporosis often remains undiagnosed in patients presenting with osteoporosis-related fragility fractures, in which, detection and early treatment are essential to decrease future risks of serious hip and spine fractures. Therefore, proper investigation and treatment of osteoporosis in patients presenting with fragility-type fractures are assessed.

Methods—All patients presenting with fractures to three Ontario community hospitals during four 1-week periods in February and November 1996 and August and May 1997 were reviewed to identify patients with apparent fragility-type fractures. The authors defined fragility-type fracture sites as distal radius, proximal femur, vertebral body, or proximal humerus. Patients less than 18 years of age, patients with underlying systemic causes of osteoporosis, and patients suffering traumatic fractures were excluded from the group. The remaining patients were informed of the study about 1 year after the index fracture, and telephone interviews were conducted for further exclusion of patients who consented to participate. Eligible patients entered information regarding prior fractures, previous diagnosis of osteoporosis, and any investigations or treatment of osteoporosis before or after the index fracture.

Results—Of the 2694 fracture clinic visits during the four periods, 228 met criteria consistent with fragility-type fractures. Of the 228 patients, 128 consented to participate, in which 20 were excluded based on their interviews. Among the 108 eligible patients, 96 (83 postmenopausal and 13 premenopausal) were women and 12 were men. Forty-three patients reported 53 prior fractures (other than the index fracture) of the fragility type. Ten patients had been diagnosed with osteoporosis before the index fracture, and 10 were diagnosed after the index fracture, all of whom were postmenopausal women. Of the 108 patients, 14 had bone densitometry before the index fracture, while 24 had the densitometry after the index fracture. Supplemental calcium had been recommended by physicians to 34 women and one man, and supplemental vitamin D to 14 women and no men. Of the 75 postmenopausal women eligible for hormone replacement therapy (HRT), only 27 had been offered HRT, of whom 15 had declined, and 12 were currently taking HRT. Of the 12 patients taking HRT, eight had been diagnosed with osteoporosis. Eight of the 20 patients diagnosed with osteoporosis were currently taking biphosphates.

Conclusion—Of the 108 eligible patients with fragility-type fractures, 20 had been diagnosed with osteoporosis, and 38 had undergone investigation of osteoporosis before or after the index fracture. These findings demonstrate the amount of undiagnosed and untreated osteoporotic patients at high risk for future fractures, and the lack of investigation of osteoporosis among patients presenting with fragility-type fractures to fracture clinics.—*M. Garrison*

♦ Although the article did not show any statistically significant data and only had 56.1% of the eligible candidates participate, I feel that it has an important message. Specifically, less than 20% of individuals with fragility-type fractures did undergo investigations or treatment for osteoporosis. As the population ages, there is an increased prevalence of osteoporosis and this study illustrates that it may often remain undiagnosed and untreated. How often do we review foot films or see reports which show osteopenia? Quite often, I am sure, these individuals may not have had a workup for osteoporosis. I think that it is important that as podiatric physicians we consider either recommending or actually ordering more investigational studies such as bone mineral densiometry in individuals with osteopenia and risk factors. In the long run, the potential alteration in this pattern of practice may allow early diagnosis and prevent bone loss and fracture.—*I. Yu, D.P.M.*

Orthopaedic Applications of Gene Therapy: From Concept to Clinic

Kang R, Ghivizzani SC, Muzzonigro TS, Herndon JH, Robbins PD, Evans CH (University of Pittsburgh School of Medicine, Pittsburgh, PA; Harvard Medical School, Boston, MA)
Clin Orthop 375:324–337, 2000

Introduction—Although gene therapy was designed to treat a variety of genetic disorders, it is now being utilized to treat musculoskeletal problems like rheumatoid arthritis, osteoarthritis, and osteogenesis imperfecta.

Principles of Gene Therapy in Orthopedics—There are several advantages to using genes instead of gene products, including being able to maintain high concentrations of gene products for long periods of time. Orthopedic gene therapy can be approached by either systemic delivery or local delivery of genes. The major advantage of systemic delivery is the ability to treat disseminated disease. The major advantage of local delivery is the ability to avoid systemic side effects. Viruses are the most efficient vectors used to deliver the gene(s), and they can be transferred to cells by either ex vivo or in vivo methods. Ex vivo transmission is safer to the patient because the vectors are introduced to cells that can be later implanted into patients after they are screened. The cells that are used are modified mesenchymal stem cells.

Gene Therapy of Rheumatoid Arthritis (RA)—RA is initiated by unknown etiologic events that trigger immune dysfunction. Thus a good site for intervention would be at the level of immune recognition and cytokine activity. This study will center around local treatment of rabbit knees (control and antigen-induced arthritis) via the synovium using an adenoviral vector for in vivo gene delivery and a retroviral vector for ex vivo gene delivery. Three different genes were used to encode for the following: IL-1 type I receptor (IL-1sRI), TNF type I receptor (TNF-sRI), and vIL-10. Individually TNF-sRI and IL-1sRI produced modest results in reducing inflammation and producing chondroprotective effects, but together they have additive effects. The vIL-10 gene produced impressive effects alone. But because of problems with the current generation of adenoviral vectors preclude their current application to human arthritis. Data collected from other studies allowed the authors to develop a human protocol for ex vivo gene transfer of IL-1Ra using a retrovirus. Nine postmenopausal women who require arthroplasty of metacarpophalangeal joints 2–5 on one hand were used. Surgical synovial biopsy specimens were taken as a source of autologous synovial fibroblasts, which were then divided into two groups. One group was transduced with the retrovirus encoding IL-1Ra (MFG-IRAP) and cultured, and the other was used as a nontransduced control. After testing the cells, they were injected into two metacarpophalangeal joints destined for total joint replacement. Two more were injected with the control. One week later all four joints underwent arthroplasty and the specimens were analyzed. This confirmed the possibility of safely transferring genes to humans and having them expressed intra-articularly.

Other Orthopaedic Applications—The methods described can also be used to treat osteoarthritis as seen with hIL-1Ra gene transferred into dog knees 2 days after they were a surgical procedure to induce osteoarthritic changes. Histopathology showed reduced size and depth of the lesions. This technology has been tested for ligamentous and tendinous injuries with some success in preliminary efforts for transfer of the genes. Gene transfer to bone can also be utilized in cases of nonunion or segmental defects, as well as in intervertebral discs.

Current Status—Development of human gene therapy has four overlapping stages. First, one must show target cells are susceptible to transduction by in vitro and next in vivo studies. The next step is successful animal models, and finally, phase I human trials. RA is currently the only indication in a human trial. Further development will require time and expenses that can only be subsidized by corporate sponsors.—*F. Nejad*

♦ This is good article which outlines some of the principles and current status of gene therapy in relationship to orthopedic applications. One should keep in mind that it may take 5–10 years (or longer) before any of these are used in clinical practice. Currently, applications in rheumatoid arthritis is the only area that has reached Phase I trials. In vitro and in vivo gene transfers, however, have been successful in areas such as osteoarthritis, bone healing, and cartilage repair, as well as ligament and tendon pathology. This is an up and coming field that may have some future applications that could improve treatment outcomes.—*I. Yu, D.P.M.*

Clinical Profile of Diabetic Foot Infections in South India—A Retrospective Study

Vijay V, Narasimham DVL, Seena R, Snehalatha C, Ramachandran A
(Diabetes Research Centre, Royapuram, Chennai, India)
Diabet Med 17:215–218, 2000

Introduction—A common cause of hospital admission of diabetic patients in India is diabetic foot infections. This study was done to determine the profile of South Indian diabetic patients with diabetic foot infections and the causative factors leading to delayed wound healing and recurrence.

Methods—This study was a retrospective study of diabetic patients with diabetic foot infections that required some type of surgical intervention between January 1994 and December 1997. Three hundred seventy-four diabetic patients were followed with a mean age of 54.9 +/− 9.4 years and a mean duration of diabetes of 10.9 +/− 7.7 years. Factors that were noted in the study included details of treatment, duration of hospital stay, history of smoking, and fasting and postprandial plasma glucose and serial glycosylated hemoglobin. Patients were considered to have neuropathy if they had a vibration perception threshold (VPT) >25 V on the biothesiometer. A patient with an ankle brachial index (ABI) >0.6 and <0.8 was considered to have peripheral vascular disease (PVD). Hypertension and ischemic heart disease were also noted. Wagner's classification was used to classify the ulcer. The surgery that was performed consisted of a major amputation (BK amputation), minor amputation, or surgical debridement. Statistical analyses were performed on the data.

Results—Data on the above parameters were collected. A majority of the foot ulcers treated were at least a grade 2. Surgical debridement was the most common surgical procedure performed. Median healing time was found to be 44 days. A shorter healing period was seen in those patients without PVD or neuropathy but the difference was not significant although delayed wound healing was found to be significantly higher in those with neuropathy. Out of the 374 patients, 198 had a recurrence of foot infection. A majority of those who relapsed had PVD and neuropathy.

Discussion—The authors felt that a lack of adequate off-loading due to available shoe material in the neuropathic patients might have contributed to the higher incidence of recurrence. Smoking and mean HbA1 were not shown to have an important association. Recurrence of foot infection was shown to have an association with neuropathy and PVD. Although patients were provided with foot infection educational materials, there was a 52% recurrence rate. The conclusion of the authors was that both neuropathy and PVD were important predictive factors for the recurrence of diabetic foot infection. It was also concluded that improvement in footwear and foot infection education in this population could be beneficial.—*L.T. Rowe, B.S.*

♦ One of the major points that this article illustrates is the importance of utilizing appropriate shoes and accommodative insoles following surgical debridement of the diabetic foot. In the South Indian society, there is a nonavailability of such special footwear which is no doubt an important factor for the high recurrence of diabetic foot ulceration. All too often we have seen transfer lesions occurring after surgical debridement of the diabetic foot. Appropriate planning of the surgical reconstructive phase following the initial debridement as well as prophylactic shoes and insoles prevent future breakdown.—*I. Yu, D.P.M.*

Bone and Joint Infections in the Elderly: Practical Treatment Guidelines

Mader JT, Shirtliff ME, Bergquist S, Calhoun JH (University of Texas Medical Branch, Galveston, TX)
Drugs Aging 16(1):67–80, 2000

Introduction—The elderly may be considered immunocompromised due to the fact that they are more susceptible to a range of infections than are younger adults. Moreover, pre-existing medical conditions result in a locally and/or systemically compromised patient, which increases the risk of infection.

Hematogenous Osteomyelitis—Twenty percent of the total number of osteomyelitis cases is due to hematogenous osteomyelitis, which is usually monomicrobic in origin. Vertebral and long bone osteomyelitis are the two types seen in the elderly.

1. *Vertebral osteomyelitis*—In the elderly population, vertebral osteomyelitis is usually hematogenous in origin, but can be secondary to trauma. Antimircobial therapy is suggested and surgical debridement is usually not necessary when the infection is diagnosed early.

2. *Hematogenous long bone osteomyelitis*—Elderly patients without implants rarely develop long bone hematogenous osteomyelitis. The most common cause is reactivation by local bone or adjacent soft-tissue trauma of a site of quiescent hematogenous osteomyelitis. Therapy should consist of adequate drainage, thorough debridement, obliteration of dead space, wound protection, and antimicrobial therapy.

Contiguous Focus Osteomyelitis without Generalized Vascular Insufficiency—Fifty percent of all cases are osteomyelitis secondary to contiguous foci of infection. This form is often difficult to treat and multiple organisms are usually the cause of the infection. Surgical debridement may hasten eradication in addition to antimicrobial therapy (broad spectrum).

Contiguous Focus Osteomyelitis with Generalized Vascular Insufficiency—Diabetic patients or patients with peripheral vascular disease from atherosclerosis account for the majority of patients with osteomyelitis in this category. There are two main types: 1) osteomyelitis involving the small bones of the feet, and 2) malignant external otitis. Treatment for osteomyelitis of the bones in the feet is centered around resection of infected bone and antimicrobial therapy that targets multiple organisms. Local debridement of the external auditory canal and aggressive antibiotics that cover *Pseudomonas* spp. comprise the mainstay of treatment for malignant external otitis.

Osteoporosis and Osteomyelitis—Age-associated osteoporosis seen in elderly patients exacerbates the fact that, during an active period of infection, surviving bone in the osteomyelitis field usually becomes osteoporotic. Hormone and vitamin supplements can be used for this situation.

Joint Infections—Septic arthritis is considered a medical emergency that is associated with serious morbidity and mortality. In addition to antimicrobials, thorough drainage in the form of needle aspiration, tidal irrigation, arthroscopy, and arthrotomy (according to the presentation) are critical.

Antibacterial Adverse Effects in the Elderly—Adverse drug reactions occur more frequently in the older patient population primarily due to decreased organ reserve capacity, altered pharmacokinetics and pharmacodynamics of drugs, and polypharmacy with associated drug–drug and drug–disease interactions.

Conclusion—Most of the cases of osteomyelitis in the elderly can be treated with adequate drainage, thorough debridement, obliteration of dead space, wound protection, and antimicrobial therapy. Septic arthritis is considered a medical emergency. In addition, decreased bone repair and adverse effects of prescribed antibacterials complicate treatment for the elderly patient.—*J.M. Dawson*

◆ This article is a good review of the management of the osteomyelitis and septic arthritis. It focuses on these conditions in the elderly and this certainly is important given the aging "baby boomers." I am not convinced that the considerations given for the elderly who are being treated for osteomyelitis are that different from the considerations for individuals who have diabetes-related osteomyelitis. Considerations regarding renal function, polypharmacy, and wound healing are mentioned. Overall, this article is a good review.—*I. Yu, D.P.M.*

Examining the Nutritional Status of Independently Living Elderly

Zulkowski K (Montana State University, Billings, MT)
Ostomy/Wound Manage 46(2):56–60, 2000

Introduction—In the American population, the fastest growing segment of society is over age 85. Moreover, 34.4 million Americans in 1998 were age 65 or older, which represented 13% of the total U.S. population. Nutritional problems defined by physical, social, and environmental factors need to be evaluated in order to maintain health, independence, and quality of life in the elderly population. Classification of the "community dwelling" elderly can be divided into those who are completely independent, those residing in assisted living centers, and those who receive home-delivered meals. Approximately 52–85% of the institutionalized elderly and more than 55% of hospitalized elderly are considered malnourished. The purpose of this study was to examine wellness behaviors, dietary practices, and nutritional lab values in the independently living elderly population.

Method—Forty-six volunteers from an area hospital over the age of 65 (mean age 74) were enrolled through their responses to a postcard mailed to them inquiring about interest in the descriptive study. Information regarding wellness behavior was collected with the use of questionnaires that contained the following categories: health screening behaviors, medication use, smoking, exercise, sleep patterns, safety practices, nutrition, and alcohol use. In addition, lab data were utilized to determine serum albumin, serum protein, and hemoglobin and hematocrit levels.

Results—See Table 1 for results.

Examination of the participants' daily food consumption revealed the following: 45% received adequate servings of milk or milk products; 26% received adequate vegetable consumption, 24% received adequate fruit or fruit juice consumption; and 14% received adequate consumption of breads, pasta, rice, or grains. The nutritional laboratory values showed a mean serum albumin level of 3.7 g/dL (normal is 3.5–5.0 g/dL), a mean serum protein level of 6.89 g/dL (normal is 6.0–8.0 g/dL), mean hemoglobin of 14.21 g/dL, and a mean hematocrit of 41.7%.

TABLE 1. Wellness behaviors

Category	%
Health Screening Behaviors	
Yearly physician visits	81%
Blood pressure checks in past 3 months	88%
Medication Use	
Take medication without assistance	100%
Taking five or more medications per day	54%
Safety Practices	
No safety concerns about home	89%
Fallen in past 6 months	89%
Smoking	
Smoke currently	0
Smoked in past	50%
Exercise	
Planned exercise program	50%
Sleep Patterns	
Get enough sleep	80%
Difficulty staying asleep	59%
Alcohol Use	
At least one alcoholic beverage per day	71%

Discussion—Overall, participants rated their quality of life as "very good" at 8.34 on a scale of 1–10. However, it was discovered that eating practices were poor for the entire sample, no one consumed nutritional supplements, and no one ate a balanced diet. Of the participants, 13.3% were below normal range for albumin levels.

Conclusion—Health care professionals need to be aware that poor nutrition in the elderly is a serious issue and, as a result, should include nutritional assessment as a component of treatment in acute and long-term care settings.—*A. Duckworth*

♦ So often wounds in the elderly take a long time to heal. Chronic wounds in the elderly may be accepted as slow healing wounds due to "old age." This study shows that health professionals need to include nutritional assessment as an important component of any examination in the community, acute care, and long-term care settings. Important factors to consider include serum albumin, serum protein, hemoglobin, and hematocrit. It should also be remembered that just because an individual may be obese, it does not necessarily mean his or her nutritional status is adequate.—*I. Yu, D.P.M.*

Healing of Diabetic Foot Ulcers and Pressure Ulcers with Human Skin Equivalent: A New Paradigm in wound Healing

Brem H, Balledux J, Bloom T, Kerstein MD, Hollier L (The Mount Sinai Medical Center, New York, NY)
Arch Surg 135:627–634, 2000

Background—Diabetic foot ulcers, pressure ulcers, and venous ulcers present considerable morbidity, mortality, and significant cost to patients and the health care system. These factors demand the best possible combination of therapies to achieve resolution. Determination of these combinations is of great importance. Physiologically active wound healing agents could show promise in the future of wound healing.

Methods—Twenty-three consecutive patients were treated with Apligraf for a total period of 10 months, with follow-up ranging from 2 to 9 months (10 diabetic foot ulcers, 13 pressure ulcers). Treatment was given after resolution of excessive drainage, infections, and the dominance of granulation tissue was established. Patient education regarding off-loading was provided and crutches prescribed. Procedurally, Apligraf was applied after excisional debridement and hemostasis were obtained, being sutured with 5-0 absorbable sutures with 1-mm space between the Apligraf edge and the skin edge. Grafts were dressed with Adaptic, followed by sterile cotton, xeroform, and Tegaderm. Pressure ulcers were staged according to National Pressure Advisory Panel Guidelines, and treated with the Renaissance zero-pressure alternating air mattress in addition to Apligraf. Healing times were based on time from placement of graft until complete epithelialization and an absence of drainage were achieved.

Results—Seven of 10 diabetic patients healed their wounds (18 consecutive wounds) with an average duration of 42 days after one application of Apligraf. Two of the three nonhealers had necrotic digital wounds. The third had a failed necrotic muscle flap that healed 50% and began healing after debridement of the remaining necrosis. Seven of 13 patients with pressure ulcers healed in an average of 29 days, all requiring only one application of Apligraf.

Discussion—The results of this study show that Apligraf helps in successfully healing diabetic foot ulcers and pressure ulcers. A limitation of this study is the absence of randomization and placebos. However, it supports evidence subsequently shown in randomized, placebo-controlled clinical trials of diabetic foot ulcers and venous stasis ulcers. These results also show that osteomyelitis near the site of the ulcer does not allow human skin equivalent to be effective. Understanding the physiology of wound healing has led to the development of new agents that actively promote wound healing. This will continue to impact wound healing treatment in the future.—*D. Clement*

♦ Although this is a good article, the authors admit that it is a nonrandomized study with no placebo group. It does reference a separate prospective, randomized, placebo-controlled study that does demonstrate how human skin equivalents can accelerate closure of chronic diabetic ulcerations. The article does not discuss rate of recurrence or plans on how to off-weight the diabetic foot ulcers to prevent recurrence. In fact, off-weighting the diabetic ulcers during the healing phase was limited to prescribed crutches which the author admits were not used with compliance. Future studies should involve the use of human skin equivalents in conjunction with proper off-weighting techniques.—*I. Yu, D.P.M.*

Topical Insulin in Wound Healing: A Randomised, Double-Blind, Placebo-Controlled Trial

Greenway SE, Filler LE, Greenway FL (Harbor-UCLA Medical Center, Torrance, CA; Northwestern University, Chicago, IL; Pennington Biomedical Research Center, Baton Rouge, LA)
J Wound Care 8(10):526–528, 1999

Introduction—In this paper, the authors presented two studies. The first was to assess the efficacy and safety of topical insulin in accelerating healing of standardized wounds in humans. The second was a pilot study to show the efficacy of insulin compared to a zinc solution in accelerating healing in standardized wounds in humans and rats. Zinc is used in the manufacturing of crystallise insulin; therefore it is not known whether the effects on wound healing are due to the insulin, the zinc, or a combination of the two.

Methods—

- *Study 1*—Five diabetics and six nondiabetics were used. A standardized wound was made on each forearm. Insulin was applied to one and saline to the other, four times a day until healed.

- *Study 2*—This study involved three separate investigations. In investigation 1, six rats were used, each given a standardized wound every day for 10 days. Saline, insulin, or zinc was applied three times a day at the time of the first cut. After 10 days, the rats were sacrificed and a pathologist analyzed the skin. In investigation 2, six rats were used, each given three standardized wounds, treated with a different solution until healed. In investigation 3, six human subjects were given three standardized wounds. Each of the cuts was treated with a different solution four times a day.

Results—

- *Study 1*—There was no significant difference in healing times between the nondiabetics and the diabetics. When the two groups were combined, those treated with insulin had a significantly faster healing time of 2.4 +/− 0.8 days.

- *Study 2*—In investigation 1, a qualitative assessment was made that showed a slower rate of healing in those rats treated with saline. In investigation 2, there was a significant difference in the healing time between those wounds treated with zinc and those treated with insulin in rats. Zinc was 1.2 +/− 0.5 days faster. In investigation 3, wounds treated with insulin were found to heal significantly faster than those treated with saline by 1.2 +/− 0.3 days. No significant difference in healing times between insulin and zinc was noted.

Discussion—In the first study, topical insulin was shown to accelerate healing in standardized wounds over the placebo. The authors assumed that if only the insulin had an effect in increasing healing time, then the zinc solution would have shown similar results to the saline, but the studies showed that was not the case. In fact, wounds treated with insulin or zinc were shown to have a faster healing time than those treated with saline.

Conclusion—Topical insulin is effective in accelerating wound healing in humans. This study did not determine if the insulin, zinc, or a combination of the two is the active factor in accelerating wound healing, but it did set some guidelines for planning a future study. The method of creating a standardized wound in humans that is accepted by the Institutional Review Board now makes future studies of wound healing in humans possible.—*L.T. Rowe*

♦ This paper presents an interesting concept. The studies seem to be very well designed and controlled. Hopefully, a delivery system can be established for this compound which make applications easier. If long-term studies prove that this is really effective in increasing the rate of healing, diabetics may be injecting insulin as well as applying it topically. The speed of healing should be tested against other growth factors. This may prove to be a more economical, readily available alternative to some of the commercially available growth factors.—*I. Yu, D.P.M.*

Primary Closure of Infected Diabetic Foot Wounds: A Report of Closed Instillation in 30 Cases

Connolly JE, Wrobel JS, Anderson RF (Dartmouth Medical School, Hanover, NH; Veterans Affairs Medical Center, White River Junction, VT)
J Am Podiatr Med Assoc 90(4):175–182, 2000

Introduction—The diabetic foot presenting with ulceration and subsequent deep-space infection or osteomyelitis, or both, is now at high-risk for amputation. Limb-salvaging procedures, most commonly combining surgical decompression with aggressive debridement of infected and necrotic tissue, are implemented to decrease bacterial load and avoid increased recovery time associated with high-level amputation. However, controversy remains in the proper management of the open wound produced from the aggressive incision and drainage. The authors used a closed instillation system near the incision and drainage site for managing infected wounds and hope to decrease the rates of higher level amputations of the at-risk infected foot.

Methods—Data were reviewed from 30 procedures performed on 29 neuropathic patients who all presented with deep-plantar-space infection of the foot, suspected acute pedal osteomyelitis, or both, between 1993 and 1998. Once the incision and drainage were completed, at the level promoting healing and minimizing the nidus for recurrent infection, the wound was prepared for closure utilizing the closed instillation system. This technique incorporated loose re-approximation of skin with no deep sutures and insertion of a 16-gauge angiocatheter through the skin at the apex of the site. This catheter allowed dependent drainage of normal saline with gentamicin solution; activity was restricted to complete bed rest while the catheter remained in place for 48 hours. Outcome measures were assessed by 1) comparing functioning and residential living status preoperatively versus postoperatively and 2) the need for re-operation or amputation.

Results—All 29 patients were male, the average age was 66 years, and 90% of patients had diabetes. Fifty-seven percent of patients had a vascular rating of "marginal" or "poor" which indicated values not consistent with those required for amputation healing. Forty-six percent of patients had hemoglobin levels below 3g/dL, and 67% of patients had total lymphocyte counts below 1500/μL. Thirty-four percent of patients had died at the conclusion of the study; however, the patients receiving the closed instillation system had a 90% success rate allowing only three patients to progress to higher-level amputations.

Conclusion—The closed instillation technique allows for promotion of wound healing, decreased tension on the wound, and decreased infection potential. Furthermore, this technique appears to be as effective as primary closure but offers decreased cost and time to surgeon and patient. The authors hope the closed instillation system will prevent higher level amputations in the at-risk infected foot, while promoting further exploration of surgical management techniques needed in this critical population.—*M. Garrison*

◆ Primary closure of an infected diabetic foot wound goes against many basic surgical principles and often many prefer a two-stage delayed primary closure approach. However, with the advent of antibiotic beads (both commercially available and self-made), the alternatives for primary closure are greater. The immediate closure of the wound may allow faster healing times. The authors describe a retrospective study in which a modified closed instillation system with a daily rate of 1 L/24 h of 80 mg/L gentamicin is delivered for 2 days postoperatively. Their success rate of 90% seems high and their parameters for a precise return-to-function time could not be determined for all patients. However, I believe that the technique described is a viable option which has similar success to other methods which allow primary closure of infected diabetic foot wounds. It is a technique which should be incorporated into the armamentarium of the diabetic foot specialist.—*I. Yu, D.P.M.*

4 Trauma

JOHN H. WALTER, Jr., D.P.M., M.S.

Osteochondritis Dissecans of the Talar Dome Treated with an Osteochondral Autograft

Chang E, Lenczner E (Montreal General Hospital, McGill University, Montreal, Quebec, Canada)
Can J Surg 43(3):217–221, 2000

Introduction—A variety of treatments, both surgical and conservative, have been used for osteochondritis dissecans of the talar dome. Osteochondral autografting is an option for lesions that are unstable, large, or when the lesion contains a small amount of subchondral bone. The authors report a case of a patient with osteochondritis dissecans of the medial talar dome treated with osteochondral autograft from the knee.

Case Report—A 35-year-old male presented with a fracture of the right fibula after an inversion ankle injury. He was treated with 6 weeks of immobilization, with satisfactory bone healing. Two months later, the patient reported pain in the ankle on walking distances, and pain and stiffness after periods of rest. Radiographs and magnetic resonance imaging revealed a superomedial talar dome osteochondral fracture ($11 \times 6 \times 11$ mm). The patient was treated conservatively for 6 months, without resolution.

Arthroscopic debridement was performed with only temporary relief. Eight months later, the patient underwent repair of the defect with osteochondral autograft from the ipsilateral knee. The patient's ankle pain had completely resolved by 6 weeks postoperatively, and by 12 months, the patient was able to resume his normal activities.—*T.C. Melillo, D.P.M.*

♦ Osteochondral autograft is indicated when there is a large cartilaginous defect with a small amount of associated subchondral bone. Hangody reported on the use of multiple small grafts to fill a large defect, while the authors of this case report harvested a single graft 10 mm wide. Both used the femoral condyle of the opposite limb of the ankle pathology as the donor site.

The benefits of using a large graft include a single harvest procedure, a greater chance of the graft taking and the cartilage surviving, less irregularity at the recipient site, and greater stability using one large graft as compared to multiple and smaller pieces of graft. A larger defect, however, is left in the femoral condyle as the result of harvesting one large osteochondral graft. In this case report the patient experienced a successful outcome and the donor site was eventually asymptomatic. Some degree of traumatic arthritis will be most likely experienced by most or all patients who have suffered an osteochondral dome fracture or lesion. Despite the use of conservative measures of care that include foot orthotics, ankle bracing, physical therapy, injection therapy, and heel lifts, surgical intervention may be necessary if symptoms continue to be more than the patient can tolerate. Osteochondral autografting is an excellent alternative in patients who have a large cartilaginous defect.—*J.H. Walter, Jr., D.P.M., M.S.*

Pilon Fractures: Treatment Protocol Based on Severity of Soft Tissue Injury
Watson JT, Moed BB, Karges DE, Cramer KE (Wayne State University School of Medicine and Detroit Receiving Hospital, Detroit, MI)
Clin Orthop 375:78–90, 2000

Methods—Treatment of 107 pilon fractures was studied, based on severity of soft-tissue injury. All pilon fractures were stabilized immediately by the application of calcaneal traction. Open fractures or fractures in patients with multiple injuries were stabilized with traveling traction that was applied in the operating room. A distraction computed tomography scan was obtained before definitive treatment. Treatment groups were based on the degree of soft-tissue compromise. Forty-one patients with Tscherne grade 0 or grade 1 injuries underwent open reduction and internal fixation using open plating and low-profile implants. Sixty-four patients with Tscherne grade II and grade III closed injuries and all patients with open fractures underwent definitive treatment with limited open reduction and stabilization using small wire circular external fixators.

Results—Clinical and radiographic evaluations were performed at an average 4.9 years after injury. For all fracture types, 81% of the patients who were treated with external fixation and 75% of the patients who were treated with open plating had good or excellent outcomes. For severe fracture patterns, type C, patients in both groups had significantly poorer results than patients with type A and B fractures. The patients in the open plating group had a significantly higher rate of nonunion, malunion, and severe wound complication compared with the patients who received external fixation for type C fractures.

Conclusions—Because of the increased incidence of bony and soft-tissue complications when treating open or closed type C fractures, use of limited exposures and stabilization with small wire circular external fixators is suggested. The lack of difference between external fixation and internal fixation for type C indicates more about the nature of the injury than about the treatment. At best, only 60% of patients with this type of fracturewill do well with the current techniques.—*A. Ghamgosar*

♦ Soft-tissue disruption or loss that commonly accompanies the more severe pilon fractures will, in many cases, necessitate the use of external fixation. Minimal soft-tissue dissection needed to apply most external fixators prevents further devitalization of both soft tissue and bone. Skin necrosis, soft-tissue infection, and fracture nonunion might be avoided if open reduction is delayed in favor of the use of external fixation.

Tscherne described a soft-tissue grading system for closed fractures. Ruedi and Allgower developed a classification for pilon fractures. Information gained by understanding and applying both of these classifications can be extremely valuable in determining the projected outcome for patients who have suffered this very disabling injury. This article provides important insight into the severity of a soft-tissue injury and the revelance it can have on the treatment of pilon fractures.—*J.H. Walter, Jr., D.P.M., M.S.*

Subtalar Arthrodesis for Complications of Intra-articular Calcaneal Fractures

Flemister AS, Infante AF, Sanders RW, Walling AK (Mary Imogene Bassett Hospital, Cooperstown, NY; The Florida Orthopaedic Institute, Tampa, FL)

Foot Ankle Int 21(5):392–399, 2000

Introduction—Subtalar arthrodesis has been advocated in the treatment of post-traumatic arthritis and as a primary treatment for highly comminuted calcaneal fractures. Studies concerning subtalar arthrodesis have thus far consisted of small patient populations and have not compared all of the indications for this procedure including the use of bone graft. This study reviewed cases of subtalar arthrodesis in a large patient population that was divided into three groups: 1) patients with calcaneal malunions, 2) patients with failed open reduction and internal fixation (ORIF), and 3) patients undergoing open reduction and primary fusion for highly comminuted fractures.

Methods—The senior author between 1985 and 1996 performed 136 subtalar fusions. Eighty-six fusions were available for the study, which included 62 calcaneal malunions (1), 16 failed ORIF (2), and 8 severely comminuted fractures (3). The operative indications for group 1 and 2 were the same; pain localized to the hindfoot with subtalar arthritis present radiographically and failure of conservative treatment. Group 3 was indicated for primary fusion due to the presence of a type IV fracture. The American

Orthopaedic Foot and Ankle Society's (AOFAS) ankle-hindfoot scale was used to score the patients' satisfaction. The authors considered a score of 69 or greater as a satisfactory result. The operative technique was basically the same within each of the groups. Three different bone grafts were used; local bone graft, autogenous iliac crest bone graft (ICBG), and freeze-dried cancellous allograft. Postoperative care consisted of 8 weeks partial weightbearing in a short leg cast followed by full weightbearing by week 12. A statistical analysis of the data was done with the statistical significance being set at $p < .05$.

Results—Eighty-three of the 86 fusions united within 4 months. In group 1, 50 of 62 patients were satisfied with their outcome. Group 2 achieved satisfactory results in all 16 patients. Six of eight were satisfied with their results in group 3. The most prevalent complication was osteomyelitits. The average postoperative talar declination angle was 14.6° with no correlation found between that and the AOFAS ankle-hindfoot score. A statistical significance was found between the length of hospital stay for patients receiving ICBG and those receiving other graft materials, with the patients receiving ICBG having a longer stay.

Conclusion—The authors results show that subtalar arthrodesis is an effective procedure following calcaneal fractures regardless of the indication. According to the talar declination angle, it was shown that complete anatomical restoration of the hindfoot is not necessary for a successful outcome. Bone graft using several different materials is recommended in subtalar fusion with the exception of ICBG, which can cause a longer hospital stay and thus increased cost.—*L.T. Rowe*

♦ Traumatic arthritis and malunion of the subtalar joint account for the majority of pain and loss of motion in patients who suffered moderate to severe intra-articular and comminuted calcaneal fractures. This is very often a career-ending injury with significant disability necessitating dramatic changes in lifestyle. Despite the recommended conservative management that includes foot orthotics, ankle bracing, injections, NSAID, pain medication, physical therapy, heel lifts, supportive shoe gear with rocker-bottom soles, and behavior modification, additional surgery is often necessary to reduce or eliminate the associated pain.

Eighty-three of 86 subtalar joint fusions that followed initial reconstructive calcaneal surgery were successfully performed with only three nonunions in this retrospective analysis. Autogenous bone grafts or bone bank cancellous allografts were used with equal success. In three fusions, in which no bone graft was used, a nonunion occurred. I will also aggressively fenestrate subchondral bone to allow for bleeding into the fusion site as well as stimulating bone formation by creating microfractures from the drilling. Painful lateral ankle impingement caused by lateral wall blowout must be eliminated at the time of the subtalar joint fusion. Triple arthrodesis is indicated when traumatic arthritis also involves the calcaneocuboid joint which is commonly associated with comminuted intra-articular fractures of the calcaneous.

Careful and accurate evaluation of all joints affected by a severe calcaneal fracture is highly recommended in order to determine which procedure will best eliminate all of the painful joints. Foot function following a fusion procedure must be a high priority. A mild valgus attitude of the subtalar and midtarsal joint is recommended. Isolated subtalar joint fusions are highly successful in the elimination of pain generated from the traumatic arthritis without drastically altering normal foot biomechanics.—*J.H. Walter, Jr., D.P.M., M.S.*

Should Calcaneal Fractures Be Treated Surgically? A Metaanalysis

Randle JA, Kreder HJ, Stephen D, Williams J, Jaglal S, Hu R (Musculoskeletal Health Status Working Group, ICES, Toronto, Ontario, Canada)
Clin Orthop 377:217–227, 2000

Introduction—Due to the small sizes in previous studies, the appropriate treatment protocol for intra-articular fractures of the calcaneus has remained a debatable topic. This meta-analysis study compares the operative versus nonoperative treatment of intra-articular calcaneal fractures.

Materials and Methods—A MEDLINE search for articles on randomized clinical trials from 1980 to 1996 was performed. Six of 1845 articles met specified criteria, three retrospective and three prospective studies. A data extraction sheet was used to review each article; pain, return to work, and range of motion (ROM) of the subtalar joint were the major outcomes common to all articles. Only "pain" and "return to work" could be summarized using meta-analysis techniques.

Data Analysis—Using the Stata statistical package, data were analyzed across the studies. Odds ratio was analyzed to determine effectiveness of certain treatments.

Results—Patients received variable postoperative care for ROM exercises and initiation of weightbearing. Pain was assessed in varying ways in all articles. In summary, pain was increased in nonoperative patients and had an odds ratio of 1.5, meaning that someone treated in this fashion was 1.5 times more likely to have pain versus operative treatment protocol. Nonoperatively treated patients were more likely to change jobs or return to the same employment with restriction after a mean duration of 38 weeks. Surgically treated patients were more likely to return to their previous occupation without restriction after only 23.8 weeks.

Nonoperatively treated patients were more likely to have an increase in heel width and gait abnormality. ROM could not be assessed using meta-analysis techniques. Patients treated nonoperatively had a mean articular step-off of 3 mm and an abnormal Bohler's angle. Surgically treated patients had complications, including infection, nerve complications, and incision problems. One surgically treated patient required subtalar arthrodesis compared to seven in the nonoperative group.

Discussion—Surgical patients seemed to fair better when evaluated for pain, return to work, heel width, gait, and radiographic findings. However, due to small patient volume, none of these figures reached statistical significance. In summary, it seems that a weak argument can be made for surgical treatment of intra-articular calcaneal fractures. To make this recommendation strong, a large randomized, treatment controlled study needs to be undertaken, where the results are measured by validated grading instrumentation.—*G. Grant*

♦ "To operate or not to operate," that is the question. As with most intra-articular fractures, anatomical reduction is usually preferred to restore joint function and to minimize the ill effects of traumatic arthritis and pain. The calcaneus with its subtalar joints and calcaneocuboid joint is no exception and, like other fractures, should be treated aggressively in most cases.

Moderate to severe comminution of the calcaneus with posterior facet depression contributing to a triplane deformity makes it, however, almost impossible to restore in all three planes. Three subtalar joints, the calcaneocuboid joint, and the numerous anatomical landmarks which are attached to tendons, ligaments, and capsules make the restoration process difficult at best. There are also major tendons that pass by and under the calcaneus whose normal functions are largely dependent on a normal calcaneus.

Small fragments of bone and cartilage from related joints of the calcaneus are always lost at the time of injury or subsequent surgery, contributing to the inevitable joint disease that will follow. Experience and surgical skill of the surgeon will give the patient the best chance of a successful outcome. Although joint pain and calcaneal widening are common complaints, I strongly believe that they can be significantly reduced relative to the degree of comminution, displacement, and joint involvement.

Foot orthotics will help to control pain in most cases. Ankle bracing and shoe modifications such as rocker bottom soles will also improve the patient's quality of life.

If an isolated subtalar joint fusion or a triple arthrodesis is performed, previous restoration of the height of the subtalar joint will help to maintain the overall length of the limb and make the fusion procedure easier. Primary fusion of the subtalar joint should be a serious consideration in all severe comminuted intra-articular joint depression fractures. When it is obvious that a calcaneal fracture is beyond repair, primary fusion will probably avoid one or more years of patient suffering and disability. Next time include the primary fusion procedure on your operative consent form just in case you choose to fuse.—*J.H. Walter, Jr., D.P.M., M.S.*

Tendo Achillis Rupture: Surgical Repair Is a Safe Option

Mellor SJ, Patterson MH (The Princess Royal Hospital, Sussex, UK)
Injury, Int J Care Injured 31:489–491, 2000

Introduction—There is a linear relationship between the recent increase in "weekend warriors" and the rise in Achilles tendon ruptures. Numerous studies quote the unpredictability of the surgical repair and its success, with the two most common sequela being infection and re-rupture. This 5-year retrospective study reviewed 67 tendo Achillis repairs in effort to judge morbidity.

Methods—Patient files were found using the Manchester database at the District General Hospital in the United Kingdom. Those who had acute tendo Achillis rupture with subsequent surgical repair were reviewed. Clinical follow-up was analyzed and further efforts were made to contact each patient via telephone questionnaire to identify any further complications.

Results—Sixty-seven patients (51 men and 16 women) were identified with mean age of 42 years. In 86% of cases, the skin was incised utilizing a medial longitudinal incision and closed with interrupted absorbable sutures with independent repair of the paratenon. The skin was generally approximated utilizing simple interrupted sutures. Postoperative care included an above-knee cast with the ankle plantarflexed for 2 weeks, progressing to a below-knee cast for 4–6 weeks until plantigrade correction was achieved. At 2 weeks postop, one superficial infection was identified and successfully treated with a short course of antibiotics. At the 30-day follow-up period, two re-ruptures had occurred and one patient developed reflex sympathetic dystrophy which resolved with guanethidine blocks.

Discussion—Nonoperative treatment of Achilles tendon rupture involves cast immobilization with the foot slightly plantarflexed and 70% of patients have complete return of function with a re-rupture rate of 8–29%. The rate of re-rupture after surgical evacuation of hematoma and repair of the tendon defect is 1–5%. With an infection rate of 1.5% in this study, previous research quoting high rates of wound infection, dehiscence, and tethering cannot be supported. According to this study, tendon apposition is best achieved by surgical intervention and with low risk of complication and re-rupture, open surgical repair should be strongly considered in the treatment paradigm.—*K. Van Voris*

♦ This British 5-year retrospective study of 67 tendon Achilles ruptures that were repaired surgically had a 3% (2 out of 67) re-rupture rate and a 1.5% (1 out of 67) infection rate. Other reports site infection rates ranging from 10% to 21%, which certainly will be a persuading factor when considering whether to operate or not.

The extremely low infection rate reported in this article might be attributed to careful patient selection, good surgical technique, infrequent use of tourniquets, minimal tourniquet time when used, and use of absorbable suture. I would also recommend the prophylactic use of antibiotics due to the dysvascular nature of tendon. Rerupture rates are higher when conservative management of Achilles tendon ruptures has been used, such as in gravity equinus casting.

Primary Achilles tendon repairs can be a relatively short procedure with minimal postoperative complications. Isometric exercises performed while in a postoperative cast as well as early rehabilitation make primary repair the treatment of choice in my opinion.—*J.H. Walter, Jr., D.P.M., M.S.*

Augmented Repair of Acute Achilles Tendon Ruptures

Zell RA, Santoro VM (Farmington, CT)
Foot Ankle Int 21(6):469–473, 2000

Introduction—Operative treatment for spontaneous rupture of the Achilles tendon in a relatively young active individual is achieved through percutaneous repair, primary repair, or augmented primary repair. One technique, in particular, that has found success is an augmentation primary repair utilizing a central slip of gastrocnemius-soleus fascia.

Methods—Twenty-five mostly male patients of an average age of 40 years were surgically treated by one surgeon for athletics-related isolated Achilles tendon ruptures. Fifty percent of these patients considered themselves well conditioned, and the other 50% were relatively nonconditioned individuals who participated in intense sporadic activities. On examination, the patients all had a palpable defect, antalgic gait, and a positive Thompson test. Open primary repair was performed within 7 days of the injury, with the major indication for the surgery being a great desire or necessity to return to work and recreation.

The surgical technique consisted of placing the patient in a prone position with a thigh tourniquet so that hemostasis was achieved. A posteromedial skin incision was made over the point of rupture and exposure of the ruptured Achilles tendon was accomplished. In neutral position the Achilles tendon was put into anatomical length as tension was felt, and nonabsorbable sutures were then tied. Ends were re-approximated using interlocking fashion followed by figure-eight suturing. By extending the incision proximally to the gastroc-soleus myotendon junction, a fascial slip was centrally marked out and created with a width of 1.5–2.0 cm and a length adequate enough to cover the repair site. The goal of this repair was to wrap and tubularize the tendon with the fascia while keeping the ankle in neutral position.

Immediately after surgery, active planterflexion and passive dorsiflexion to 0° was encouraged. At 2–3 weeks postoperatively, weightbearing was allowed as tolerated; 3–4 weeks postoperatively, active stretching of the Achilles tendon was allowed; 4–6 weeks postoperatively, leg toe rises and passive resistive exercises were begin; at 8 weeks, low impact activities were allowed; and finally at 4–6 months postoperatively, competitive high-impact sports were allowed.

Results—All patients completely healed their repairs. No ruptures recurred. There was, however, one infection which required plastic reconstruction with skin graft. At 6 months, edema was noted, and the calf of the surgical side was within 1 cm of the contralateral limb. All the patients were able to return to full preinjury activities by 4–6 months after the surgery, with no loss or disruption of fixation.

Discussion—It is obvious that the traditional postoperative management of 3–4 weeks of immobilization in equinus followed by 2–3 weeks of immobilization in neutral position, and weightbearing in 6–8 weeks in a walking cast is not going to be adequate or acceptable for those patients who demand a short rehabilitation time. Because augmentation adds collagen to the repair site and gives biomechanical stability, patients can be encouraged to initiate early weightbearing and range-of-motion exercises. All patients also stated that they would choose to have this same type of surgery done again if the contralateral Achilles tendon ruptured.—*S.B. Heninger*

♦ Augmenting a primary repair of an acutely ruptured Achilles tendon will no doubt ensure a stronger repair and significantly reduce the risk of re-rupture. Reinforcement of the end-to-end anastomosis of the Achilles tendon is most often performed by utilizing the gastrocnemius-soleus fascia (aponeurosis).

The 25 patients in this study ranged in age from 24 to 66. All were male except one. Twenty-three ruptures occurred during athletic activities such as basketball, tennis, softball, karate, racquetball, and running. The other two were the result of a fall. Fifty percent of the patients would be considered athletic and well conditioned with the other 50% only occasionally athletically active.

Extending the incision to the myotendinous junction allows for adequate exposure of the aponeurosis. A single flap of aponeurosis from 1.5 to 2.0 cm in width was freed from the underlying muscle extending from the myotendinous junction to the most proximal origin of the combined tendon. This single flap is reflected distally and rotated 180° to keep the smooth aponeurosis on top and next to the peritenon. Holding the ankle in neutral, the aponeurosis is laid over the primary repair or rupture site and sutured in place. Utilization of a single strip of aponeurosis is known as the Silfverskiold procedure. When two strips are used for repair, it is called the Lindholm procedure. Widening of the heel cord following augmented repairs is to be expected. Although the re-rupture rate following primary repair is already low, adding a secondary and augmenting procedure that will further lower the re-rupture rate makes good sense for the majority of patients, especially those who are athletically active. —*J.H. Walter, Jr., D.P.M., M.S.*

Arthroscopic findings in Acute Fractures of the Ankle

Hintermann B, Regazzoni P, Lampert C, Stutz G, Gächter A (University of Basel and the Kantonsspital, St. Gallen, Switzerland)
J Bone Joint Surg 82-B(3):345–351, 2000

Objective—Ankle fractures are often accompanied by persistent disabling pain despite the restoration of joint stability and congruity. Articular cartilage lesions, undetectable by plain radiographs at the time of injury, may be the source of pain. This article aims to assess prospectively the role of arthroscopy for evaluating acute fractures of the ankle.

Methods—The authors evaluated 288 consecutive acute ankle fractures requiring surgical treatment between July 1993 and November 1997. Fractures in 148 men and 140 women were classified according to the Danis-Weber system: 14 type A, 198 type B, and 76 type C. Arthroscopy, followed by open reduction and internal fixation, was performed within 72 hours of injury.

Results—Cartilage lesions were found in 228 ankles (79.2%): 200 on the talus (69.4%), 132 on the distal tibia (45.8%), 130 on the fibula (45.1%), and 119 on the medial malleolus (41.3%). Lesion frequency and severity increased from type B to type C fractures. Lesion subgroups increased from 1 to 3 within each fracture type. Lesions were worse in all patients under 30 and over 60 years. Lesions in men were more prevalent and severe; men were affected at younger and older ages compared with women. Lateral ligament injuries were seen more often in type B than type C fractures. Deltoid ligament injuries were more frequent in type B.1 fractures. Anterior tibiofibular ligament damage increased from type B.1 to type C.3 fractures. Arthroscopy was successfully used to assist in debris removal and fracture repair in 81 patients. Nineteen complications included transient impaired nerve function (13), scar irritation (4), local pain (1), and synovial cyst (1).

Discussion—Talar rotational or translational forces impacting the malleoli cause ankle fractures, and forces on talar collateral ligaments can avulse the malleoli. Treatment to date has been determined by injury classifications based on simple hinge mechanics and plain radiographs. The high incidence of cartilage lesions demonstrated by this study may explain why treatment results do not always correlate with osseous damage or achieved reduction and stability. Further studies must determine the effects of intra-articular lesions as predictors of fracture outcome.

This study demonstrates that cartilage lesions secondary to ankle fractures appear most often on the talus regardless of fracture type, and supports the belief that the severity of talar and malleolar lesions is dependent on fibular fracture height. Pronation and rotational forces cause talar cartilage lesions, particularly in type-C fractures and less so in type-B fractures. Local stresses from supination forces in type-A fractures may cause more lesions on the distal medial tibia than on the medial talus. Study results are consistent with the belief that higher fibular fractures are met with more extensive anterior tibiofibular ligament damage. This study suggests that arthroscopy via an anterocentral portal is a reliable means to diagnose intra-articular lesions and some ligament injuries in acute ankle fractures, and may also advance our understanding of injury mechanisms.—*D. Collman*

♦ Traumatically induced chondral lesions of the ankle joint are a common occurrence with ankle injuries such as in sprains or fractures. Inversion, eversion, supination, and pronation mechanisms of injury that affect the ankle joint can lead to damage of cartilage which many times goes undetected at the time of open reduction.

Of the 288 arthroscopic procedures performed in acute ankle fractures, cartilaginous defects were found in 79.2% of them. On the talar dome, 69.4% lesions were found; the distal tibia plafond had 45.8%, the fibula 45.1%, and the medial malleolus had 41.3%. The more severe lesions were associated with higher lateral malleolar fractures and distal fibular diaphysis fractures. Chronic ankle pain post fracture repair is usually associated with traumatic arthritis. Chondral or osteochondral ankle joint lesions can also be a source of chronic ankle pain, which may necessitate MRI or arthroscopic evaluation.

The incidence of cartilaginous or osteochondral defects is significant as substantiated by recent literature. Careful intraoperative evaluation of joint cartilage is warranted and highly recommended.—*J.H. Walter, Jr., D.P.M., M.S.*

Closed Ankle Fractures in the Diabetic Patient

Flynn JM., Rodriguez-del Rio F, Pizá PA (University of Puerto Rico School of Medicine, San Juan, Puerto Rico)
Foot Ankle Int 21(4):311–319, 2000

Introduction—Diabetes mellitus (DM) is known to affect patients' ability to heal as well as their renal, vascular, and nervous system functions. Although the diabetic foot is a known entity, there are no clear guidelines for management of ankle fractures in the diabetic population. Past studies have suggested that this population is at higher risk for infection, and, when they have associated neurovascular impairments, stand a higher risk of postsurgical complications. This retrospective study compares closed ankle fracture management in diabetic versus nondiabetic patients.

Methods—Ninety-eight patients were studied, 25 of whom were diabetics. Study variables included but were not restricted to duration of DM, DM treatment compliance, associated neurovascular impairments, grade of ankle fractures, alcohol and tobacco use, and fracture management regimen. Fracture management was either closed reduction with immobilization (casting) or open reduction with internal fixation (ORIF). Conservative management included long leg cast for 4 weeks followed by weightbearing (WB) cast for 2 weeks. ORIF management included non-WB short leg cast for a total of 6 weeks and then followed with WB as tolerated.

Results—Diabetic patients <45 years old have a higher risk of infection than nondiabetic patients of the same age group. Diabetic patients who present with swollen/ecchymotic skin are also at higher risk than nondiabetics. Within the diabetic population, fracture treatment/regimen and infection were noted to be statistically significant ($p < .05$). Diabetics treated conservatively were at higher risk than those treated surgically ($p = .059$) as well as nondiabetics also treated conservatively ($p = .045$). Patients with poor DM treatment compliance and neurovascular compromise were at higher risk for development of infection.

Conclusion—There is limited literature dealing with ankle fracture management in the diabetic patient. This study suggests that regardless of treatment, diabetics with ankle fractures are at higher risk of infection than nondiabetics ($p = .003$). This is especially true when accompanied with ankle soft-tissue swelling, ecchymosis, neurovascular compromise, and so forth. In this high-risk population group, it is advised that a multidisciplinary team approach be adopted to manage these individuals.—*D.D-Q. Tran, D.P.M.*

♦ Diabetic patients, especially those who smoke, are at a significantly greater risk for infection. This study found that 32% of the 25 diabetic patients treated for ankle fractures developed an infection whether they had concurrent diabetic ulcers or not.

Compliance is always a concern especially in the higher risk groups that include the diabetic or the smoker. Neuropathy and peripheral vascular disease are two additional compromising factors when contemplating surgery, which may very well be the deciding factor not to operate. Closed reduction can produce satisfactory results when properly performed, eliminating the risks of surgery. Cessation of smoking, control of blood sugars, the use of prophylactic antibiotics and the control of swelling can be helpful to lessen the risk of infection. —*J.H. Walter, Jr., D.P.M., M.S.*

Calcaneal Fractures in Children: Long-Term Results of Treatment

Brunet JA (Ottawa Hospital, Canada)
J Bone Joint Surg 82-B(2):211–216, 2000

Background—Long-term follow-up of 19 childhood calcaneal fractures managed with conservative care showed excellent results. The outcome gives validity to conservative treatment for such a problem, and suggests that open reduction may only be indicated in adolescents with severe displacement of their os calcis.

Methods—Old charts, x-rays, and follow-up notes were reviewed and, of the 34 patients with calcaneal fractures under the age of 14, 17 were available for interview and examination; two had bilateral fractures. Displacement of calcaneal fragments were considered minimal if 1–2 mm on x-ray, moderate if 3–4 mm or with a loss of Bohler's angle of 7° or less, and gross if more than 5 mm or with a loss of 8° or more of Bohler's angle. Five fractures were extra-articular with minimal displacement. Of the 14 intra-articular fractures, six showed gross, two moderate, and six minimal or no displacement. These intra-articular types can be further subdivided: two tongue types, two centrolateral, one at the sustentaculum tali, and six grossly comminuted. Two of these children also had talar neck fractures, two had Lisfranc fractures or subluxations, and one also fractured the lateral cuneiform. Without regard to the type of fracture, all of these children were treated conservatively in a cast without manipulative reduction; one exception required open wound debridement. Patients were followed for at least 10 years.

The final follow-up covered inquiries about function (namely restrictions from discomfort with work or sports, and a subjective score of residual pain), physical exam, and x-rays. Results were impressive as all could walk comfortably on uneven ground and few had serious complaints: four had mild cramps with abrupt barometric changes, two had cold sensitivities, two had mild discomfort, and two had reduced range of motion. None were aware of any functional restrictions and many were involved in competitive or high-impact sports. All but the two with talar neck fractures displayed full or only slightly reduced subtalar joint mobility. None required any special accommodations or inserts in their shoes, and all worked without complication. Clinical scoring using the AOFAS rating system averaged 96.2. Radiographic analysis did show common rearfoot abnormalities. Four patients showed reductions of Bohler's angle between 10° and 30°, five showed calcaneal widening up to 7 mm, and one showed arthritic changes.

Discussion—The severity of the injury did not seem to correspond to the functionality of the patients' lifestyle; in fact, many who had sustained joint depression or comminution were still involved with demanding sports activities. This retrospective study suggests that conservative treatment of calcaneal fractures has a good prognosis, at least 16.8 years after the insult. Many authors have recommended open reduction in the face of joint displacement or when the injury is bilateral. However, it is suggested here that children have great potential to remodel damaged articular surfaces and achieve congruency and normal function, making conservative management a rewarding alternative.—*C. Jacka*

♦ Children who suffer intra-articular calcaneal fractures fortunately do not experience the same devastating sequelae as adults do in the vast majority of pediatric calcaneal trauma. This long-term follow-up evaluated calcaneal fractures in patients who ranged in age from 2.5 to 13.5 years of age. Fractures were both intra-articular and extra-articular. Nineteen calcaneal fractures in 17 children were largely caused by falls, jumps, or crush-type injuries. All but one of the 19 fractures were treated conservatively with immobilization. Closed reduction and percutaneous pinning utilizing the Essex-Lopresti method was performed in only one of the worst intra-articular joint fractures.

Almost 17 years after injury, each patient was again evaluated for residual effects of their particular calcaneal fracture. These included an achy feeling with low barometric pressure or bad weather systems, reduced subtalar joint mobility, mild to moderate discomfort with sports-related activities, and widened heels.

Joint adaptation with bone and cartilage repair after injury is one of the privileges of childhood. Mother Nature is very forgiving with pediatric fractures in general, although closed or open reduction is still recommended in severe cases. In pediatric intra-articular calcaneal fractures, subtalar joint arthrosis is not nearly as devastating and disabling as with adults.

Foot orthotics should be the very minimum used in the treatment of healed calcaneal fractures with any age patient in order to limit subtalar joint motion, improve foot mechanics, and slow the joint disease process. Ankle bracing can also be of value, supplying ankle support and strength needed for the reduction of secondary knee, hip, and back pain commonly associated with compensating for the painful foot.—*J.H. Walter, Jr., D.P.M., M.S.*

Competence of the Deltoid Ligament in Bimalleolar Ankle Fractures After Medial Malleolar Fixation

Tornetta P (Kings County Hospital, New York, NY)
J Bone Joint Surg 82-A(6):843–847, 2000

Introduction—The ankle joint consists of the medial and lateral malleolus and the associated ligamentous structures. When these structures are interrupted as seen with bimalleolar fractures, talar subluxation often occurs resulting in ankle joint instability. Past studies suggest that medial ankle stability can be restored with reduction and fixation of the medial malleolus. Very little emphasis, however, has been put on the medial collateral ligaments. The purpose of this study was to assess the integrity of the deltoid ligament after reduction of the medial malleolus in patients with bimalleolar fractures.

Methods—Twenty-seven patients were diagnosed with bimalleolar fractures according to the Lauge-Hansen classification scheme. In all cases the medial malleolus was fixated first using strict dissection to avoid disrupting any ligamentous attachments. At no time were the deep fibers of the deltoid evaluated for injury. Stress radiographs were then taken to assess the medial clear space and talar subluxation. The lateral malleolus was then anatomically reduced and fixated. Postoperative radiographs were taken in all patients.

Results—Seven (26%) of the stress radiographs taken after medial malleolar fixation showed an abnormally widened medial clear space with talar subluxation indicating deltoid incompetence. Because the lateral malleolus was correctly reduced and fixated, the medial clear space and talus were restored in all patients postoperatively.

Discussion—The strongest portion of the deltoid ligament is the deep fibers that originate on the posterior colliculus and insert on the talus. The weaker, superficial fibers originate from the anterior colliculus and insert on the talus and navicular. In patients with fractures involving the anterior colliculus, the deep fibers of the deltoid were injured posteriorly. Even after medial fixation, the superficial fibers were not sufficient enough to restore medial ankle stability. Conversely, in patients with supracollicular fractures, the deltoid ligament remained intact and medial fixation was adequate in restoring medial ankle joint stability.

Conclusion—In bimalleolar fractures, the injury may be strictly osseous, or it may be a combination of an osseous injury with ligamentous disruption involving the deep fibers of the deltoid ligament. In the latter, medial fixation alone may be insufficient in restoring medial ankle stability.—*D. Carmack*

♦ Ankle trauma must be carefully evaluated radiographically for both osseous and associated soft-tissue pathology. Anatomical restoration of fracture fragments is essential if near normal function is desired. Unfortunately, proper evaluation and repair of the ligamentous structures do not receive the same attention during surgery. They are often overlooked, which could account for less than satisfactory results when not repaired. Osteochondral fractures of the talar dome should also be ruled out during intraoperative evaluation of the ankle joint. Radiographic evaluation of the ankle under stress or MRI may prove valuable in those cases that have a high suspicion of occult osseous or ligamentous damage.—*J.H. Walter, Jr., D.P.M., M.S.*

Complications After Treatment of Tibial Pilon Fractures: Prevention and Management Strategies

Thordarson DB (University of Southern California School of Medicine, Los Angeles, CA)
Am Acad Orthop Surg 8(4):253–265, 2000

Background—Nonoperative treatment of displaced pilon fractures (>2 mm) has been plagued by poor results. However, high rates of complications occur in tibial pilon fractures treated with classic open reduction and internal fixation due to the complexity of the periarticular injury and the limited nature of the soft-tissue envelope of the distal tibia. This report reviews complications that occur with pilon fractures and strategies to avoid or treat them.

Pilon fractures most often occur after high-energy trauma due to axial compression. High-energy injuries are often open fractures and compromise the soft tissues resulting in higher rates of complications.

Ruedl and Allgower developed the first widely accepted fracture classification systems for tibial pilon fractures. Type I is a cleavage fracture of the distal tibia with a nondisplaced articular surface. Type II has mild-moderate displacement of the articular surface with minimal to no comminution of the joint surface or metaphysis. A type III fracture shows comminution of the articular surface and metaphysis with significant impaction of the metaphysis. The AO group developed a more detailed classification system for pilon fractures.

Surgical Planning—Preoperative templating can help in fixation placement. Plate fixation is used for buttressing rather than compressing fractures.

Open fractures require emergent irrigation, debridement, and fracture stabilization with external fixation. Soft-tissue coverage of open fractures should be done early along with fixation of the fracture.

Closed fractures with significant swelling may need a waiting period of 5–14 days before surgery. The goal in the interim is to reduce swelling and stabilize the fractures. A closed reduction with splinting may be necessary in stable fractures.

In unstable fractures, limb length should be restored with a calcaneal traction pin or joint-bridging external fixator if surgery needs to be postponed. Staging surgery can beneficial in the presence of swelling.

Fracture blisters occur in high-energy pilon fractures due to the soft-tissue injury and rapid swelling. It is best to leave the blisters intact and avoid placement of surgical incisions through fracture blisters.

Surgical Pearls—Indirect reduction technique relies on ligamentotaxis to reduce fracture fragments without excessive soft-tissue stripping. A distractor is placed between pins in the tibia and the neck of the talus. With distraction, the comminuted areas disimpact and facilitate indirect and direct reduction of the articular fragments.

If tension-free closure cannot be achieved, the wound should be left open and closed secondarily or closed with a skin graft or muscle flap. When two incisions are needed, there should be a 7- to 10-cm skin bridge to reduce the risk of skin necrosis.

Treatment of Wound Complications and Infections—A full-thickness skin slough requires aggressive debridement in the operating room with soft-tissue coverage as soon as possible. The hardware may need to be removed if a deep space infection occurs. A course of intravenous antibiotics is recommended for 3–6 weeks in these situations.

Conclusion—Complications are frequently encountered in pilon fractures. Proper preoperative planning can minimize intraoperative complications. Wound problems can be prevented or minimized with delayed surgery, temporary traction, indirect reduction techniques, appropriate soft-tissue management, and the use of smaller implants or external fixation.

Late complications such as stiffness can be reduced with early mobilization. Nonunion and post-traumatic arthritis can be salvaged with bone grafting and ankle fusion, respectively.—*O.T. Wang, D.P.M.*

♦ In 1999, Drs. Ruedi and Allgower published a classification of intra-articular tibial pilon fractures, which today bears their name. Three types of pilon fractures where described:

Type I has minimal comminution and a nondisplaced articular surface. Alignment is good to fair.

Type II also has minimal comminution; however, displacement is mild to moderate. Alignment is fair to poor.

Type III presents with severe comminution, severe articular disruption, and metaphyseal impaction. Alignment is poor.

The more severe the comminution, the more difficult the restoration is. Hopes of approaching anatomical alignment are usually slim to none. MRI or CT can help in the planning for these difficult surgical reconstructions.

Massive bleeding as a result of the injury causes gross swelling and severe pain. The skin becomes shiny and taut. Deeper tissues appear devitalized. Delaying surgery 5–14 days to allow the skin and deep tissues to return to normal will dramatically reduce the infection and dehiscence rate.

External fixation can be used to supplement the use of other forms of internal fixation, adding more stability. Rigid internal fixation, although difficult to achieve in severely comminuted fractures, will allow for early rehabilitation, which is essential during the remodeling process of the ankle joint.

Since this injury occurs mostly in the highly osteogenic cancellous bone of the distal tibial metaphysis, nonunions are uncommon. Malunions, however, are not uncommon largely due to the severity of the comminution and metaphyseal impaction.

Traumatic arthritis of the ankle joint is inevitable, as is its altered mechanics. Limited ankle joint motion significantly changes the gait pattern to avoid stressing the ankle in the dorsiflexed position. Compensatory gait changes will quickly generate numerous other postural complaints which should be minimized with the use of ankle bracing, foot orthotics, heel lifts, and rocker bottom soled shoes.—*J.H. Walter, Jr., D.P.M., M.S.*

Evaluation and Management of Common Running Injuries
Browning KH, Donley BG (Cleveland Clinic, Cleveland, OH)
Cleveland Clin J Med 67(7):511–520, 2000

Introduction—Greater than 25% of adult runners suffer musculoskeletal injury. The history of a running injury is critical. Questions concerning changes in running terrain, pre- and postrunning routine, intensity, and change in distance are important. A sudden significant change in training routine is the most common cause of injury. Many running injuries are due to overuse and therefore duration and frequency are critical clues. Shoes should be inspected for they lose shock-absorbing capacity and functional stability by 300 miles. The physical exam should focus on gait, scoliosis, genu valgum/varum, leg length discrepancy, muscle atrophy, and muscle spasm to gain insight into the pathomechanics.

Discussion—Apophysitis of the iliac crest, anterior superior iliac spine, and anterior inferior iliac spine, and ishial tuberosity are problems commonly seen in younger runners. Secondary to overuse, these occur at tendon insertion sites and will respond to icing, analgesics, and protection with full recovery to exercise.

Trochanteric, ishial, and pes anserinis bursitis are common overuse complaints and respond well to corticosteroid injection. Stress fracture of the hip, pelvis, and thigh usually occur when excess stress is applied to normal bone. Pain is exacerbated with weightbearing. Stress fracture of the femoral neck carries a risk avascular necrosis, delayed union, and nonunion and should be carefully managed by a specialist. Radiographs are usually not positive for 2–4 weeks and a MRI should be used with a high index of suspicion. In most cases, protected weightbearing, and a change to low-impact exercise are appropriate. Osteoarthritis of the hip usually presents as pain in the groin area and is treated with nonsteroidal anti-in-flammatory drugs (NSAID) and low-impact training.

Anterior knee pain is the most common complaint of runners, accounting for 29% of all injuries. The differential diagnosis is patellofemoral syndrome (PFS), chondromalacia, plica syndrome, bursitis, and tendonitis. PFS contributing factors are abnormal tracking of the patella secondary to biomechanical and/or anatomical abnormalities. Evaluate the entire lower extremity for anteversion of the femur, tibial torsion, subtalar joint pronation, and a widened Q angle. Treatment consists of ice, muscle rebalancing, and avoidance of squatting exercises. Plica syndrome presents as anterior-medial knee pain and a snapping sensation during range of motion. The plica is a medial synovial fold present in about 60–80% of the population. Excessive friction over the medial femoral condyle may lead to pain and fibrosis. Surgical arthroscopic excision is appropriate if conservative measures fail.

Iliotibial band syndrome occurs due to friction over the lateral femoral condyle in patients with calcaneal varies, tibial varum, and hip abductor weakness. Treatment consists of ultrasound, ionophoresis, corticosteroid injection, and surgery for intractable cases.

Tibial stress fracture and medial tibial stress syndrome (shin splints) often present similarly. Shin splint pain usually resolves with running and after the run, whereas with stress fractures the pain is worse with running and persists through the night. Diagnosis is made by radiograph looking for periosteal reaction and callous formation. Fracture of the anterior middle third of the tibia has a risk of nonunion, delayed union, and displacement and should be treated carefully. Shin splints are associated with excessive pronation and respond well to rest, ice, and anterior muscle strengthening.

Achilles tendonitis occurs with repetitive loading, foot pronation, and Achilles tendon tightness. Treatment consists of heel lifts or a walking cast.

Plantar fasciitis is an overuse injury, which occurs as a result of microtrauma to the fascia at its origin. Heel pain with the first step of the day is a classic presentation. Conservative treatment is 95% effective, with surgery indicated for intractable cases. Calcaneal stress fracture pain is exacerbated with medial-lateral compression.

Metatarsalgia is a synovitis most commonly of the second or third metatarsophalangeal joint, which can easily be confused for a neuroma, which is commonly seen in the third web space and presents with burning and stabbing pain. A fifth metatarsal fracture should be investigated as a Jones fracture, which occurs at the metaphyseal–diaphyseal junction. Jones fractures carry a risk of nonunion or delayed union and should be treated by a specialist.

Conclusion—The list of running injuries is great and, when injured, the runner should follow a general guideline, dependent upon the injury as to when to return to running. Returning to a normal running routine is dependent upon the number of weeks missed. The longer the runner has been away from running, the more rehabilitation and low-impact training should be performed before resuming running again.—*K. Carriero*

♦ Overuse injuries or syndromes are usually caused by an increase or sudden change in a runner's routine. A detailed history of a runner's previous injuries along with specifics of the chief complaint with any and all changes in daily activities will usually lead to an accurate differential diagnosis.

Common running injuries include stress fractures of the metatarsals, the calcaneus, the tibia and fibula, shin splints, plantar fascitiis, Achilles tendonitis, and chondromalacia patella (runner's knee). Serious runners will keep a log of their mileage, types of running shoes worn, and where the running occurred with type of surface. It is not unusual to have a runner present with six or more pairs of running shoes for you to evaluate. Of course, excessive or abnormal wear can be helpful in evaluating biomechanical problems that may be directly relate to the injury in question.

Cross training with cycling or swimming will help to maintain a runner's stamina and strength. Following a serious injury, the runner should be guided by his or her physician, who will recommend a safe and gradual return to a full running schedule. Ankle bracing and foot orthotics are very beneficial in the treatment and prevention of many running injuries.—*J.H. Walter, Jr., D.P.M., M.S.*

5   Sports Medicine and Related Conditions

STEPHEN M. PRIBUT, D.P.M.

Current Issues in the Design of Running and Court Shoes

Reinschmidt C, Nigg BM (Human Performance Laboratory, The University of Calgary, Calgary, Canada)
Sportverl Sportschad 14:71–81, 2000

Introduction—Athletic shoes are designed based on functional and nonfunctional factors. The nonfunctional factors include price, fashion, style, and durability. More importantly, however, are the functional factors. These include the shoe's ability to prevent injury, to enhance performance, and to provide comfort during activity. Since different sports execute different movements, each sport requires a uniquely designed athletic shoe to support the athlete. Athletic shoes can be divided into running shoes and court shoes. Court shoes refer to footwear worn by basketball, volleyball, and tennis players.

Methods—The three main functional factors in sport shoes include injury prevention, performance, and comfort. Since running shoes are more widely studied than court shoes, more information has been gained about that type of footwear.

1. Injury prevention
   A. *In runners:* Pronation control and cushioning are still believed to be the essential factors preventing injury in these athletes. Earlier studies have shown that excessive pronation and excessive impact forces are primary causes of running injuries. Therefore, controlling pronation and reducing impact forces should prevent injury.
      - *Pronation control*—Excessive pronation has by been linked to overuse injuries like Achilles tendinitis, shin splints, plantar fasciitis, iliotibial band syndrome, and patellofemoral pain syndrome. In addition, many injured runners appear to have slightly more foot eversion. Alterations of the midsole (dual density midsoles, round

81

and flared heels), the insole (orthotics, medial supports), the heel counter (heel stabilizers, heel caps), and the upper (medial and lateral reinforcements) have been designed to control pronation. A flexible midsole is an important design feature for running shoes because it allows the forefoot and rearfoot to maintain its natural torsion about the longitudinal axis. A current proposal states that the skeleton has a preferred path for any activity and if something supports this pathway, then muscle activity can be reduced, thereby decreasing fatigue and increasing comfort.

- *Cushioning*—Cushioning is the ability to reduce a runner's impact forces during heel strike. High-impact activities involving running and jumping tend to increase bone density while low-impact activities like swimming do not. Epidemiological studies have shown that there is no relationship between impact forces and frequency in running injuries. Also, maximum impact forces occur during midstance and take-off (active phase) instead of during heel strike (impact phase). The newly proposed muscle tuning paradigm suggests muscles maintain a preactivated state to decrease impact forces. All of this suggests that cushioning is more useful for comfort rather than to decrease the incidence of stress fractures.

B. *In court shoes:* Court shoes support movements like forward, backward, and sideward movements as well as jumping, landing, rotations, and stopping. They have to support the foot by providing lateral stability, cushioning, and traction control. Of these three factors, traction control is the most important.

- *Lateral stability*—Inversion sprains are common ankle injuries in court sports like basketball. A shoe with lateral stability has the ability to prevent excessive supination. The most common shoe modification to prevent these injuries is increasing the shaft length (hi-tops), but studies have shown that they do not reduce the incidence of ankle sprains.

- *Torsional stiffness*—The degree of torsional stiffness is inversely proportional to the amount of movement between the forefoot and rearfoot. A low torsional stiffness allows the forefoot to move independently from the rearfoot, thereby increasing lateral stability during toe strike in landing. The best way to create lateral stability in a shoe is to have low torsional stiffness and a special rearfoot construction.

- *Cushioning*—Heel-cushioning ability of court shoes is similar to that of running shoes. Players have been shown to prefer thicker soled shoes because they like the heel and forefoot cushioning for protection and comfort.

- *Traction*—A high translational traction at the shoe–surface interface lets the player change directions rapidly without slipping and injuring him/herself. Rotational traction needs to be minimized in functional courts shoes. Traction can be altered by changing the outer sole material as well as by adding treads and cleats.

2. Performance enhancement—
   A. *In runners:* For runners, enhancing performance is measured by time to finish a race or energy required to achieve a distance goal. The main factors influencing a runner's performance are shoe weight, efficiency, and energy return.
      - *Shoe weight*—As a shoe increases in weight or density, more energy is needed to carry that shoe through the motions of running. The variables affecting this added energy requirement are the maximum speed of the foot during the swing phase as well as the extra weight of the shoe. Shoe weight increases quadratically with increased running speed. Thus, shoe weight plays a big factor for high performance sprinting, long-distance running, and middle-distance running.
      - *Efficiency*—Changing the construction of a shoe can alter the kinematics of running, thereby differing the muscles used. However, if no differences in kinematics result, then the runner will change muscle activity to compensate for the changes in the shoe. Either way, muscle activity changes.
      - *Energy return*—In order for energy return to be efficient, the energy must be returned to the forefoot, where take-off is occurring at the right time. By this reasoning, energy would have to be transferred from the rearfoot to the forefoot for heel-toe runners. It has been proposed that minimizing energy loss would be more useful. This can be done by reducing the weight of a shoe as well as reducing the energy needed for muscle stabilization while running.
   B. *In court shoes:* The most important factors for enhancing performance of court shoes are traction, dynamic stability, and muscle fatigue. Adequate stability and support from a shoe reduces energy requirements and reduces muscle fatigue.
      - *Traction*—High translational traction allows quick changes in movement but increases the risk of injury. Experiments have shown that there is an optimal coefficient of friction between the shoe and surface to balance between traction and injury. Special outsole patterns exist to decrease rotational friction.

3. Comfort—in running and court shoes
   Comfort depends on the fit, climate, and cushioning ability of a shoe. Studies have not been done to distinguish these factors between each shoe type.

- *Fit*—Since shoes are made around one type of last, the shoe fit is not optimal for every athlete. Strategies like lacing patterns, air compartments, padding, varying widths, and sock-liners help to make the fit more individualized.
- *Climate*—Sock fabrics, ventilation systems, and breathable materials help make the uncomfortable hot and humid environment within the shoe more tolerable.
- *Cushioning*—Cushioning decreases total plantar force and increases comfort. The stiffest insoles were the most uncomfortable.

Discussion—Injury prevention, performance, and comfort are not independent of each other. For example, alterations promoting stability often increase shoe weight and vice versa. Although the most optimal shoe would be a customized shoe, a realistic goal would be to know the demands of a special group and to build that design.—*G.H. Jhala*

♦ The athletes we treat usually recognize the importance of wearing different athletic shoes that specifically meet the requirements of their individual sports. In the abstract, most of us realize this also. However, on occasion I have seen media interviews in which the requirements of athletic shoes for different sports have been reviewed and the person interviewed has essentially stated the same requirements for every type of shoe and sport that they were asked about. This article would be an excellent cure for that type of interview. This article details a variety of types of shoes from court shoes to running shoes, discussing several different sports and the specific types of requirements that each sport places upon the shoe and the foot. Shock absorption, motion control, lateral stability, traction, shoe weight, and energy return are discussed in detail. Also reviewed is the role of climate and comfort and fit in the selection and design of athletic shoes.—*S.M. Pribut, D.P.M.*

Energy Aspects Associated with Sport Shoes

Stefanyshyn DJ, Nigg BM (Human Performance Laboratory, The University of Calgary, Calgary, Canada)
Sportverl Sportschad 14:82–89, 2000

Introduction—During gait, energy is transferred from the athlete to the given surface and is lost due to surface deformation and friction. The deformation energy can be returned to the athlete by the surface. Athletic footwear, like a sport surface, can have its own exchange of energy with the athlete. This paper concentrates on maximizing energy return and minimizing energy loss in sport shoes.

Methods and Discussion—

1. *Maximizing energy return*: Upon ground contact, energy is stored in the sole as it is compressed. In order for the absorbed energy to be exerted as a force on the athlete during sole expansion, the following conditions must be fulfilled. The energy returned from the sport shoe must have a notable influence on the athlete's performance. The energy should be returned from the shoe to the athlete during the second half of the contact phase, exerting a force that contributes to the vertical and forward acceleration of the athlete. To aid in athletic performance, there must be expansion of the sole vertically and anteriorly. However, conventional materials allow as much decelerating posterior expansion as anterior. The appropriate stiffness of the midsole according to the mass of the athlete ensures a correct force frequency. This optimal stiffness is two to four times that of lower leg stiffness (~80 kN/m). Energy return must be exerted where propulsion occurs, at the forefoot, rather than the rearfoot.

2. *Minimizing the loss of energy:* By decreasing the amount of energy exerted for aspects not directly related to performance, more energy would then theoretically be available to enhance performance. Described below are some of the means to reduce the expenditure of unnecessary energy. A reduction of shoe mass would require less oxygen consumption and would allow for greater speed and acceleration. An increase in shoe cushioning decreases the energy needed for the muscles to absorb impact and reduce motion and vibrations. Increasing shoe stability, such as in high-top shoes, reduces the need for muscular stabilization. Much energy is absorbed when the shoe bends at the metatarsophalangeal joint, but little energy is produced during take-off since the joint is only minimally extended. However, a stiffer midsole could minimize energy loss.

Conclusion—Through improving the timing, frequency, direction, and location of the force exerted on the athlete by the shoe, it is possible in principle to maximize energy return. However, the actual influence it has on performance is most likely minimal. In improving the lightness, cushioning, stability, and stiffness of the shoes, the energy spared can be applied to and yield a measurable influence in athletic performance.—*J.M. Dawson*

♦ The concept of energy return or minimizing the loss of energy and sporting activities has not yet yielded satisfactory results that have improved the manufacture of sporting shoes. Over the past year this concept has been at the forefront of advertising and appeared in many media articles, some of which were derisive in nature. However, this concept has been researched for several years. This article reviews some of the thought processes and science that have gone into attempts to minimize energy loss within the running gait cycle. It is noted that tendons and quite possibly ligaments are 88–95% efficient at returning energy. Shoe midsoles, in contrast, are only 60–70% efficient.

Some of the means detailed in this article include mass reduction, time of force exertion, vector of force exertion and force return, tuning and dampening of forces, midsole compressibility, stability of the shoe and other factors. This is a good overview of current thought on the concept of energy return in athletic shoes.—*S.M. Pribut, D.P.M.*

Calcaneal Loading During Walking and Running

Giddings VL, Beaupré GS, Whalen RT, Carter DR (Stanford University, Stanford, CA; Veteran Affairs Health Care System, Palo Alto CA; NASA Ames Research Center, Mountain View, CA)
Med Sci Sports Exerc 32(3):627–634, 2000

Objective—This study uses experimentally measured kinematic and kinetic data with a numerical model to evaluate in vivo calcaneal stresses during walking and running.

Methods—External ground reaction forces (GRF) and kinematic data were determined for a normal subject during walking and running using cineradiography and force plate gait measurements. Data were acquired from one male subject. Metal reference markers, attached to the force plate and visible in each x-ray image, allowed the study to transform GRF and the center of pressure (COP) data from the force plate reference frame to the image and the foot reference frames. A contact-coupled approach was used to model the calcaneus with the inclusion of the hindfoot and the forefoot.

Results—They found that the calculated-force time profiles of the joint contact, ligament, and Achilles tendon forces varied with time-history curve of the moment of the ankle joint. The Achilles tendon, the plantar fascia, and the plantar ligaments show similar patterns of force development, with peaks for walking and running. The model predicts peak loads for the Achilles tendon of 3.9 body weights (BW) during walking and 7.7 during running. The load for the plantar fascia and plantar ligaments of 1.8 and 2.2 BW during walking and 3.7 and 4.8 BW during running, respectively. Talocalcaneal joint reached 5.4 BW during walking and 11.1 BW during running. The calcaneocuboid joint load was 4.2 during walking and 7.9 BW during running.

Conclusion—The study demonstrates that the magnitude of loading in the hindfoot increases throughout the gait cycle, peaking in the later portion of stance, and that large magnitude forces and calcaneal stresses are generated late in the stance phase, with maximum loads occurring at 70% of the stance phase during walking and 60% of the stance phase during running, for the gait velocities analyzed.—*Q. Solomon*

◆ The authors considered their study to be an important step in the systematic study of loading on the calcaneus and forced distribution within the calcaneus during walking and running. They appear to be correct in their judgment of the value of their work. Among the many significant findings in this study was that, contrary to common font and much current teaching, vertical impact loading on the calcaneus was not considered to play an important role in stress generation within the calcaneus itself. The authors detailed their thoughts on what contributes to forces within the calcaneus. Some of these factors include the balance of impact, the pull of the Achilles and triceps surae, the anatomical bony connections of the forefoot and midfoot, and the soft-tissue connections about the calcaneus.

Load forces between walking and running usually doubled in amounts. The loads in the plantar fascia were noted to be to be 2.2 times body weight in walking, while they were 4.8 times body weight and running. Maximum total strain was noted to occur at 70% in walking, while it occurred earlier at 60% of stance and running. This article can be read to detail the many differences between walking and running in your foot forces, force production, and force curves.

While not studied, orthotics might be thought to impact the timing of the application of forces, the rate of force application, and the magnitude of the forces generated. Future studies may lead to alterations in the orthotic conception and design. This study points to the significance of the soft-tissue attachments into the calcaneus as playing the major role in force production and tensile stress forces within the calcaneus. Clinically it has been found that Achilles tendon stretching has been effective in the treatment of heel pain. This study demonstrates the impact that the pull of the Achilles tendon may have on the development of forces within the calcaneus.—*S.M. Pribut, D.P.M.*

In Vivo Studies of Peritendinous Tissue in Exercise

Kjaer M, Langberg H, Skovgaard D, Olesen J, Bülow J, Krogsgaard M, Boushel R (Bispebjerg University Hospital, Copenhagen, Denmark)
Scand J Med Sci Sports 10:326–331, 2000

Introduction—Overuse injuries of the tendon can lead to pain, inflammation, and degenerative tissue changes. However, the knowledge of the physiological mechanisms that lead to injury is very limited. In vivo studies have been done to look at the changes in tissue concentrations and release rates of substances involved in metabolism, inflammation, and collagen synthesis in the peritendinous region around the Achilles tendon in humans during exercise. Tissue blood flow and oxygenation in this region were taken as well.

Objective—The study was conducted to answer the following questions using in vivo methods:

1. Is blood flow in the peritendinous region increased in response to exercise? If so, how is it regulated?
2. To what extent is the peritendinous tissue metabolically active during muscular contraction, and does it influence inflammatory mediators?
3. Does acute exercise cause any tendon-related collagen type I formation? If so, what is the time pattern of this?

Radiolabeled ^{133}Xe-washout placed immediately ventral to the Achilles tendon was done to measure the blood flow in the peritendon region during dynamic heel-raising exercise and static intermittent calf muscle exercise. Near infrared spectroscopy was used to measure tissue oxygenation. The use of the microdialysis technique allowed for a detailed study of the peritendon tissue metabolites, prostaglandin E_2 (PGE$_2$) and thromboxane B_2 (TXB$_2$).

Results—It was found that blood flow in the peritendinous region increased with exercise in an intensity-dependent manner. In addition, oxygen extraction and total hemoglobin volume increased in both the muscle and peritendinous regions at the same rate. This represented an increase in tissue oxygenation.

The study showed that the metabolic activity in the region surrounding the Achilles tendon increased several folds during exercise. There was an increased rate of both lipolysis and glycolysis. It was found that lipolysis was only elevated for the first 10 minutes of a 30-minute bout of exercise, whereas glycolysis ended just prior to the termination of the exercise. This observation supports the idea that there is a down regulation of lipolysis in the area since the adipose tissue is important as mechanical support for the tendon and bone tissue. Loss of the fat stores around the tendon may put the tendon at higher risk for injury.

There was also an increase in the release of both prostaglandin and thromboxane. The PGE$_2$ concentrations in the interstitial space were also elevated in the peritendinous tissue during early recovery.

Acute exercise can stimulate the formation of type I collagen in the Achilles tendon region. The release of prostaglandins could be involved in the conversion to type I collagen due to mechanical stress. This coupling is suspected due to the time frame of increases in both substances. Other factors are likely to play a role as well.

It has also been recently demonstrated that a negative pressure of 150 mmHg can be found in the epitenon and peritendon during intense exercise. The role of these changes is unknown, but it is speculated that this negative pressure may counteract the negative effects of compression on the tendon.

Conclusion—The changes in blood flow, oxygenation, metabolism, inflammatory mediators, and collagen turnover in response to exercise can help build a foundation to better understand the pathophysiology of tissue injury. In return, there can be improvements made in training and treatments of injury based on these findings.—*S. Patel*

♦ Much basic research remains to be done in the area of tendon physiology and metabolism. This excellent article reviews many recent research efforts in the field of tendon and peritendinous tissue physiology. The review of current areas and future areas of research gives insight and provides much to think about regarding function and physiology of tendons and the surrounding tissues. The topics covered include summaries of research on tissue oxygenation, circulation, collagen turnover, and many other areas. This article should be read to update your knowledge in this important area.—*S.M. Pribut, D.P.M.*

Lateral Ankle Sprains: A Comprehensive Review. Part 1: Etiology, Pathoanatomy, Histopathogenesis, and Diagnosis

Safran MR, Benedetti RS, Bartolozzi AR, Mandelbaum BR
Med Sci Sports Exerc 31(7 Suppl):S429–S437, 1999

Introduction—Lateral ankle sprains are the most common injuries found among athletes. The purpose of this article is to discuss the anatomy and biomechanics of the lateral ankle, mechanism of injury, histopathogenesis, clinical diagnosis, and the factors involved in recurrent ankle sprains.

Discussion—A sprain is defined as an injury that stretches the fibers of a ligament. O'Donoghue staged ligament sprains. Grade I is described as a mild sprain with some fibers being torn and minimal hemorrhage. Full function and strength are maintained, with no subsequent instability. Grade II is a moderate sprain that is characterized as an incomplete tear of the ligament, with mild instability, a slight reduction in function, a possible decrease in strength, and the potential loss of proprioception. A third-degree sprain is severe, with a complete disruption of the ligament, gross instability, and possibly a complete loss of full function, strength, and proprioception. Grade I sprains require an average of 11.7 days before resuming athletic activities, while grade II sprains take about 2–6 weeks. Grade III sprains, however, take more than 6 weeks to return to full function. Additionally, there is a residual functional instability found in a percentage of patients with grade III sprains, which is not found in those individuals with grade I and II sprains. Functional instability can lead to chronic ankle injury and early arthritic changes.

Ligaments serve three major functions. They provide proprioceptive information, prevent excessive motion, and act as guides to direct motion. The lateral ligament complex of the ankle is made up of the anterior talfibular ligament (ATFL), the calcaneofibular ligament (CFL), and the posterior talofibular ligament (PTFL). The ATFL is an intracapsular structure. It is the most important ligament in preventing talofibular instability. It is taut in plantarflexion and inversion. Despite ankle position, it is the first ligament to be torn in inversion injuries due to its low maximal load to failure. The CFL is an extra-articular structure, and is larger and stronger than the ATFL. The PTFL is the strongest of the complex and is rarely injured. It is taut only in severe dorsiflexion. Ankle injuries of the lateral ligaments result from supination and inversion of the foot and external rotation of the leg on the foot. The sequence of injury begins with the ATFL, the anterolateral capsule, and the distal tibiofibular ligament. Further inversion strain results in a CFL tear, followed by the PTFL. PTFL ruptures are associated with ankle dislocation, distal lateral malleolar avulsion or spiral fracture, medial malleolar fracture, or talar neck or medial compression fracture.

Injury to ligaments show the normal histologic changes of inflammation which progresses to scar tissue formation. Ligaments with interposed scar tissue have loads to failure and energy absorbing capacities of only 60% of normal.

When treating an individual with an ankle sprain, it is important to ascertain a good history. The physician should inquire about the time of injury, the position of the foot, onset and location of swelling, history of previous sprains, and the patient's goals of recovery.

On physical exam, areas of tenderness and swelling should be identified. Areas of tenderness can correlate to specific ligament injury. Passive inversion of the ankle should reproduce the symptoms. Neurovascular status should also be assessed. The structures in question include the dorsalis pedis, posterior tibial artery, and the sural nerve. The anterior drawer test checks for the integrity of the ATFL. Attenuation of the ligament results in 4 mm of displacement, while normal displacement is 2 mm. The inversion stress maneuver tests for CFL integrity.

Radiographs are ordered based on the guidelines set by the Ottawa Ankle Rules. These rules require x-rays to be ordered if there is bone tenderness in the posterior half of the lower 6 cm of the tibia or fibula, tenderness over the navicular and/or fifth metatarsal, and the inability to bear weight. Views to look at the ankle include the AP, lateral, and mortise views. If there is tenderness in the foot, AP of the foot is recommended. Stress views can also be useful. The stress views include inversion to assess talar tilt and the anterior drawer. These should be performed under local anesthesia and compared to the contralateral side. The talar tilt is thought to be more reliable. A difference of more than 10° between the injured and normal ankle is indicative of a torn ATFL and CFL. Other imaging studies include arthrography, peroneal tenography, and MRI.

Conclusion—Many individuals have functional instability after an ankle sprain. They complain of frequent sprains, difficulty running on uneven surfaces, difficulty in cutting and jumping, recurrent pain and swelling, and weakness. There are many causes of chronic disability after an ankle sprain. These include an osteochondral fractures of the talus, post-traumatic degenerative arthritis, peroneal tendon dislocation, chronic lateral pain and tenderness (i.e., chronic sprain), recurrent sprains due to instability, tibiotalar impingement, injury to the syndesmosis, subtalar instability, sinus tarsi syndrome, cuboid subluxation, and fracture of the anterior process of the calcaneus or the fifth metatarsal. The etiology of recurrent ankle sprains is unknown, although it is believed to be due to one or more of the following: 1) healing of the ligaments in a lengthened position, 2) weakness due to presence of scar tissue, 3) peroneal muscle weakness, 4) distal tibiofibular instability, 5) hereditary hypermobility, 6) loss of proprioception, 7) impingement of the distal fascicle of the anteroinferior tibiofibular ligament, and/or 8) impingement of meniscoid tissue in the talofibular joint.—*S. Patel*

♦ This article is part 1 of a multipart series on lateral ankle ligamentous injuries. It is well worth reading for a comprehensive review of lateral ankle injuries. The biomechanics, anatomy, injury mechanisms, diagnosis, physical examination, and x-ray examination are discussed in preparation for part 2 of this series, which delineates therapy and rehabilitative regiments for lateral ankle ligamentous injuries.—*S.M. Pribut, D.P.M.*

The Gender Issue: Epidemiology of Ankle Injuries in Athletes Who Participate in Basketball

Hosea TM, Carey CC, Harrer MF (UMDNJ—Robert Wood Johnson Medical School, New Brunswick, NJ)
Clin Orthop 372:45–49, 2000

Introduction—In 1972, Title IX caused an increase in the participation of females in athletics. This produced studies that compared the injury pattern among males and females. Initial reports have shown similar rates, except in injuries involving the patella and other knee injuries that require surgery (anterior cruciate ligament). Ankle injuries are the most common type of injury in athletes who participate in basketball, which has not had much attention in regards to a gender difference or risk associated with level of competition (high school versus college athletics).

Methods—A total of 125 high schools, colleges, and universities in New Jersey that had men's and women's basketball teams that had a common practice court were used as the subjects. The study was conducted over a 2-year period, documenting each injury affecting the ankle and knee. The severity of the injury was also recorded. The data were then compiled and compared the relative risk between male and female, and level of competition.

Results—Among the 11,780 athletes who participated, 6840 were male (of those, 504 were college athletes and 6336 were high school athletes) and 4940 were female (of those 364 were college athletes and 4576 were high school athletes). The difference in male and female participation is due to higher participation at the freshman and junior varsity level. A total of 1384 injuries to the knee and ankle were documented. Among these injuries, 76% involved the ankle; 72% of the ankle injuries were grade I sprains for male and female athletes. Females in high school had a 24% greater relative risk for grade I ankle sprains compared to males. There was not a significantly increased risk for more severe ankle sprains between males and females. Ankle sprains when compared to high school and collegiate level showed a relative risk that was doubled. This study found that females had three times the risk for suffering an anterior cruciate ligament injury compared to the male athletes. A 3.66:1 increased risk of anterior cruciate ligament was found in females who competed at a collegiate level. The males had no increase in risk of anterior cruciate ligament injury when competing at a higher level of competition.

Conclusion—There is a difference in injury rates among males and females. Further, there is a difference in the level of competition that increases the risk of injury. The differences between male and female strength and physiology have been well studied. Further investigations need to address the differences that cause the injuries, in order to determine the best training programs to decrease the risk of injuries in both high school and college athletes.—*T. Marshall*

◆ Many recent studies have highlighted differences in injuries, injury rates, and maladies that female athletes may suffer. While the study demonstrated an overall increase of nearly 25% in relative risk for female athletes in the incidence of ankle injuries, the authors noted that this risk was attributable to the increased incidence of grade I ankle sprains. There is no significant difference in overall incidence of grade II or grade III ankle sprains or other types of ankle injuries.

The authors concluded that the relative risk of serious ankle injuries was not higher for women than for men. This differs considerably from the reported differences that have been observed in the relative risk rate of anterior cruciate ligament injuries in women versus men basketball players. One possible reason, not mentioned by the authors, for the observed overall difference caused by the reporting of grade I injuries might be a different threshold used by the women in reporting the grade I injuries. The female athletes may have been more honest and forthright in reporting the grade I injuries than their male counterparts. This gender difference in reporting would more likely be revealed in personality inventory studies than in a mechanical study.—*S.M. Pribut, D.P.M.*

Chronic Achilles Tendinosis: Recommendations for Treatment and Prevention
Alfredson H, Lorentzon R (Umeå University and National Institute for Working Life, Umeå, Sweden)
Sports Med 29(2):135–146, 2000

Introduction—Chronic Achilles tendinosis is considered to be an overuse injury; however, this condition is associated with and affects both active and sedentary individuals. Alterations of collagen fibers with increased interfibrillar glycosaminoglycans are present histologically, but no evidence of inflammatory cells are noted. The level of chronic pain is most often located at the midportion (1.5–7 cm proximal to the insertion in the calcaneus) and proximal and distal (tendon–bone junction) parts of the tendon. Achilles tendinosis is a difficult entity to treat with about 25% of patients requiring surgery. Poorly defined terms reflecting the tendon's pathology may contribute to this difficulty. Therefore, this review focuses on treatment and prevention in patients with long duration of symptoms from a painful midportion of the Achilles tendon.

Methods—Conservative treatment modalities and recent studies with strength training programs were reviewed for efficacy. Surgical techniques and indications, postoperative rehabilitation, and complications associated with the surgery were reviewed among patients not responding to conservative treatment. Identification and correction of preventable risk factors were also mentioned.

Results—Studies revealed little to no correlation of tendinopathy with biomechanical etiologies; one study questioned orthotic value as a conservative treatment modality. Rest, stretching, strength training, proper shoe gear, local cold therapy, heat, massage, ultrasound, electrical stimulation, and laser therapy are all suggested components in conservative therapy; however, NSAIDs and corticosteroid injections may have limited use. Athletes with chronic Achilles tendinosis responded well to specially designed heavy load eccentric calf muscle training programs (after a 2-year follow-up, only 1 out of 15 patients required surgery). The straight longitudinal incision medial to the Achilles tendon for excision of adhesions and abnormal sections of the paratenon and tendon is most used; the excision area is repaired by a side-to-side absorbable suture. The return of muscle strength is found to be independent of short (2 weeks) postoperative immobilization time compared to long (6 weeks). Complications to surgery included skin edge necrosis and superficial infection; however, few complications were reported. Essential components for prevention are strength training and stretching.

Conclusion—Chronic Achilles tendinosis primarily affects middle-aged male recreational runners, but sedentary individuals experience the same tendinopathy. Combination therapy of multiple conservative modalities is used for initial management and possible treatment. Surgical intervention is required in 25% of patients with excellent short-term results and acceptable long-term results. The Achilles tendon is the strongest tendon in the body; therefore, patients should be aware of the lengthy rehabilitation period. Prevention of Achilles tendon injuries mainly resides in maintenance of strength and flexibility. Furthermore, promising results following calf-strengthening programs may lead to a decrease in patients who will require surgical intervention.—*M. Garrison*

◆ This is a must-read article for those dealing with Achilles tendon injuries. The term tendinosis is one that has come upon the scene within the last few years. This term should have greater recognition within the sports medicine community. For years the terms tendonitis and tendinitis have been used exclusively to represent most of the painful conditions of tendons. In reference to the Achilles tendon, studies have shown that inflammatory cells are not usually noted on biopsy. In fact, what is present is often the condition of local degenerative changes that are called tendinosis or tendinopathy. This condition includes significant changes in collagen fiber structure and an increase in intrafibrillar glycosaminoglycans.

This article details much of the recent thought on Achilles tendon pain. It focuses on pain and injury to the area 1.5–7.0 cm proximal to the insertion of the tendon. The concepts in this article are spreading to the sports medicine community. The article offers an approach to pain in this area that consists of attempting to strengthen the tendon and calf muscle group by performing eccentric loading exercises. This is in contrast to the usually employed stretching and concentric loading and contracture of the muscles. The patient gently lowers his or her heel while standing on a stair; weights are then added to increase the tension and load borne by the muscle and tendon group. Normally when individual perform calf raises, they will lift themselves back up again; however, that is not the case in the study. The emphasis is solely on eccentric exercise.

I do not normally recommend the stair stretch or calf raises when the patient has acute pain with Achilles tendon injury. This study does present an interesting approach and one should consider employing these exercises in difficult cases. It is important to note that the study performed by these authors only details the results on 15 athletes.—*S.M. Pribut, D.P.M.*

Pelvis and Sacral Dysfunction in Sports and Exercise

Prather H (Washington University School of Medicine, St. Louis, MO)
Phys Med Rehabil Clin North Am 11(4):805–836, 2000

Introduction—With the current exercise and sports activity rave, pelvic injuries and dysfunction are becoming more and more prevalent not only in men, but in women as well. As a result, this article focuses on the etiologies of injuries at the pelvis and also provides a complete knowledge of the differences between the genders in regards to specific anatomic, physiologic, and biomechanical differences. The health care provider can now take this into account for a therapeutic approach to decrease the number of injured female athletes.

Discussion—Injuries involving the pelvic region are due to multifactorial causes from overuse injuries dealing with the bony, ligamentous, joint, and muscle structures surround the area. Due to the considerable amount of spine, hip, and lower extremity support to the central pelvic region, there must be significant consideration of the direct and indirect synergistic activation to the pelvis from these neighboring anatomical regions in regards to pelvic pain. Also, one must keep in mind that the pelvic floor and structures are comprised of gender-specific differences. This encourages the health provider to implement a comprehensive evaluation when providing therapeutic care for the female athlete.

This article extensively defines the plethora of etiologies and also denotes the different chronological stages of treatment for each specific cause. The etiologies include soft tissue, nerve, osseous, and muscle. This article also defines the particular, acquired adaptive changes with aging. Women athletes are predisposed to experience hormonal changes, pregnancy, and pelvic surgery, which put them at a greater risk for pelvic pain, both floor and general, and urinary problems once they return to exercise and sports participation.

Conclusion—The provider's success in making a good diagnosis, and subsequently, appropriate care for the pelvic injuries, is not only dependent upon acquiring a thorough history and the ability to isolate the pain and structures involved, but the need to consult with additional physicians in other areas of medicine who provide special treatment for women, such as gynecologists and urologists.—*R.L. Childers*

♦ As podiatric sports medicine practitioners, we are often called upon to evaluate and treat biomechanically related injuries from the foot up to the back. In order to understand biomechanics of the lower extremity, the anatomy and biomechanics of the hip, sacrum, and pelvis must also be understood. The foot and lower leg do not function in isolation from the structures above. This article was included in a special issue on "Tough Topics in Sports Medicine." This indeed is a tough and complex topic; however, this article covers the anatomy, function, and biomechanics of this region in great detail. This article should well serve to update your knowledge in this anatomical region that is little understood by sports medicine practitioners of all specialties. — *S.M. Pribut, D.P.M.*

Asymmetrical Strength Changes and Injuries in Athletes Training on a Small Radius Curve Indoor Track

Beukeboom C, Birmingham TB, Forwell L, Ohrling D (The University of Western Ontario, London, Ontario, Canada; Sudburg Regional Hospital, Sudburg, Ontario, Canada)
Clin J Sport Med 10(4):245–250, 2000

Introduction—Track and field athletes have traditionally performed on various sizes of indoor and outdoor tracks in a counterclockwise direction. The outdoor tracks now have a standardized 400-m length. The indoor tracks, however, have many variations; a circular 200-m track with constant radius, a 160-m oval with banked curves, and a flat 200-m oval with unbanked curves. These differences alter an athlete's normal linear running biomechanic, changing it to curvilinear running. This curvilinear running adds moment of supination and pronation to a normal linear gait and sets up a potential increase in the force exerted by the posterior muscle groups acting to stabilize the subtalar joint. This consequently could cause a muscle imbalance between the evertors and invertors, and a difference in strength between the two legs, which potentially could cause injuries.

Methods—The subjects were on the 1996 University of Western Ontario track and field team, 7 males and 18 females who ran long sprints, 200–600 m, or middle distance, 80–3000. These athletes were not injured at the beginning of the season and competed for a season that was 10–12 weeks on the indoor track. The track had 45-m straightaways and 55-m unbanked curves with a curve radius of 17.5 m. The strength of the subjects was assessed using a Cybex 6000 isokinetic dynamometer model that tested invertor and evertor ankle strength bilaterally, both concentrically and eccentrically, and velocity at the beginning of the season and end of the season. The athletes had similar training programs and filled out questionnaires that had data regarding previous injuries, weight training regimens, orthotic usage, training foot wear, on-track training days, and off-track training distance. In addition, any injuries were reported.

Results—The left invertors increased in strength more than the right invertors and the right evertors increased in strength more than the left evertors. Twenty-four total lower extremities injuries were recorded in 17 athletes (68% of athletes in study). Among the 17 athletes who were injured, 15 had reported a history of injury; four of the noninjured athletes during this study had reported a history of injury. There was no difference in the strength component between injured and noninjured athletes. When the results of this study are compared with those of studies that have analyzed outdoor track athletes, the injury rate in this study higher (0.75 injuries per 100 person-hours vs. 0.58 injuries per 100 person-hours).

Discussion—This study does not prove that the indoor tract is the sole cause of this difference in injuries; further studies are needed. In addition, the testing of the invertors and evertors with the Cybex does not simulate running exactly; therefore, a closer evaluation of the invertors and evertors needs to be conducted with a more biomechanical true design. This study does show that the biomechanics of linear running are altered to a curvilinear running pattern.—*T. Marshall*

♦ It is well known that training errors are considered to be the most significant cause of running-related injuries. Training and racing around circular tracks has often been thought to contribute to injury. This study documents asymmetrical changes in muscle strength that occur following training around a small circumference indoor track over the course of one season. The inside limb demonstrated an increase in inverter strength, while the outer limb demonstrated an increase in everter strength. This study did not document a correlation between the amount or asymmetry of muscle strength changes and that of injury occurrence. However, this training change can be one of the causal factors and further study is warranted.

The study demonstrated a high rate of lower extremity injury occurrence of 68%. While this study is limited to track athletes, other studies of both track athletes and long distance runners also noted injury rates that varied between 66% and 77%. This high figure among competitive athletes may be due to their attempt to approach peak performance by training close to their personal red line.—*S.M. Pribut, D.P.M.*

Measures of Functional Limitation as Predictors of Disablement in Athletes with Acute Ankle Sprains

Wilson RW, Gansneder BM (University of South Florida, College of Medicine, Tampa, FL; Curry School of Education, University of Virginia, Charlottesville, VA)
J Orthop Sports Phys Ther 30(9):528–535, 2000

Objectives—The goals of this study were to evaluate the validity of clinician observed activity scores, self-reported athletic ability, and measurements of physical impairment to predict the disability duration for collegiate athletes with acute ankle sprains.

Methods—The authors observed 21 voluntary intercollegiate athletes (13 men, 8 women) who compete in NCAA Division I sports. Each athlete suffered a grade I or II ankle inversion injury. Any athlete with one or more torn lateral ligaments or a syndesmosis sprain was excluded from the study. Each athlete described a history of inversion injury and had local tenderness and swelling around the injury site. The same investigator took all of the measurements. Joint swelling was measured using the water displacement technique and the data were recorded to the nearest 5 mL. Bilateral passive ankle dorsiflexion was measured to the nearest degree. Any pain felt during this measurement was used as the indicator for end of range of motion. Subjects were then asked to perform six weightbearing activities with one point awarded for each successful completion and zero points for any tasks aborted or not performed. Using a visual analog scale, the subjects were asked to compare their athletic ability to normal, ranging from no limitation to severe limitation. The disability duration was calculated to be the time from the injury date to the athlete's full participation in practice or competition.

Results—Physical impairment accounted for one-third of the disability duration. Adding the functional limitation measures significantly increased the proportion of disability duration. Therefore, including the functional limitation measurements improved the accuracy of the estimates of disability duration compared to measuring the physical impairments alone.

Discussion—The data from this study show that it is possible to calculate the disability duration of an acute ankle sprain 72 hours after the injurious event. Calculation of the physical impairments offered somewhat accurate estimates of disability duration, but the addition of functional limitation measurements increased the accuracy. The degree of functional limitation and disability from the acute ankle sprains was not directly proportional to the severity of the athlete's physical impairment. Since functional limitation had such an effect on disability duration, behavioral factors like motivation, confidence, and stoicism may have also played an influencing role. These traits were not measured directly in this study but may be reflected in the self-reported athletic ability answers. In summary, although subjects who experienced more involved physical impairment had longer disability durations, the clinician-observed and self-reported measures of functional limitation were stronger predictors of disability duration.—*G.H. Jhala*

♦ This study was done in an attempt to define the parameters that might be measured following ankle ligament injury to predict how quickly an athlete may return to activity and competition. Physical impairment, limitation of activity, and disability duration were measured using a multivariate design. Impairment of activity was found to be responsible for one-third of the variance in the duration of disability.

When measurements of activity limitation were added, the predictive models were improved. Activity limitation alone was found to account for 67% of the variance in days until return to participation. The article studied grade I and grade II ankle ligament injuries.

Some of the activities measured included a 40-m walk or running 40 m, figure 8 run, single foot hop, crossover hop, and 14-step stair hop on the injured extremity. The concepts and purposes of this article are laudable. The authors of the study were physical therapists with Ph.D.s who worked in an academic setting. Their writing style belies this fact. The first sentence of the article is a quote that states "one of the primary tasks of researchers is to provide clinicians with valid tools that can be used to do clinically useful things." While the concepts included within this article are important and the testing mechanisms or modifications of these testing mechanisms may be useful, a more straightforward writing style by these researchers would be appreciated. Researchers looking to provide clinicians with useful tools should be able to write in a clear manner using the language of clinicians. This article needed to move somewhat more in the direction of plain speaking in order to meet the demands of their target audience. For further details on practical determination of fitness for return to activity following ankle ligament injuries, I suggest reading the recent writings or attending the lectures of Doug Richie, D.P.M., in a variety of publications and forums. His premises, analysis, measurement techniques, and rehabilitative suggestions are clearly laid out.—*S.M. Pribut, D.P.M.*

Midterm Effects of Ankle Joint Supports on Sensomotor and Sport-Specific Capabilities

Jerosch J, Schoppe R (Johanna-Etienne Hospital, Neuss, Germany)
Knee Surg Sports Traumatol Arthrosc 8:252–259, 2000

Introduction—The most common sports-related injury is ligamentous disruption of the ankle. It is estimated that approximately 23,000 ankle injuries occur per day in the United States and in 8–40% of reported cases this type of injury results in recurrent instability and chronic pain. Stability of the ankle joint is dependent upon proprioception and coordination. In two studies, one with cadets and one with football players, it was found that the incidence of ankle joint injury was 2–3 times higher in those subjects without bracing or stabilization aids.

Methods—Twenty-one subjects with clinically defined post-traumatic functional ankle instability participated in a 3-month period of standardized tests. The subjects consisted of 18 males and 3 females with a mean age of 30.2 ± 10.1 years and an average sporting activity of 3 hours per week. All subjects were given an epX Ankle Dynamic (Lohmann-Rauscher), a flexible ankle wrap. Static and dynamic balance indices were measured using the KAT-2000. In timed trial, subjects also ran a 16-m roundtrip course by side stepping. An angle reproduction test measured the subjects' proprioception and ability to re-establish position of both the injured and uninjured ankle joints in 30° plantarflexion, neutral position, and 10° extension. Isokinetic force was tested via the Cybex 6000 in five repetitions at both 50°/s and 100°/s to determine maximum force and elastic force, respectively. Quality of life from the patient's viewpoint was evaluated with the health questionnaire SF-36 and each subject was assigned a Weber ankle score.

Results—The support brace had a positive effect on sport-specific abilities necessary for side stepping. During the active angle reproduction test, dorsal extension was reproduced more accurately with the use of the brace than without. The Weber score did improve over 3-month period from an average of 4 ± 2.357 to 2.6 ± 2.573, while the SF-36 showed no significant improvement

Discussion—The goal of the epX Ankle Dynamic is to improve the neurophysiologic feedback mechanism of ankle joint mechanoreceptors, thereby improving stabilization and increasing proprioception of injured ankles. Bracing provides compression of the ankle while allowing minor limitation in the range of plantarflexion and dorsiflexion and increasing sensomotor abilities. Frequent, long-term usage of the support was not shown to negatively impact athletic performance. Both coaches and athletes generally approve a support if no detrimental effect is seen on athletic performance. Therefore it is recommended that the prophylactic use of braces for a period of 3 months be considered in treatment of a functionally unstable ankle joint.—*K. Van Voris*

♦ It has been reported that nearly 23,000 ankle injuries occur each day in the United States. Ankle ligament injuries are the most frequently reported injury in both sporting activity and leisure. Studies that demonstrate means of prevention of ankle injuries and prevention of recurrence of ankle injuries are important to both athletes and practitioners. Athletes are often concerned about the impact of any therapy or prophylactic treatment upon performance. This study addresses that concern. Bracing is one of the components of successful treatment of ankle sprains. Studies previously performed have shown bracing to be effective as prophylactic treatment for ankle ligament injuries. This article demonstrated an improvement in function and no decline in performance over the study period of 3 months. This supports the concept that it is prudent to wear an ankle brace for an extended period of time following ankle ligament injury and that it will improve function and not inhibit performance.—*S.M. Pribut, D.P.M.*

6 Radiology of the Foot and Ankle

Kenneth Bloom, D.P.M., and G. Adam Shapiro, D.P.M.

Avulsion Fracture of the Base of the Fifth Metatarsal Not Seen on Conventional Radiography of the Foot: The Need for an Additional Projection

Pao DG, Keats TE, Dussault RG (University of Virginia Medical System, Charlottesville, VA)

AJR 175(2):549–552, 2000

Introduction—There are two classic fractures of the proximal fifth metatarsal: the Jones fracture and an avulsion fracture of the tuberosity. A third type of fracture has been observed, an avulsion fracture of the proximal tip of the tuberosity. This fracture is only seen on radiographs of the ankle, due most likely to the difference in positioning of the patient and projection of the central ray.

Materials and Methods—Using a computer database, it was determined that of the 443 patients who had regular foot and ankle radiographs taken, 26 had fractures of the proximal fifth metatarsal. All 26 patients had the three standard views of the foot and two standard views of the ankle taken on the same day. Two radiographers independently reviewed the radiographs and without disagreement categorized fractures as present or absent.

Results—Anteroposterior ankle radiographs revealed six avulsion fractures of the proximal fifth metatarsal tuberosity that were not visible on foot films. Sixteen of the 26 patients had foot and ankle radiographs that revealed avulsion fractures of the expanded portion of the tuberosity. Only 4 of the 26 patients were diagnosed with Jones type fractures that could be seen on both foot and ankle views. In summary, all 26 fractures could be seen in the AP projection of the ankle, but only 20 could be visualized with the standard foot films.

Discussion—Based on our findings not all fractures of the fifth metatarsal can be seen using the standard views of the foot. If no fracture is seen with the standard three views, then the radiologist should consider recommending

101

an AP view of the ankle that includes the proximal fifth metatarsal to rule out an avulsion fracture of the proximal tuberosity. The film cassette should be centered on the fifth metatarsal base instead of the standard location for the ankle film.

It has been proposed that the lateral cord of the plantar aponeurosis causes this type of avulsion fracture. The fracture is proximal to most, if not all, of the broad insertion of peroneus brevis.

The ability to see the fracture on ankle films is most likely due to patient positioning. Position the patient with the knee extended and the heel resting on the cassette so that the long axis of the foot is vertical. Position the central ray equidistant from the malleoli.—*G. Grant*

♦ This report recommends obtaining AP and AP oblique radiographs in the detection of fifth metatarsal base avulsion type fractures when conventional foot views are negative. The authors attribute the ability of the ankle views to detect the avulsion fractures to the change in foot position (more dorsiflexed than in foot views) and the more proximal location of the central beam. The authors present a thorough review of the proposed pathomechanics in fifth metatarsal base fractures. Before one incorporates these views in their fifth metatarsal base fracture protocol, I would like to see a larger retrospective study.—*K. Bloom, D.P.M.*

Sonography of Morton's Neuromas

Quinn TJ, Jacobson JA, Craig JG, van Holsbeeck MT (University of Michigan Medical Center, Ann Arbor, MI; Henry Ford Hospital, Detroit, MI)
AJR 174(6):1723–1728, 2000

Introduction—Morton's neuroma has been well described and clinically characterized, which allows for relatively automatic diagnosis. There are, however, times when presentation becomes more atypical and allusive, which calls for imaging correlation to specify the cause of the presenting metatarsalgia.

Sonography has emerged as a successful modality in the diagnosis of Morton's neuroma. Although sonographic appearance of Morton's neuroma has been described as a hypoechoic intermetarsal mass, variability in this description warrants further characterization and determination of sonography's effectiveness in imaging this pathology.

Methods—Both prospective report review and retrospective image review were utilized to evaluate 30 intermetatarsal spaces that were plantarly imaged with ultrasound, using a 7.5–10 MHz linear array transducer. Information in the original sonographic reports were blindly reviewed in a prospective fashion and then compared to the surgical results for Morton's neuroma. A retrospective review of the sonograms was then accomplished in order to complete the characterization of the Morton's neuromas and other intermetarsal abnormalities that were discovered at surgery. This retrospective review was not blinded.

Results—In the prospective sonographic reports, 85% of the cases were correctly identified with neuromas. Retrospectively, 79% of the neuromas were characterized as what has been previously described as hypoechoic mass; 12.5% were of mixed echotexture and 8.3% were anechoic. Additionally 50% of the neuromas were located dorsal to the plantar aspect of the metatarsal heads. In three surgically positive cases, no mass was retrospectively identified in the sonographic reports.

Of the three dimensions measured (width, length, height), only the difference in length was statistically significant between neuromas and non-neuromal masses. All Morton's neuromas were less that 20 mm in length. Plantar digital nerve continuity with the interdigital mass was present in 15 neuromas.

Conclusion—Because ultrasound can reveal Morton's neuroma in 85% of cases, this imaging modality proves to be a valuable tool in the diagnosis of such pathology. Common plantar intermetatarsal nerve continuity with a hypoechoic mass, particularly in the third interspace, greatly increases diagnostic confidence. Masses greater than 20 mm in length should direct one toward possibilities other than Morton's neuroma in the differential.—*S.B. Heninger*

♦ The authors found an 85% success rate in the prospective diagnosis of Morton's neuroma using sonography. They provide a comprehensive overview of its pathology and anatomy. The success rate in detecting neuromas using sonography remains high with the primary limiting factors being the technique and experience of the sonographer, as well as the size of the neuroma. This modality is a useful adjunctive tool for localizing the neuroma and searching for neuromas in adjacent interspaces.—*K. Bloom, D.P.M.*

The Association Between Heel Ultrasound and Hormone Replacement Therapy Is Modulated by a Two-Locus Vitamin D and Estrogen Receptor Genotype

Giguère Y, Dodin S, Blanchet C, Morgan K, Rousseau F (Centre de Recherche de l'Hôpital Saint-François d'Assise du CHUQ; Université Laval, Quebec, Canada; McGill University and General Hospital Résearch Institute, Montred, Quebec, Canada)
J Bone Miner Res 15(6):1076–1084, 2000

Introduction—Postmenopausal women are at risk of developing osteoporosis. In addition to environmental factors, a genetic component has been linked to the role of estrogen deprivation in the process of bone remodeling and increased risk of fracture in postmenopausal women. A common *Bsm* I polymorphism at the vitamin D receptor (*VDR*) gene and *Pvu* II polymorphism in the estrogen receptor (*ESR1*) gene have been elucidated as two of the many susceptibility genes involved. The interaction between hormone replacement therapy (HRT) and the receptor genotypes on bone mineral density was the focus of this study.

Methods—Four hundred twenty-five ambulatory postmenopausal French-Canadian women (age range, 42–85 years old) were recruited through voluntary response to a local newspaper advertisement for the study. Each participant underwent heel ultrasound, determined by right calcaneal quantitative ultrasound (QUS), and the results were expressed as an age-and-weight adjusted stiffness index (heel SI z score). In addition, each participant was genotyped for both VDR *Bsm* I and ESR1 *Pvu* II polymorphisms.

Results—Of the subjects, 19.8% carried the *VDR-BB* genotype, 43.0% the *VDR-Bb* genotype, and 37.2% the *VDR-bb* genotype. The *ESR1 Pvu* II genotypes were in Hardy-Weinberg equilibrium ($X^2 = 0.01$; df $= 2$; $p = .99$). VDR *Bsm* I and *ESR1 Pvu* II genotypes were distributed independently ($X^2 = 2.18$; df $= 4$; $p = 0.70$). It was determined that a 20.8% difference existed in heel SI z score between women bearing the *VDR-bb/ESR-PP* genotype who received HRT for ≥5 years and those who received no HRT or HRT for <5 years. It was shown that of the women who received HRT for ≥5 years, those carrying the *VDR-bb/ESR-PP* genotype had a significantly higher heel SI z score than those carrying other *VDR/ESR1* genotypes.

Discussion—There is a definite positive impact on heel SI with the use of HRT, for women who received HRT for ≥5 years had an 8% greater heel SI than those who received HRT for <5 years. However, it is still controversial as to whether the contribution of common variants of candidate genes such as *VDR* and *ESR1* to bone marrow density is significant. The magnitude of benefit of HRT use ≥5 years is heterogeneously distributed in postmenopausal women and depends in part on the *VDR/ESR1* two-locus genotype.

Conclusion—The two-locus genotype (*VDR-bb/ESR1-PP*) is present in 9.5% of women and accounts for over 30% of the total HRT-related heel SI differences found in the sample of postmenopausal women. HRT for more than 5 years in the women bearing this genotype had a 21% greater heel SI than those with the same genotype who received HRT for less than 5 years. Ultimately, this represents a 2- to 3-fold difference in the risk of fracture in these women.—*A. Duckworth*

♦ The authors' study shows that those women with the combined *VDR/ESR1* genotype taking HRT for more than 5 years have a significantly greater stiffness index than women taking hormone replacement therapy for less than 5 years. The variance between the two groups of women, those with the genotype taking HRT for more than 5 years versus less than 5 years and those without the genotype taking HRT for more than 5 years versus less than 5 years is 6-fold. Future studies linking genotypes to the success of HRT in the treatment of osteoporosis will help us to better understand and reduce the risks of fractures in this population. — *K. Bloom, D.P.M.*

Biomechanical Assessment of Plantar Foot Tissue in Diabetic Patients Using an Ultrasound Indentation System

Zheng YP, Choi YKC, Wong K, Chan S, Mak AFT (The Hong Kong Polytechnic University, Hong Kong, China; Queen Mary Hospital, Hong Kong, China)
Ultrasound Med Biol 26(3):451–456, 2000

Introduction—Foot complications of diabetes mellitus (DM) stem primarily from peripheral neuropathy and the associated musculoskeletal and skin pathologies that result from it. These lead to increased plantar pressures. As footwear and other modalities are sought to lower plantar pressures, investigations into the effects of bony structure and biomechanical forces on soft-tissue properties are underway to help in this effort. Plantar tissue thickness and Young's modulus can be measured by ultrasound (US) indentation.

Materials and Methods—Four neuropathic DM patients and four healthy subjects were tested. Testing consisted of US plantar tissue thickness assessment in three different postures: supine–knee flexed–ankle neutral, prone–knee extended–ankle 5° dorsiflexed, and prone–knee extended–ankle 20° plantarflexed. The probe was placed with minimal pressure and gradually loaded. This was repeated five times for each posture. Sites tested were under the first metatarsal head, second metatarsal head, big toe, and heel.

Results—Tissue thickness in elderly DM patients was significantly thinner than in young healthy subjects in four testing sites. Young's modulus at four sites was significantly higher in DM subjects. In DM patients, Young's modulus was greatest at the first metatarsal head. Site differences in healthy subjects were small. Postural differences with Young's modulus were significant in healthy subjects, but insignificant in DM subjects. No significant postural differences in tissue thickness were observed in either group.

Discussion—Plantar soft tissues were stiffer, and Young's moduli were greater in DM subjects. This could be due to skin changes secondary to neuropathy. Site dependence of the stiffness of DM tissues could be due to the musculoskeletal deformity. For example, toe deformity could lead to reduction of the fat pad under the metatarsal head, which creates more pressure. The already stiff, hard skin reacts by building up more callus than normal skin would, thus increasing pressures more.

Limitations of the study include those inherent with nonmatched, small sample size groups. Age differences between groups represent a potentially significant variable. Overall it was shown that US indentation is an effective tool for assessment of plantar soft-tissue properties.—*D. Clement*

◆ This is an interesting study using an ultrasound indentation system to assess plantar soft-tissue thickness in elderly diabetic patients. However, as the authors point out, because the diabetic and healthy group of patients used for this study was not age-matched, the effect of age as well as diabetes could not be distinguished from their results. A future study of the plantar tissues of elderly nondiabetic patients should be included to differentiate if the thinner and stiffer plantar soft tissues are diabetes or age related.—*G.A. Shapiro, D.P.M.*

Distribution of Sonographically Detected Tendon Abnormalities in Patients with a Clinical Diagnosis of Chronic Achilles Tendinosis

Gibbon WW, Cooper JR, Radcliffe GS (The General Infirmary at Leeds, Leeds, UK)
J Clin Ultrasound 28(2):61–66, 2000

Introduction—This is a retrospective study to determine the possible mechanical processes involved with Achilles tendon pathology. Sonographic studies were conducted to view any detectable abnormalities in patients clinically diagnosed with Achilles tendinitis.

Patients and Methods—All patients were examined by the same sonologist (W.W.G.). Patients with inflammatory arthropathy and possible tears in the soleus or gastrocnemius muscle, close to the myotendinous junction, were excluded from the study. There totaled 118 symptomatic heels on 73 patients with a mean age of 45.3 years.

Results—Of the patients included in the study, 45 (62%) had abnormalities detected bilaterally. Abnormalities were confined in 96 (81%) of the 118 heels to the proximal two-thirds of the tendon, 9 (8%) to the distal third, and 13 (11%) to both locations. Of the 109 abnormalities detectable in the proximal two thirds of the tendon, 99 (91%) were on the medial side, and 22 (20%) in the transverse plane, no isolated lateral tendon cases were seen. Of the 22 abnormalities in the distal third of the tendon, 18 (82%) had retrocalcaneal bursitis, 14 (64%) had Achilles paratendinitis detected, and 13 (59%) had Achilles tendinitis. Of the 14 patients with detectable Achilles paratendinitis, 13 (93%) had concomitant retrocalcaneal bursitis.

The deep surface was primarily involved in all cases of distal one-third tendon injury. The superficial segment of mid-Achilles was at least partly involved in the 13 tendons that had pathology in both sections of the tendon.

Discussion—Due to the high incidence of concomitant distal third tendinopathy and retrocalcaneal bursitis, we conclude there is either a link in the mechanism of injury or a common causal relationship.

It was further noted that the high incidence of medial tendon involvement is in large part due to hyperpronation of the foot. Poor ankle dorsiflexion and/or impingement of the tendon by footwear might be attributed to pathology seen superficially on the tendon.

Conclusion—The pathology and possible mechanism of injury can be diagnosed using sonography. There are limitations to the study, which can be eliminated in future studies to more definitively outline the role of sonography in evaluation of the relationship between chronic Achilles tendinitis and the biomechanical process involved with the injury.—*G. Grant*

♦ This retrospective study describes the distribution of Achilles tendon disease and its relationship to biomechanics. Compared to MRI, sonography allows real-time examination of the Achilles tendon and is generally more cost-effective than MRI. However, an experienced sonologist is required if sonography is to be of clinical benefit for this condition.—*G.A. Shapiro, D.P.M.*

Intertarsal Ligaments: High Resolution MRI and Anatomic Correlation

Rand T, Frank L, Pretterklieber M, Muhle C, Resnick D (Veterans Affairs Medical Center, San Diego, CA; University of Vienna, Vienna, Austria)
J Comput Assist Tomogr 24(4):584–593, 2000

Background—MRI has become the imaging method of choice for analysis of most tendons and ligaments. While MRI has been shown to be useful in the evaluation of ankle joint ligaments, very few studies have been published on the role of MRI in the evaluation of ligaments of the intertarsal and tarsometatarsal joints. High-resolution MRI can now be obtained using a new local gradient coil and this may allow viewing of the ligamentous structures of the distal tarsus and tarsometatarsal junction. In this study, the authors attempted to correlate the MR images of these ligaments with the images derived from inspection of gross anatomical dissections.

Methods—Four human cadaveric feet were used in this study (derived from two men and two women, 65–87 years old at the time of death, mean age 75.7 years). Images were obtained using a 1.5-T MR unit using a local gradient coil, which was optimized for high resolution of the lower extremities. Images were obtained in all three planes.

Specimens were deep-frozen and then cut into 2-mm slices along one of the imaging planes. Each slice was examined and photographed for correlation with the MR images. One radiologist and one anatomist evaluated the MR images to determine the visibility of the desired ligaments: Visualization was judged in all planes using four grades (0 = not visible; + = partially visible; ++ = comply visible without delineation of internal structure; +++ = completely visible with delineation of internal ligamentous structures).

1. Talocalcaneonavicular (cervical ligament, ligament of the tarsal canal, lateral, medial, and posterior talocalcaneal ligaments, talonavicular ligament)
2. Calcaneonavicular joint (superomedial calcaneonavicular ligament, inferior and lateral calcaneonavicular ligaments)
3. Calcaneocuboid joint (medial and dorsolateral calcaneocuboidligaments, long plantar and short plantar ligaments)
4. Cubonavicular joint (dorsal, plantar, and interosseous ligaments)
5. Ligaments of the cuneonavicular joint (dorsal and plantar medial ligaments)
6. Cuneocuboid joint (dorsal, plantar, and interosseous ligaments)
7. Intercuneiform joints (dorsal, plantar, and interosseous ligaments)
8. Tarsometatarsal ligaments (dorsal, plantar, and interosseous ligaments)

Results—The results and analysis of the ligaments are listed in Table 1

Conclusion—High-resolution imaging can provide detailed anatomic information about portions of most of the ligaments of the tarsus and tarsometatarsal region. However, it is not yet known if it will provide useful information concerning pathologic alterations in these ligaments.—*B. Hoffman*

TABLE 1. Best visulation of individual ligaments of the midfoot in the coronal, sagittal, and axial plane

	Coronal	Sagittal	Axial
Talocalcaneonavicular joint			
Cervical ligament	++	+++	+
Ligamentum of tarsal canal	+	+++	+
Lateral talocalcaneal ligament	+	0	0
Medial talocalcaneal ligament	++	0	0
Posterior talocalcaneal ligament	0	0	0
Talonavicular ligament	0	++	0
Calcaneonavicular joint			
Superomedial calcaneonavicular ligament (neglectum)	0	0	0
Inferior (plantar/spring) ligament	++	+++	+
Lateral ligament (medial part of bifurcate ligament)	0	++	+

(continued)

TABLE 1. *(continued)*

	Coronal	Sagittal	Axial
Calcaneocuboideum			
Medial calcaneocuboid ligament	0	0	++
Dorsolateral calcaneocuboid ligament	0	0	0
Inferior calcaneocuboid ligament	++	+++	+++
Long plantar ligament	++	++	+++
Short plantar ligament	++	++	+++
Cubonavicular joint			
Dorsal ligament	++	0	0
Plantar ligament	0	0	0
Interosseous joint	+	+	0
Cuneonavicular joint			
Dorsal cuneonavicular ligaments			
Nav-C1	+	++	+++
Nav-C2	0	++	+
Nav-C3	0	+	+
Plantar cuneonavicular ligaments			
Nav-C1	0	+	+
Nav-C2	0	+	+++
Nav-C3	0	+	+
Medial cuneonavicular ligaments			
Nav-C1	0	+	++
Cuneocuboid joint			
Dorsal ligaments: C3-Cub	0	+	0
Plantar ligaments: C3-Cub	0	+	0
Interosseous ligaments: C3-Cub	+	+	++
Intercuneiform joints			
Dorsal ligaments: C1–C2, C2–C3	+	0	+
Plantar ligaments: C1–C2	+	0	+
Plantar ligaments: C1–C2	+	0	+
Interosseous ligaments: C1–C2, C2–C3	+	0	++
Tarsometatarsal joints			
Dorsal ligaments:			
Cub-M4, Cub-M5, C1-M2, C2-M2, C3-M2, C3-M3	0	0	+
Plantar ligaments			
C1-M2	0	++	+
C1-M2, C1-M3, C3-M3/4, Cub-M4, Cub-M5	0	0	+
Interosseous ligaments			
C1-M2 (ligament of Lisfranc)	0	++	++
C1-M1, M1-M1	0	0	++

♦ The authors present a detailed review of the anatomy and magnetic resonance imaging of the intertarsal ligaments of the foot. For sinus tarsi syndrome, high-resolution MRI is an excellent method to evaluate the ligaments of the talocalcaneal joint.— *G.A. Shapiro, D.P.M.*

Morton's Neuroma: Is It Always Symptomatic?

Bencardino J, Rosenberg ZS, Beltran J, Liu X, Marty-Delfaut E (Massachusetts General Hospital, Boston, MA; Hospital for Joint Diseases, New York, NY; Maimonides Medical Center, Brooklyn, NY; Long Island Jewish Medical Center, New Hyde Park, NY)

AJR 175(3):649–653, 2000

Introduction—MR imaging was used to determine the prevalence of clinically silent Morton's neuroma. It was also used to search for distinguishing features between symptomatic and asymptomatic patients.

Methods—Eight-five MR images of the foot were reviewed retrospectively. The MR images were analyzed for the presence of a low to intermediate signal intensity soft-tissue mass in the intermetatarsal space. The size, location, and signal intensity, as well as the presence of any intermetatarsal bursae, were recorded for each image. The patients were classified as symptomatic or asymptomatic according to a questionnaire, which allowed the patient to document any symptoms as well as their location. Each of the referring physicians was also contacted and their clinical findings were reviewed. Eight of the 25 symptomatic patients were confirmed to have had surgery.

Results—Nineteen of the 57 (33%) patients who did not have any clinical complaints were shown to have a Morton's neuroma upon review of the MR image. Twenty-five patients had signs of neuroma on the MR image as well as symptoms, while 41 had no clinical or imaging signs. The authors found that the symptomatic Morton's neuroma were slightly larger than the asymptomatic ones. The mean transverse diameter of the symptomatic neuroma was 5.3 mm, while the asymptomatic neuroma had a mean diameter of 4.1 mm. The difference in the two was found to be marginally significant.

Conclusion—Patients without any clinical symptoms were found to have Morton's neuroma as well as the patients with symptoms. Therefore, the presence of Morton's neuroma on a MR image does not imply that the patient will have symptoms. The authors suggest that a correlation between clinical signs and MR imaging findings be made before the diagnosis of Morton's neuroma is confirmed.—*L.T. Rowe*

♦ If one is using a MRI to confirm the diagnosis of Morton's neuroma prior to surgical planning, it is important to review the imaging center's protocol. It should be similar to that of the authors. Specifically, a 3-mm slice thickness with a 1-mm interslice gap. Thinner slices of less than 3-mm often result in signal and noise problems. Helpful images are both fat-saturated T1-weighted images and STIR images in the short axis. A post-Gadolinium study enhances the neuroma and provides a higher sensitivity. The diagnosis of this pathology rremains primarily clinical and based upon the patient's symptoms.—*K. Bloom, D.P.M.*

Characterization of Patients with Primary Peroneus Longus Tendinopathy: A Review of Twenty-Two Cases

Brandes CB, Smith RW (University of California at Los Angeles, Long Beach, CA; Bellevue Orthopaedic Associates, Inc., Bellevue, WA)
Foot Ankle Int 21(6):462–468, 2000

Introduction—The function of peroneus longus is threefold: to plantarflex the first ray, pronate the foot, and act as a secondary plantarflexor of the ankle. The short tendon excursion and bipennate nature of the muscle limits the ability to compensate for changes in its resting length. As a result, a small amount of lengthening secondary to a partial tear or a frank rupture will significantly affect its function. The lateral malleolus, the lateral calcaneal trochlear process, and the cuboid notch are the three anatomic zones where the peroneus longus changes direction in the hindfoot; noncoincidentally, this is also where injury to the peroneus longus may occur. The goal of the study was to identify any common clinical characteristics in the 22 patients with peroneus longus tendinopathy, describe any shared MRI and surgical findings, and propose a classification of peroneus longus pathology.

Methods—The authors defined the lateral malleolus, the calcaneal trochlear process, and the cuboid notch as zones A, B, and C, respectively. They further defined MRI changes into three grades. Grade 1 displays an increased signal around the tendon, the loss of signal planes between the tendons or tendon sheaths, or a change in thickness of the tendon without internal signal changes. Grade 2 changes are defined by an increased signal within the tendon with some normal tendon signal remaining. Grade 3 MRI changes represent complete loss of normal signal with the tendon. Finally, the surgical findings were classified into three grades. Grade 1 changes are defined as scarring, adhesions, or a change in thickness without tears or degeneration. Grade 2 changes are longitudinal splits, tears, or degeneration, but with some normal tendon continuity. Grade 3 changes are complete tears represented by rupture or scarring with loss of continuity of normal tendons.

Results—Of the 22 patients with peroneus longus tendinopathy, 21 underwent surgery and of those, 12 were studied with MRI. The following surgical changes were noted: two patients had normal findings, four patients had grade 1 changes, nine patients had grade 2 changes, and six patients had grade 3 changes. The grade 3 MRI changes all took place in zone C. All ruptures occurred in zone C, and eight of nine partial tears involved zone B. The two patients with normal findings in surgery were both found to have grade 2 changes by MRI. Interestingly, grade 2 surgical changes appeared to be associated with a more cavus foot. Upon clinical and radiographic evaluation, 18 of the 22 patients had a cavo-varus hindfoot position.

Discussion—The authors feel that the cavo-varus foot position is a predisposing factor to peroneus longus tendinopathy by placing the tendon at a mechanical disadvantage, reducing its moment arm, and increasing frictional forces at the lateral calcaneal process and cuboid notch. The MRI and surgical grading systems did not significantly correlate; however, there was a tendency for the MRI to diagnose a more severe level of pathology. The findings of this study showed that ruptures were more likely to occur at the cuboid notch and that partial tears were more apt to occur at the lateral calcaneal process. The results confirm that peroneus longus teninopathy should be suspected in patients with lateral hindfoot pain and a cavo-varus foot position.—*J.M. Dawson*

♦ MRI is an excellent method for diagnosing peroneal tendon pathology. However, there is the possibility that because the peroneus longus makes two angular turns in the rearfoot, a false increase in signal intensity could occur and be mistakenly read as an abnormal finding.—*G.A. Shapiro, D.P.M.*

Bizarre Parosteal Osteochondromatous Proliferation (Nora's Lesion) of the Sesamiod: A Case Report

Harty JA, Kelly P, Niall D, O'Keane JC, Stephens MM (Cappagh Orthopaedic Hospital, Dublin, Ireland)
Foot Ankle Int 21(5):408–412, 2000

Introduction—A case of bizarre parosteal osteochondromatous proliferation, aka Nora's lesion, is presented along with the radiographic and histologic data and differential diagnoses.

Case Report—A 32-year-old woman presents with a large painless mass under her first metatarsophalangeal joint (MPJ) which occurred suddenly and enlarged over a 2-year period. Past medical history was unremarkable with no history of trauma or athletic involvement, but she indicated recent discomfort and problematic shoe gear. Clinically, the 3 × 4 cm² solid mass was fixed to the first MPJ; and the overlying skin was mobile without callus. Both active and passive range of motion were available, and blood labs and systemic parameters were all normal. On plain radiograph, the well defined mass had a diffuse, mottled, calcified look and was indistinguishable from the tibial sesamoid. A bone scan revealed a hot spot under the first MPJ and CT showed evidence of avascular necrosis of the tibial sesamoid with periosteal spicules. MRI displayed its pedunculated shape, its tibial sesamoid origin, and suggested a breach into an adjacent metatarsal. Core-needle biopsy allowed histology to report the appearance of a benign growth of reactive mature bone and marrow-cavity fibrosis. Excisional biopsy was performed, the lesion was clearly defined and encapsulated, and was indeed attached to the tibial sesamoid with no nerve involvement. The specimen was sent to pathology and the patient made an uneventful recovery free of complications at 1-year follow-up.

Results—Grossly the circumscribed mass measuring 4×2 cm^2 included an irregular, fibrous capsule. Cross-sections revealed areas of fibrous tissue, cartilage, and solid bone. Under the microscope, the lesion was seen to have a mixed lobular pattern of cartilaginous proliferation, with areas of increased cellularity and distinctly enlarged chondrocytes. Seen peripherally were regions of fibroblastic propagation and areas of disorganized bone with endochondral ossification, lamellar thickening, and remodeling; more centrally was an organized collection of mature bone.

Discussion—This irregular pattern, of multiple lobules of proliferating cartilage and bone with no continuity with the sesamoid's actual cortex, led to the benign diagnosis of osteochroma; however, a differential diagnosis must be considered. Peripheral chondrosarcoma, rarely in hands and feet, appears on x-ray as ring-like or "popcorn" calcification. Parosteal osteosarcoma, also rare in the hands and feet, presents radiographically as a saucer-shaped diaphyseal lesion with central perpendicular streaks of periosteal new bone; most are low- to moderate-grade chondrosarcomatous growth with a small foci of definite osteosarcoma. Myositis ossificans shows ossification peripherally and has no cartilaginous cap. Florid reactive periostitis is usually related to trauma and reveals laminated or mature periosteal reaction. Soft-tissue chondroma is a slow-growing focus of cartilage appearing spottily opaque on x-ray and moderately cellular under the microscope with calcified areas likely to necrose. Giant cell tumor of tendon sheath, aka localized nodular tenosynovitis, often presents in fingers as a firm and compact, lobulated mass. The sesamoids could simply be hypertrophied, either congenitally (acromegaly) or secondary to trauma, and fracture can lead to hyperostosis, but not to the extent seen here. Finally, chondromyxoid fibroma is predominantly found in the metaphyseal region of long bones in young males.

Bizarre parosteal osteochondromatous proliferation, although rare, usually is seen in young adults with no previous trauma, typically presenting as a slow-growing mass causing mechanical irritation rather than pain. Nora and colleagues first defined the benign lesion in 1983 as an ossified mass best seen on CT, but also on x-ray. With well defined borders, the lesion arises from the cortex of the affected bone without medullary continuity. Once excised, Nora's lesion recurs in more than half of affected patients within the next 2 years. With the above information, this bizarre parosteal osteochondromatous proliferation can be accurately diagnosed.—*C. Jacka*

♦ Tumors of the sesamoids are rare. The authors present an interesting case study and an excellent review of their differential diagnoses: giant cell tumor, soft-tissue chondroma, myositis ossificans, parosteal osteosarcoma, hypertrophied sessamoids, and chrondrosarcoma. In this case, excisional biopsy was necessary to confirm the diagnosis of bizarre parosteal osteochondromatous proliferation.—*G.A. Shapiro, D.P.M.*

7 Forefoot Surgery

Thomas J. Chang, D.P.M.

Combined Cuboid/Cuneiform Osteotomy for Correction of Residual Adductus Deformity in Idiopathic and Secondary Club Feet

Schaefer D, Hefti F (University of Basel, Switzerland)
J Bone Joint Surg 82-B(6):881–884, 2000

Introduction—Recurrent metatarsus adductus is commonly seen after correction of idiopathic clubfoot. A combination osteotomy that shortens the cuboid and lengthens the first cuneiform, as described by McHale and Lenhart, has the potential to correct the deformity with minimal additional scarring. It is not known whether it will maintain the correction during growth. This study examines outcomes with a mean follow-up of 5 years.

Methods—Average age for subjects was 9.5 years. Twenty-seven clubfeet were operated on. Twenty-two were idiopathic and four were secondary to amniotic band syndrome. The procedure consists of removing a laterally based wedge out of the cuboid and placing it into the medial first cuneiform, with its base medial. The wedge is approximately one-third the width of the cuboid laterally. Follow-up consisted of questions regarding pain, ankle joint mobility, sports activity and footwear. Radiographically, the talocalcaneal angle, talar–first metatarsal angle, and calcaneal–second metatarsal angle were measured.

Results—All osteotomies healed within 3 months. No idiopathic clubfeet needed further surgery. All secondary clubfeet needed further surgery. At 5 years, all patients with idiopathic clubfeet were pain free and could walk at least 5 km. All but one could wear normal shoes, and all but two could participate in sports. The average calcaneal–second metatarsal angle changed from 20.7° to 4.6° at 3 months to 8.9° at 5-year follow-up. Four of 22 idiopathic clubfeet had recurrence. In secondary clubfeet, three of four patients suffered pain and two were unable to walk 100 m. All required insoles, and two required custom shoes.

Discussion—The problem of recurrence of adductus deformity in treated clubfeet is observable after every form of treatment. The recurrence rate increases with time following the procedure. It has been suggested that over correction may prevent recurrence, but the authors do not advocate this. The goal is to get complete correction by osteotomy, with medial soft-tissue release as needed.

Secondary clubfeet did not benefit from this procedure. The Ilizarov technique seems to be the most efficacious treatment for these, although the procedure itself is complex, requiring external fixation for several months.

Idiopathic clubfeet appear to benefit from this procedure, even after 5 years. The recurrence rate for this study is nearly the same as for the original study by McHale and Lenhart (4:22 vs. 1:7). In the present study, all patients with idiopathic clubfeet were pain free, satisfied with the outcome, and neither patient nor surgeon felt the need for further operations at 5 years. This implies that recurrence does not necessarily imply pain, difficulty shoeing, or decreased activity. Overall, this is a safe procedure that allows satisfactory correction of the residual adductus deformity in treated idiopathic clubfeet.—*D. Clement*

♦ The technique described in this paper can also be useful in other situations with forefoot adductus or metatarsus adductus. It does address the deformity at the region where the apex often resides, behind the tarsometatarsal joint, rather than performing panmetatarsal base osteotomies. We have performed this on a fair number of patients presenting with a cavo-varo-adductus deformity, one which the forefoot deformity was adequately addressed with this exact approach. It is often necessary to make the medial osteotomy well into the intermediate cuneiform in order to completely reduce the clinical adductus in surgery. Internal fixation of the medial wedge is usually not necessary.

Radiographic measurement of this correction should be performed utilizing the calcaneal–second metatarsal bisection rather than the traditional measurements described for metatarsus adductus. The traditional measurements (Engel's angle, etc.) evaluate the relationship of the metatarsals with respect the midfoot (cuneiforms). When this procedure is performed, the alignment of the metatarsals to the cuneiforms is not significantly altered since the osteotomy lies behind Lisfranc's joint.—*T.J. Chang, D.P.M.*

Distal Oblique Osteotomy of the First Metatarsal for the Correction of Hallux Limitus and Rigidus Deformity

Ronconi P, Monachino P, Baleanu PM, Favilli G (Foot Medical Hospital, Rome, Italy)
J Foot Ankle Surg 39(3):154–160, 2000

Introduction—Hallux rigidus/limitus is a common forefoot pathology that is not effectively treated with conservative measures. Several structural and biomechanical etiologies are responsible for this disorder, including first-ray elevation and hypermobility, metatarsal length abnormalities, extrinsic muscle imbalance, and uncompensated forefoot and rearfoot deformities. Trauma, postoperative complications, and several arthrities may also contribute to deviating the rotational axis position of the first metarsal–phalangeal–sesamoid joint, thereby causing progression to a hallux limitus. The staging of this condition is primarily based on the amount of degenerative and arthritic changes observed at the first metarsophalangeal joint (MTPJ). Both conservative and surgical treatments aim to reduce or eliminate symptoms, while attempting to preserve or improve the function of the first MTPJ.

The distal oblique osteotomy, a triplanar shortening decompression osteotomy, is indicated for the correction of stage 1 and stage 2 hallux limitus (Drago et al. classification). The osteotomy cut is performed from dorsal-distal to plantar-proximal with a 35°–45° angle in the sagittal plane. Following the proximal and plantar displacement of the capital fragment, two screws are used for fixation and the metatarsal head is remodeled.

Methods—There were 26 patients (mean age, 54 years) who underwent 30 distal oblique osteotomies with a mean follow-up period of 21 months. Following the procedure, 95% of the patients were allowed immediate limited weightbearing with a postoperative shoe and crutches. Postoperative evaluation was achieved through patient satisfaction rating, along with clinical and radiographic examination.

Results—Using the modified University of Maryland 100-Point Painful Foot Center Scoring System, 84% of the patients related their satisfaction as good to excellent, 7% as fair, and 9% as poor. Radiographic examination revealed a decrease in the postoperative first intermetarsal angle and proximal articular set angle means, while clinical examination showed an increased range of motion (ROM) of the first MTPJ.

Discussion—The distal oblique osteotomy allows for elevation of the rotational axis, thus decompressing and preserving the first MTPJ. Function of the joint is not sacrificed, and a significant gain in ROM is attained. This procedure, when performed in stage 1 and 2 hallux limitus, restores joint mechanics and function, while eliminating or reducing symptoms.—*E. Zarutsky*

♦ This paper presents a surgical approach to the hallux limitus deformity which has been reported previously. The osteotomy is essentially a modified Hohmann technique of a through-and-through cut with tremendous positional versatility and also mimics the Mau osteotomy described for hallux valgus. The main goals of any osteotomy for limitus surgery should be to achieve decompression and some plantarflexion. The most important component appears to be decompression or shortening. Due to the dorsal shelf of this osteotomy, there is some inherent stability imparted to weightbearing, but I would recommend at least an aperture under the metatarsal head or heel weightbearing for 3–4 weeks.

The authors also report less hallux purchase power and also increased lesser metatarsal pressure after the surgery. Unfortunately, their reasons for this are not explained. Overjudicious shortening will often lead to continued lesser metatarsalgia even if the sagittal plane position of the metatarsal is restored with plantarflexion. Overjudicious shortening can also lead to more relaxation in the physiologic tension of the plantar tendons and affect hallux purchase.—*T.J. Chang, D.P.M.*

Plantarflexion Torque Following Reconstruction of Achilles Tendinosis or Rupture with Flexor Hallucis Longus Augmentation

Monroe MT, Dixon DJ, Beals TC, Pomeroy G, Crowley DL, Manoli A (Las Vegas, NV; Wayne State University, Detroit, MI; University of Utah School of Medicine, Salt Lake City, UT; South Portland, ME; Warren, MI; University of South Alabama, Mobile, AL)
Foot Ankle Int 21(4):324–329, 2000

Introduction—Most Achilles tendon ruptures occur 2–6 cm from the tendon's calcaneal insertion. Studies have shown this area to have a decreased blood supply. It has been demonstrated that a flexor hallucis longus (FHL) muscle–tendon transfer can provide additional mechanical support to the pathologic tendon. However, healing of a repaired Achilles tendinosis or rupture may be improved by providing an additional vascular supply from transferring the low-lying FHL muscle belly.

Methods—Thirteen patients were surgically treated for Achilles tendon ruptures or tendinosis. Each patient had either an inadequate primary repair, or a debridement and augmentation with the FHL musculotendinous unit. Ankle plantarflexion was tested in nine patients using the Cybex 2+ Isokinetic Dynamometer at an average of 19 months postoperatively, and from this a peak plantarflexion torque was calculated.

Results—The mean American Orthopaedic Foot and Ankle Society Ankle Hindfoot score was 90. Subjective assessment showed a satisfaction rate of 9.8 out of 10. The most common complaint was postoperative pain. Most reported no limitation of function nor weakness. Cybex testing showed a mean plantarflexion peak torque of 28 foot-pounds for the operative side and 35 foot-pounds for the nonoperative side at 120° per second. At 30° per second, the operative side mean plantarflexion peak torque was 55 foot-pounds and the nonoperative side was 74 foot-pounds.

Discussion—The intention of this study was to describe the functional outcome of patients who have been treated with FHL augmentation for rupture or tendinosis of the Achilles. The patient satisfaction rate was high and functional limitations were low. In addition to the obvious mechanical advantage of the FHL transfer, delivery of a vascularized soft-tissue bed to the area of rupture or degeneration would theoretically strengthen the healing potential in the region.—*J.M. Dawson*

♦ This study supports the functional outcomes we have observed in patients with this procedure. The FHL tendon complex is an excellent option for augmentation in the difficult population who experience pain and weakness with tendinosis or rupture. Although the belief in the ability of the tendon to provide enhanced vascularity to the repair is still theoretical, the distal muscle belly does seem to provide clinical confidence that this occurs.

Depending on the level of injury within the tendon, it may not be necessary to harvest the tendon at the Master Knot region which is described within the article. The tendon can be harvested from the posterior ankle and very nicely augment a repair of a more proximal lesion. Tendon surgery of this type, however, does have prolonged disability and patients should be aware that the rehabilitation period may be upwards to 1 year before full recovery or return to preoperative activities.—*T.J. Chang, D.P.M.*

Salvage First MTP Arthrodesis Utilizing ICBG: Clinical Evaluation and Outcome

Brodsky JW, Ptaszek AJ, Morris SG (Lackland AFB, TX; Birmingham, AL; Baylor University Medical Center, Dallas, TX)
Foot Ankle Int 21(4):290–296, 2000

Introduction—Surgical failure of the first metatarsophalangeal (MTP) joint secondary to implant arthroplasty, avascular necrosis (AVN), and bone loss after an infection is a challenging problem to correct. Restoration of forefoot biomechanics with first MTP arthrodesis via the use of corticocancellous iliac bone graft is reported by the authors both clinically and radiographically.

Methods—Twelve women underwent this salvage procedure with autologous iliac crest bone graft (ICBG). Patients with rheumatoid arthritis or diabetes mellitus were excluded. Eight patients had failed arthroplasties for hallux abducto valgus or hallux rigidis, one patient had a Keller, two patients had AVN of the first metatarsal head, and one patient had osteomyelitis. Indications for the salvage procedure are intractable pain, deformity, intractable plantar karatosis, and a short first ray.

Operative Technique—A dorsal longitudinal incision is placed through the previous incision site, EHL is retracted laterally, and a dorsal longitudinal capsulotomy is made. Implant removal and synvectomy were performed if indicated. Debridement and curettage of cystic and intermedullary bone were done. ICBG was inserted and held in place with a smooth K-wire. The hallux was positioned at 10°–15° valgus and 20°–30° dorsiflexion. Eleven grafts were secured with a dorsal plate while one was stabilized with dual dorsal and medial plates. All lesser digital deformities were corrected. Patients were non weightbearing in dressings 10–14 days and then placed in a short leg cast for about 4 weeks.

Results—Eleven of the 12 patients returned for follow-up clinical and radiographic exam. Radiographically, union was achieved at an average of 15 weeks. Clinical union was apparent at an average of 12 weeks. The average IM achieved was 7.2 (range 5–10) and the average HA was 14.1 (range 7–25). The average dorsiflexion at the MTP joint was 22 (range 13–38), and the average increase in metatarsal length was 7.5 mm. Five patients had mild pronation of the hallux, six in neutral, and one in supinatus. The salvage procedure resulted in three excellent, four good, four fair, and one poor result. None of the patients were pain free after the surgery, yet all but one could walk greater than a mile without difficulty. Patients were able to carry out activities of daily living without difficulty. Three patients required hardware removal.

Conclusion—Arthrodesis with structural bone graft provides a stable, weightbearing first ray. Arthrodesis with ICBG is a reliable salvage technique when confronted with a functionally limited, painful MTP joint with shortening. Limited motion at the inerphalangeal joint is a relative contraindication to this procedure. The length of time needed to achieve radiographic and clinical union is prolonged, yet in face of the difficulty of restoring first ray function, the time is justified. It is found that a failed Keller bunion procedure, as well as the others mentioned, leave the surgeon with few options and a difficult task. In these cases, arthrodesis with ICBG is indicated.—*K. Carriero*

♦ The options for a shortened, degenerative first MTP joint are few. The goals are to alleviate pain, provide first ray weightbearing stability, and attempt to achieve hallux position. If restoration of length can be achieved, then lesser metatarsalgia can also be treated. A recent paper by Myerson et al. stated allogenic bone grafting can also be utilized with good success in this procedure, but my experience has primarily been with autogenous grafting. The calcaneus can also provide a nice bicortical segmental graft for this procedure and is an excellent option to the iliac crest.

In situations where significant soft-tissue contracture is present, from long-standing deformity or prior infection, there may be difficulty in getting length to the hallux with an interpositional bone graft. Skin necrosis and wound breakdown have both been reported. Callous distraction techniques can be utilized at the proximal metatarsal to get length back to the metatarsal before moving to an in situ fusion at the MTP joint. This will avoid the need for bone grafting and potential concerns of soft-tissue contractures and wound breakdown. These are technically difficult procedures with prolonged weightbearing, yet they can provide a very acceptable result in a difficult clinical setting.— *T.J. Chang, D.P.M.*

Traumatic Hallux Varus Repair Utilizing a Soft-Tissue Anchor: A Case Report

Labovitz JM, Kaczander BI (Botsford General Hospital, Farmington Hills, MI)
J Foot Ankle Surg 39(2):120–123, 2000

Introduction—Hallux varus is characterized by a triplaner deformity with a medially deviated, varus-rotated, hammered hallux. Classification is divided into congenital and acquired, but the most common etiology is iatrogenic overcorrection of hallux abductovalgus. In addition, and although rare, traumatic hallux varus can result from a disruption in the normal function of adductor hallucis and abductor hallucis, which creates a transverse plane deformity.

Case Report—A 38-year-old male presented to clinic with a chief complaint of a medially deviated left hallux. The patient described falling down three to four stairs 9 days ago. Physical exam revealed an adducted and nonreducible hallux with ecchymosis present in the first interspace. A small avulsion fracture fragment at the lateral base of the proximal phalange of the hallux was discovered with a radiograph and the hallux abductus angle was found to be $-11°$. Surgery was rendered 25 days following the injury. Following a U-shaped capsular lengthening incision just proximal to the metatarsophalangeal joint (MTPJ), a T-shaped capsulotomy was performed laterally, and a soft-tissue anchor (Mitek Mini G2) was used to correct the varus instability that remained. To tighten the lateral aspect of the first MTPJ capsule, the anchor was inserted into the lateral aspect of the MTPJ capsule. Lastly, both the extensor hallucis longus and abductor hallucis tendons were lengthened using a Z-lengthening procedure.

Results—The hallux abductus angle was reduced to $-0.5°$, following surgical treatment. Ultimately, transverse plane stability was attained and the use of the soft-tissue anchor allowed a more rapid postoperative period. The patient was immobilized nonweightbearing for only 4 weeks, return to activity was achieved 7 weeks postop, and all types of shoe gear were worn comfortably at this time. The Mitek anchor significantly reduced the postoperative recovery period.

Conclusion—In the case presented here, traumatic hallux varus, a subtype of acquired hallux varus, developed secondary to adductor tendon rupture. This etiology is rare, for iatrogenic overcorrection of hallux abductovalgus is the most common cause of hallux varus. In order to recreate joint stability, the MTPJ capsule was tightened using a soft-tissue anchor. In this case, special interest was paid to the short postoperative period and full return to activity without complications accomplished with the soft-tissue anchor.—*A. Duckworth*

♦ This case illustrates the versatility of soft-tissue anchor systems. In a recent article, I found over 20 types of anchor systems and the majority of them have sizes compatible with foot and ankle bones. The anchors with diameters under 2.0 mm can be placed easily within the phalangeal bones for delicate tendon-balancing procedures.

The good outcome in this case again demonstrates the significant contributions of soft-tissue to hallux and digital deformities. Soft-tissue releases (capsulotomies and capsulorrhaphy) should be a part of most approaches to capsule tendon balancing at the MTPJ. We all have seen the dramatic cases of a McBride or a Keller in achieving excellent correction of the bunion deformity in significant intermetatarsal angles of 16 or greater. — *T.J. Chang, D.P.M.*

Interdigital Neuroma: Intermuscular Neuroma Transposition Compared with Resection

Colgrove RC, Huang EY, Barth AH, Greene MA (Kaiser Permanente, San Diego, CA; Scripps Mercy Hospital, San Diego, CA)
Foot Ankle Int 21(3):206–211, 2000

Introduction—Persisting pain is a common complaint following interdigital neuroma resection. One of the explanations for incomplete pain relief is the development of a symptomatic transection neuroma. A transection neuroma is especially likely to be symptomatic if it is fixed to the skin or joint capsule in a weightbearing area. The implantation of the end of a transected nerve into muscle in order to produce a smaller and moreorganized transection neuroma has been tried with clinical success. Implantation into muscle is also appealing because it directs the transected nerve away from the plantar skin and weightbearing surfaces, and it cushions the transection neuroma from trauma.

Methods—During a 1-year period, 45 neuroma operations were performed on 44 patients who were unresponsive to conservative care. Only patients with primary interdigital neuromas were included in the study. Two types of operations were performed: standard resection of the interdigital neuroma (22 operations in 22 patients) or intermuscular transposition of the interdigital neuroma after distal release (23 operations in 22 patients). Patient selection was random and an independent interviewer who was blinded to the surgical procedure performed follow-up. Telephone interviews were conducted at 1 month, 3 months, 6 months, 12 months, and 36–48 months postoperatively. Patients were asked to rate pain on a scale of 0–100.

The surgical technique used for both procedures involved a linear incision over the appropriate interspace. The transverse metatarsal ligament was identified and transected, and the interdigital nerve was transected at the digital branches. The nerve was then isolated proximally. At this point the two procedures diverged. For the resection procedure, the nerve was transected proximally. In the transposition procedure, the distal epineurium was tagged with suture and threaded between the adductor hallucis and the interossei muscles. The suture was then passed through a nonweightbearing area of the plantar skin. Routine closure was performed. Skin sutures were removed at 10–14 days, and the plantar suture was removed at 3–4 weeks postoperatively.

Results—Preoperative pain levels were similar for both groups: transposition 78 versus resection 77. At 1 and 6 months postop, the average pain level in the transposition group was higher: transposition 22 and 11 versus resection 19 and 8. However, at 12 months and at final follow-up, the average pain level in the transposition group was lower: transposition 4 and 2 versus resection 6 and 9. Furthermore, at final evaluation 18% of the resection group had worsened when compared to their 12-month findings; none of the transposition group had deteriorated.

At the final evaluation, patient outcomes were graded as excellent, good, fair, and poor based on the percentage of pain relief from preoperative values. The resection group contained 86% excellent results, while the transposition group contained 96% excellent. The transposition group also contained a larger percentage of asymptomatic patients (96% vs. 68%).

Discussion—Assuming that patient selection and diagnosis are correct, the most likely cause of recurrent pain after resection of an interdigital neuroma is the formation of a symptomatic transection neuroma. The data from this study support the contention that transposition of the interdigital neuroma produces better long-term results with a greater number of asymptomatic patients. These findings are consistent with the hypothesis that the neuroma formed following the transection of a sensory nerve is less likely to be symptomatic if it is smaller, better organized, and less exposed to the irritations of weightbearing.—*T.C. Melillo, D.P.M.*

♦ This is an interesting approach and a critical look at the contribution of the actual visible neuroma to the pain experienced in patients. Not surprisingly, maintaining the visible neuroma within the foot, but transplantation of the nerve end into skeletal muscle showed tremendous results. This has been described by several plastic surgeons over the past decade and is my standard approach to revisional neuroma surgery. Since the reported technique is easily performed from a dorsal approach, it makes clinical sense to attempt this for better outcomes while still allowing patients early weightbearing.

Over the years, surgeons have tried different approaches to slow down the regeneration of nerve tissue after neurectomy. We have experimented with fibrin glue techniques, tying off the epineurium over the end of the nerve and nerve caps. The most consistent approach always seems to come back to burying the nerve into skeletal muscle or bone. The placement of the nerve end into a richly innervated skeletal muscle will chemically inform the nerve that the tissue it is lying in is already well innervated and appears to turn off nerve regeneration.

Also of interest is the isolated release of the deep transverse ligament without nerve resection. Advocates of the EDIN procedure or open techniques in which the nerve is maintained have reported good results as well.— *T.J. Chang, D.P.M.*

Rheumatoid Forefoot Reconstruction: A Long-Term Follow-up Study

Coughlin MJ (Boise, ID)
J Bone Joint Surg 82-A(3):322–341, 2000

Background—Chronic metatarsophalangeal joint inflammation due to rheumatoid arthritis is believed to result in capsular distention, and eventual loss of capsular and ligamentous integrity. With repetitive ambulation, hallux valgus, fixed hammering of the lesser toes, and subluxation or dislocation of the lesser metatarsophalangeal joints can occur.

This study presents long-term results of reconstruction of the rheumatoid forefoot with arthrodesis of the first metatarsophalangeal joint, resection arthroplasty of the lesser metatarsal heads, and open hammertoe repair with arthrodesis of the proximal interphalangeal joint of the lesser toes.

Methods—A retrospective study on 32 patients was conducted between January 1988 and January 1995. Indications for surgery included disabling foot pain secondary to intractable plantar keratoses, painful hallux valgus deformities, and pressure over the lesser toes with hammertoe deformities.

Each patient returned for an interview and clinical examination. A postoperative forefoot score was calculated, based on data derived during the interview and physical examination. This 100-point scale includes items related to pain, level of activity, deformity, and motion. A Harris-mat pressure study was performed and evaluated for all feet.

Surgical Concepts—Exposure was achieved through three dorsal linear incisions. The metatarsal parabola was maintained by using the length of the remaining second metatarsal as the reference. The goal is to transect the metatarsal heads so that each metatarsal was left slightly shorter than the next medially adjacent metatarsal.

The first metatarsophalangeal joint was fused at $15°-20°$ of valgus, $20°-30°$ of dorsiflexion, and neutral rotation. The first ray should be equal to or slightly (2–4 mm) longer than the second ray.

Results—All first metatarsophalangeal joints fused in the subjects with an average hallux valgus angle of $20°$. All subjects left a positive imprint of the hallux on the Harris-mat study.

The average postoperative score from the American Orthopaedic Foot and Ankle Society was 69 points. Postoperative pain was rated as absent in 18 feet, mild in 25, moderate in 4, and severe in none.

Conclusions—The key to a successful reconstruction of a rheumatoid forefoot is stable realignment of the first ray. Fusion of the first metatarsophalangeal joint increases weightbearing along the medial column as shown by the Harris-mat study, minimizes stress on the lateral metatarsophalangeal joints, and keeps the plantar fat pad relocated.

Excessive valgus angulation leads to widening of the forefoot and less pleasing cosmetic appearance. In the sagittal plane, insufficient dorsiflexion may cause increased pressure at the tip of the toe on the ground. In converse, too much dorsiflexion may lead to increased pressure under the first metatarsal head or pressure over the dorsal aspect of the interphalangeal joint. The recommended dorsiflexion angle of arthrodesis varies depending on the degree of pes planus, the presence of hypermobile first ray, and the desire to wear an elevated heel.—*O.T. Wang, D.P.M.*

♦ This is an excellent study and Dr. Coughlin should be applauded for a very thorough long-term (6 years) follow-up. The approach of panmetatarsal head resection with first metatarsophalangeal joint (MTPJ) fusion, and lesser digital proximal interphalangeal joint arthrodesis has been performed in podiatric and orthopedic communities for years and I encourage more follow-up studies. First MTPJ arthrodesis seems to be more predictable in the long-term than implant arthroplasty or resection arthroplasty at this joint. Arthrodesis also provides added stability to the medial column which we appreciate from medial column procedures in general and will add to better long-term outcomes.

We have also recognized that dorsal plate fixation with interfragmental screw fixation provides significant stability at the first MTPJ. Utilization of this technique may possibly give the surgeon more confidence in allowing early weightbearing in this difficult population and provide for a much easier postoperative course. Any technique modifications to improve mobility in the rheumatoid patient should be considered seriously.—*T.J. Chang, D.P.M.*

Gait Analysis After Ankle Arthrodesis

Wu W-L, Su F-C, Cheng Y-M, Huang P-J, Chou Y-L, Chou C-K (National Cheng Kung University, Taiwan; Kaohsiung Medical College, Kaohsiung, Taiwan)
Gait Posture 11:54–61, 2000

Introduction—To the author's knowledge, a similar study of three-dimensional gait analysis of the foot and ankle, post ankle arthrodesis, has not been documented. The purpose of this study was to evaluate forefoot and rearfoot motion along with muscle activity during level walking using computer analysis.

Methods—Ten unilateral solid ankle joint arthrodesis subjects were enrolled in the study, along with 10 "normal" subjects serving as controls. Markers were placed on the foot to measure motion in all three planes. The rectus femoris, vastus lateralis, vastus medialis, tibialis anterior, and soleus were evaluated with surface EMG and force plates. Motion was determined from a neutral position of standing at rest.

Results—No statistically significant difference was noted in the cadence of the two groups. However, swing phase time was decreased and stance phase was increased on the affected side. The sound limb had an increase in swing phase and decrease in stance phase time. Motion in the frontal plane of the affected side was within normal ranges but larger than the control group. There was increased transverse plane motion of the hindfoot, but sagittal plane motion of the hindfoot was significantly decreased in the arthrodesis group, along with an increase in forefoot motion. This is easily explained as compensation of surrounding joints for motion lost by fusion of the ankle. All patients showed marked calf atrophy with an additional change in firing of the soleus muscle on the fused side.

Discussion—The study showed increased motion in surrounding joints following ankle joint fusion despite the follow-up time of 1.7 years. This is presumed to result from compensation required after ankle fusion. While ankle arthrodesis can have a clinically satisfactory outcome, predisposing midtarsal arthritis decreases the likelihood of this outcome. Increased frontal plane motion was seen as increased eversion of the hindfoot, supporting the notion that eversion of the hindfoot follows internal rotation of the leg. The study also showed a girth reduction of 1.5 cm in the calf after ankle fusion. These results may help find a more optimal position in which to fuse the ankle and aid in rehabilitation postoperatively.—*G. Grant*

♦ Due to the well understood mechanics of compensation in adjacent joints around an arthrodesis site, surgeons have tried to focus on both joint position and preservation of joint architecture during these procedures. An attempt to approximate a neutral subtalar joint position in hindfoot arthrodesis seems to make a difference in minimizing increased stress to adjacent joints. Patients with a proximal contribution of varus or valgus will require additional subtalar joint manipulation to get the heel to a good vertical position. Proper positioning coupled with joint curettage techniques (preservation of architecture) will better preserve the height and width of the foot. These two principles have been applied to isolated fusions of the hindfoot with early reported success.

Curettage of the ankle will also better preserve the height of the limb, yet will not suffice in cases of extreme frontal plane deformity. Sagittal and transverse plane deformities are easier to accommodate with curettage and release of the Achilles tendon may be helpful in cases of significant preoperative equinus. A posterior rocker (Sach heel) placed onto the shoe will also help minimize stresses to the midtarsal during ambulation.— *T.J. Chang, D.P.M.*

Effects of a Tendo-Achilles Lengthening Procedure on Muscle Function and Gait Characteristics in a Patient with Diabetes Mellitus

Hastings MK, Mueller MJ, Sinacore DR, Salsich GB, Engsberg JR, Johnson JE (Washington University, School of Medicine, St. Louis, MO; University of Southern California, Los Angeles, CA)
J Orthop Sports Phys Ther 30(2):85−90, 2000

Introduction—High plantar pressures in combination with deformity and neuropathy constitute the primary factors leading to plantar ulceration in patients with diabetes mellitus (DM). Although there are studies that describe short-term gains in ankle joint range of motion and peak pressure reduction following tendo-Achilles lengthening (TAL), there are none that look at long-term changes. This case study sought to describe the results of TAL after 7 months in a patient with the above factors.

Case Report—The subject was a 42-year-old male with a 20-year history of type I DM and a history of foot ulceration. He had no history of peripheral vascular disease, Charcot arthropathy, or other comorbidities. He had a 6-week-old ulceration at the right fourth metatarsal head. Objective measures were applied to the subject pre-TAL, 8 weeks after TAL, and 7 months after TAL. The measures included palpation of foot structure, prone ankle joint dorsiflexion, plantar flexor torque, and in-shoe and barefoot plantar pressures. The operative procedure followed the Hoke triple hemisection technique. Postoperative management included total contact cast for 6 weeks, and a walking boot for 2 weeks. At 8 weeks, the patient began physical therapy and wearing extra-depth rocker shoes with custom-made two-layer plastizote inserts.

Results—The ulcer healed in 6 weeks, but opened up 2 weeks after the patient returned to shoe gear, remaining open through 7 months (HbA1c 9.2% at 7 months). Plantar flexor torque decreased 21% at 8 weeks but returned to baseline by 7 months. Initial dorsiflexion range of motion (DFROM) was 0° with the knee extended, 10° with the knee flexed. At 8 weeks postoperatively, DFROM was 18° both extended and flexed. At 7 months, they were 18° and 24°, respectively. In-shoe peak plantar pressures postoperatively and at 7 months were decreased by 83% and 55%, respectively. Barefoot pressures had a postoperative decrease of 46% postoperatively and 14% at 7 months. Peak plantar flexor moment during gait was decreased 68% at 8 weeks and 33% at 7 months. Hip flexor moment increased 64% at 7 months over pre-TAL values.

Discussion—Short-term gains in dorsiflexion are similar to those reported in other studies. Immediate loss of plantar flexor torque with regaining of it was also similar to other studies. The recurrence of the forefoot ulceration is a negative outcome. Decrease in barefoot pressure was less than for in-shoe pressure. This supports the need for proper shoe gear even after TAL. The recurrence of the ulcer demonstrates the multifactorial approach necessary in wound healing and prevention. Overall, evidence is provided for the utilization of TAL to improve DFROM and peak plantar pressures in both the short and long term.—*D. Clement*

♦ The significant role of equinus in both hindfoot and forefoot deformities continues to surface in the literature. As the care of the foot and ankle continues to expand into more specialties, we will continue to see well established principles revisited in new publications. Although the role of Achilles lengthening in effecting forefoot pressures was recognized many centuries ago in the European literature, it still appears to be forgotten today in many treatment centers. Other surgeons have elected to perform percutaneous tenotomies as their solution to minimizing forefoot pressures with dramatic results in classically nonhealing forefoot ulcerations.

I have found this to be essential in surgical management of the diabetic Charcot deformity. Most of the classic collapse noted at the tarsometatarsal joint and proximal have a significant Achilles contracture as either a primary or a secondary component. If the Charcot foot is reconstructed without attention directed at the Achilles contracture, then often the outcome is doomed to failure.— *T.J. Chang, D.P.M.*

Surgical Treatment of Hallux Valgus Deformity in Rheumatoid Arthritis: Clinical and Radiographic Evaluation of Modified Lapidus Technique

Shi K, Hayashida K, Tomita T, Tanabe M, Ochi T (Osaka University Medical School, Osaka, Japan)
J Foot Ankle Surg 39(6):376–382, 2000

Introduction—Hallux valgus deformity is often experienced in the rheumatoid foot, in which, the deformity is commonly corrected surgically through joint destructive procedures [arthrodesis and resection arthroplasty of the first metatarsophalangeal (MTP) joint]. However, radiographic evidence leads the authors to believe rheumatoid feet in the early and intermediate stages exhibit normal joint space and subchondral bone of the first MTP joint with hallux valgus deformities. Therefore, the modified Lapidus technique, a first MTP joint-preserving procedure indicated for idiopathic hallux valgus, is studied in the treatment for hallux valgus deformities in rheumatoid feet.

Methods—The modified Lapidus technique and resection of the lesser metatarsal heads were performed on 21 feet of 16 patients (15 females and one male) with rheumatoid arthritis between 1988 and 1995. The modified Lapidus technique utilizes three skin incisions, in which the adductors of the hallux were cut first. A lateral base wedge was then removed from the first tarsometatarsal joint and fused in the corrected alignment. Capsulorraphy was performed on the medial side of the first MTP joint. Lastly, Kirschner wires were used to secure the correction of the hallux and the lesser toes. Postoperative management allowed partial weightbearing at 6–10 weeks and full weightbearing at 10–14 weeks. Patients classified their pain relief, footwear comfort, and overall outcome of the surgery as three separate categories. The hallux valgus angle (HVA), the first and second intermetatarsal angle (M1/2), and the first and fifth intermetatarsal angle (M1/5) were evaluated radiographically before and after surgery.

Results—Pain relief was great in seven feet, moderate in 10, minimal in two, and none in two. Footwear comfort was viewed as improved in 16 feet and not improved in five. The overall satisfaction with the outcome of the surgery showed six were satisfied, 11 were satisfied with some reservations, one was satisfied with major reservations, and three were unsatisfied. Although the HVA and the M1/5 had increased at the last follow-up, there was still a significant difference between preoperative assessment and the last day of follow-up assessment for the HVA, M1/2, and M1/5.

Conclusion—Arthrodesis and resection arthroplasty of the first MTP joint both limit the function of the hallux. This study shows similar overall results using a modified Lapidus technique as compared to the commonly used joint destructive and hallux limiting procedures for hallux valgus deformities in rheumatoid feet. Therefore, the modified Lapidus technique allows preservation of first MTP joint motion and corrects the hallux valgus. Radiographic examination correlated the recurrence of hallux valgus deformity with splay deformity; however, there was no significant difference with the deterioration of the HVA and the M1/5.—*M. Garrison*

◆ Procedural selection for the deformity of hallux valgus still should be considered an individual process and not necessarily one approached with generalizations. Although many authors have advocated first MTP joint destructive approaches in the rheumatoid patient, it really should still depend on the disease process evident at the time of surgery. To believe all rheumatoid patients should undergo joint destruction is similar to saying all rheumatoid patients with forefoot deformity require a panmetatarsal head resection or all patients with a flatfoot should undergo a talonavicular fusion.

When the disease process is well controlled and both clinical and radiographic evaluation of the deformity leads to a joint preservation procedure, then this approach is appropriate. I have performed distal osteotomies in certain rheumatoid patients and proximal procedures in others. The criteria used are similar to those used for the nonrheumatoid patient and I believe patients still deserve this approach. Of course, they should be educated again to their overall disease process and aware that further surgery may be necessary in the future. — *T.J. Chang, D.P.M.*

A Retrospective Analysis of Swanson Silastic® Double-Stemmed Great Toe Implants with Titanium Grommets Following Podiatric Surgery for Arthritic Joint Disease

Ashford RL, Vogiatzoglou F, Tollafield DR, Casella JP (University of Central England, Birmingham, UK; Thessaloniki, Greece; Walsallmanor Hospital, Walsall, UK; University of Derby, Derby, UK)
Foot 10:69–74, 2000

Introduction—Since 1977, the double-stemmed implant has been used in patients with severe hallux valgus associated with arthritic destruction of the first metatarsophalangeal joint (MTPJ). In 1985, titanium grommets were introduced to shield and improve long-term durability of the silastic joint prosthesis. In studies done it has been determined that the implant is efficient in eliminating first MTPJ pain, while preserving length and proper alignment. Implant arthroplasty also allows for a shorter period of recovery time. This study retrospectively analyzes pain, physiological function, and quality of life in patients with Swanson total implant arthroplasty.

Methods—Twenty-one patients took part in the study, 12 female and nine males, ages 48–85 years. An interview was given to evaluate pain, and a clinical exam was performed to access joint movement and hallux purchase.

Results—Sixteen patients responded to a foot surgery questionnaire. Ten patients were very satisfied with the implant procedure, four patients rated the result good, and two patients were fairly satisfied. Most patients reported a significant decrease in pain, and 14 of 16 patients would repeat the procedure with their current knowledge. On clinical exam, the average joint dorsiflexion was 21° (range, 6°–46°). Hallux purchase averaged 254.32 (range, 110–460) as compared to a normal group sample of young females, which averaged 392.15 (range, 196.67–570). On interview, five patients had pain in the implant site and nine patients had pain elsewhere.

Discussion—The major objectives of the Silastic double-stem flexible-hinge implant arthroplasty are to relieve pain, allow shorter periods of recovery, preserve length and proper alignment of the great toe, and provide a stable first MTPJ. This study found that there was a significant decrease in pain, and activity levels were increased after implant arthroplasty. Joint dorsiflexion and hallux purchase were found to be decreased as compared to normal values, yet inconsistencies in measurement may have occurred. These patients are compared to patients with normal first MTPJ as opposed to their preoperative values that may show more dramatic improvement. The authors found that flexible implant arthroplasty has been successfully utilized in a particular patient population to provide pain relief, get them ambulating faster, and provide a stable platform from which to propulse.—*K. Carriero*

♦ This study reports similar results to many studies over the years on the use of the silicone implants in hallux limitus/rigidus. The inclusion of the titanium grommets may play a role on survival of the implant from osseous ingrowth, but their use does not seem to dramatically improve the patient satisfaction parameters measured and reported in numerous articles. The issues of transfer metatarsalgia and loss of hallux purchase and function are well noted and again reported in this paper. Reattachment of the long flexor tendon to the remaining base of the proximal phalanx has provided improved hallux purchase from anecdotal observation. Although most implants boast they can re-establish first MTPJ function, we are still far away from designing an implant that comes close. Most patients, however, still report a very high acceptance rate with the utilization of current models.

If silicone implantation is still chosen as a choice in joint replacement, then the patients may require a revisional implant in a period of 5–15 years. Our orthopedic colleagues often will replace a hip or knee prosthesis in this time frame with high patient acceptance and we should not feel uncomfortable discussing this same approach with our population.—*T.J. Chang, D.P.M.*

8 Rearfoot Surgery

STEPHEN H. SILVANI, D.P.M.

MR Imaging of Overuse Injuries of the Achilles Tendon

Karjalainen PT, Soila K, Aronen HJ, Pihlajamaki HK, Tynninen O, Paavonen T, Tirman PFJ (Helsinki University Central Hospital, Helsinki, Finland; Mt. Sinai Medical Center, Miami Beach, FL; University Hospital of Kuopio Kuopio; Finland; San Francisco MR Imaging Center, San Francisco, CA)
Am J Radiol 175:251–260, 2000

Background—The Achilles tendon is a common site of overuse and athletic injuries. Injuries can occur around the peritendinous tissue, or structural degeneration of the tendon itself may be incurred, or the tendon can partially tear or rupture completely. Clinical distinction is difficult, so this study relates findings from Magnetic Resonance (MR) imaging to clinical presentations.

Methods—One hundred patients (75 men) from ages 15–58 with 118 chronically painful Achilles tendons were evaluated. None had systemic disease which might affect the Achilles tendon and none had acute injury or sudden onset of symptoms; all were involved with competitive or recreational sports. MR imaging utilized a 1.5-T magnet and the following pulse sequences: sagittal T1-weighted (TR/TE, 460/14) and fast short tau inversion recovery (STIR) with 3-mm sections; axial T1-weighted spoiled gradient-echo fast low-angle shot (FLASH) with a short TE (600/10) with 4-mm sections; and axial fast STIR (4700/30) and dual spin-echo images (2100/20) with 4-mm sections. Sixty-two asymptomatic heels were also imaged. Abnormal was defined as follows: >6 mm of anteroposterior diameter or ≤2 mm thicker than the asymptomatic side; convex anterior border on axial or anterior bulging on sagittal images; and a focal intratendinous lesion of >3 mm on axial FLASH images. Peritendinous tissue like pre-Achilles fat pad and retrocalcaneal bursae as well as calcaneal marrow deep to the insertion were also analyzed.

Results—One hundred eleven of 118 symptomatic and 12 of 62 asymptomatic imaged tendons showed abnormalities. Abnormal thickening in symptomatic tendons averaged 7.6 mm, and 5.2 mm in asymptomatic. Anterior bulging was seen in 67 tendons, and convexity of the anterior margin in 77. Forty-five percent of tendons showed intratendinous lesions from as far as

8 cm proximally; 14 were found at the insertion itself. FLASH images allowed the most clear shot of these lesions, especially the small ones, and showed a range of 5–90% of the cross-sectional area, most often situated anteriorly. The height of the lesions ranged from 5 to 100 mm. Twenty-eight abnormalities were noted at the insertion of the Achilles tendon, 10 of which were signal intensities in the marrow of the calcaneus, ranging from 3 to 20 mm in diameter. Eighteen showed tendon abnormalities 0–2 cm from the insertion, mostly at the anterior margin at the level of the retrocalcaneal bursa. In 23 cases, the retrocalcaneal bursa was enlarged, and in eight, this was the only abnormality. Three patients showed increased signal intensity in the soleus muscle. Sixty-nine percent of tendons showed abnormalities in the peritendinous tissue: 48 show signal intensities at the medial, lateral, or posterior aspect of the paratenon, and the anterior fat pad was abnormal in 12. Thickening of the paratenon, also best visualized with the FLASH sequence, was found in 32 cases. In 64% of cases, both the tendon and its surrounding tissue were abnormal.

Only 30 of 54 tendons with an intratendinous lesion on MR had clinically palpable nodules. Four tendons were thickened on palpation, and this correlated with the level of thickening on MR, but none of these had focal lesions. Palpable tenderness did correlate well with MR findings; all 28 with abnormal findings at the insertion also had maximum pain and tenderness at that level. Patients with enlarged retrocalcaneal bursae faired better with an average of 3.2 symptomatic months, compared to those with abnormal tendon insertions or marrow who suffer on average 10.2 months. The same averages held true for those with (12.1 months) and without (6 months) thickened paratenons.

Of the 21 surgically detected intratendinous lesions, 20 were spotted on MR; three proved to be smaller than depicted on FLASH images. Each case of true positive MR findings showed disorganized fiber structures intraoperatively. six showed partial rupture; of these, four had an intratendinous lesion on STIR and three on T2 images. Fifteen of the 21 surgically detected intratendinous lesions were deranged fiber nodules, suggesting healed partial tears. Three cases with thickened tendon on MR were found to be swollen intraoperatively without fiber disturbances. Of the 19 thickened paratenons found in surgery, 12 were detected on FLASH images. Pathology reported fiber disturbances, lack of collagen continuity, capillary proliferation, a correlation between severity and MR signal intensity, some hemosiderin deposition, but no inflammation.

At follow-up, two patients had poor results, both with intratendinous lesions. All with normal MRIs fully recovered. Those patients with a high-intensity signal on STIR images did significantly worse than those without. Those with abnormalities limited to peritendinous tissue had significantly better long-term results than those with combined abnormalities.

Discussion—Similar clinical scenarios can have different etiologies which surface on MR imaging. High-resolution T1-weighted FLASH and fluid-sensitive STIR sequences were compared with conventional settings: FLASH proved superior in detection of intratendinous lesions and in visibility of the paratenon, most likely a result of the high-resolution matrix and short TE. STIR and proton density-weighted images accurately predicted the macroscopic size of the lesion. Pathology reports confirmed MR-detected abnormalities. Surgically treated patients with intratendinous lesions had better long-term results, giving credence to surgical intervention for these types. The elucidation of pathology location can better predict prognosis; case in point, insertional tendinosis had the worst prognosis in this study and isolated retrocalcaneal bursitis, had the best. This highlights the prognostic and diagnostic value of MR imaging.—*C. Jacka*

♦ Overuse injuries are very commonly seen in the Achilles tendon. They vary from peritendinitis to tendinosis to complete rupture, which can be difficult to clinically differentiate. MRI has been shown to definitively distinguish whether the cause of pain is intratendinious or not. Small lesions have been found before they are palpable. Histologic examinations very closely correlated with the MRI appearance of these lesions.

The prognostic value of MRI was demonstrated in the worse long-term outcomes with those lesions that were insertional and those with high-intensity intratendinious appearance. Patients with isolated retrocalcaneal bursitis, isolated peritendinitis, or normal findings on MRI had a good prognosis. Therefore, this technique not only makes the diagnosis, it also helps determine treatment and predicts outcome.—*S.H. Silvani, D.P.M.*

Avascular Necrosis of the Talus Following Subtalar Arthrorisis with a Polyethylene Endoprosthesis: A Case Report

Siff TE, Granberry WM (St. Luke's Hospital, Houston, TX)
Foot Ankle Int 21(3):247–249, 2000

Background—Smith and Millar originally developed the polyethylene peg implant (STA-Peg) for pediatrics with flexible flatfoot. The peg was inserted into the lateral aspect of the subtalar joint (STJ) and designed to eliminate excessive pronation. They conducted a study in the 1970s in which the STA-Peg was used for 27 patients with flexible flatfeet. After a 3-year minimum follow-up, a success rate of 96.2% was reported with the only complication being STJ synovitis. At no time was avascular necrosis (AVN) of the talus reported.

Case Report—In 1987, a 22-year-old female was treated for bilateral pes planus deformity with a tendo Achillis lengthening and a STJ arthrorisis using the polyethylene STA-Peg implant. Within 5 years, she began to experience significant rearfoot pain despite normal radiographs. By 10 years, her pain had progressively worsened and her clinical exam revealed a significant planovalgus deformity with an exceedingly limited STJ range of motion. Radiographs featured osteosclerosis of the talus while MRI revealed AVN of the talus. Talar dome biopsies revealed focal necrosis with empty lacunae and a stromal infiltrate consisting of multinucleated giant cells. The synovium also demonstrated fibrosis consistent with chronic synovitis. Upon implant removal and synovectomies, the patient was able to return to normal activities within 6 months without any major sequelae. Although her planovalgus deformity went unchanged, she did regain a significant amount of STJ range of motion.

Discussion—Polyethylene implants have been shown to cause an immune complex response as well as chronic inflammatory changes. One theory is that microscopic fragments of polyethylene are deposited within the body of the talus causing a foreign-body reaction as demonstrated by the presence of multinucleated giant cells. Eventually, this leads to chronic fibrosis and ultimately avascular necrosis.

Conclusion—Although polyethylene implants are an acceptable protocol in the treatment of pes planus deformity, they are not without complications. Several studies have reported complications such as improper pistoning, implant failure and fragmentation, peroneal spasticity, STJ arthritis, and osteomyelitis.—*D. Carmack*

♦ Flatfoot surgery is classically fraught with complications of short- and long-term nature. Just deciding which patients would benefit from a repair is difficult, but not as confusing as to what type of procedure should be attempted and its timing. Controversy and poor outcomes surround flatfoot surgery, especially in young, flexible feet.

Therefore, great interest was generated when the polyethylene endoprosthesis for extra-articular arthroresis was introduced. It was supposed to be joint sparing, nonreactive, minimally invasive, and reversible. However, as time wore on and so did the implants, a myriad of complications arose. Many were due to poor patient selection, such as adults, since the implant was designed for children. Significant reactive synovitis and foreign-body immune responses were common. Degenerative arthritis and peroneal spasms were created. I have performed more than my share of subtalar arthrodesis as salvage after a STA-Peg procedure.

This case report is the first one involving avascular necrosis of the talus many years after an adult implant. It was postulated that a foreign-body chronic inflammatory reaction caused the AVN. It behooves the surgeon to wait for some outcome studies to determine the efficacy and complications associated with new procedures, especially those involving new materials or applications.—*S.H. Silvani, D.P.M.*

Isolated Subtalar Arthrodesis

Easley ME, Trnka H-J, Schon LC, Myerson MS (Duke University Medical Center, Durham, NC; Orthopaedic Hospital Gersthof, Vienna, Austria; The Union Memorial Hospital, Baltimore, MD)
J Bone Joint Surg 82-A(5):613–624, 2000

Background—Although triple arthrodesis has been favored for treatment of talocalcaneal ailments, advocates of isolated subtalar arthrodesis cite the advantages of preserved hindfoot motion, a lower risk of arthritis of adjacent joints, a less complex operative procedure, and elimination of the risk of nonunion or malunion of the transverse tarsal joint.

The outcomes of this procedure have been favorable in the current literature. The purposes of this retrospective study were to review the results of isolated subtalar arthrodesis in adults and to identify factors influencing the union rate.

Methods—Between January 1988 and July 1995, 184 isolated subtalar arthrodeses were performed in 174 adults. Eighty patients (46%) were smokers. The indications for the procedure were post-traumatic arthritis secondary to a rearfoot trauma. Bone graft (cancellous autograft, structural autograft, cancellous allograft, and structural allograft) was used in 145 feet. A preoperative score according to American Orthopaedic Foot and Ankle Society was used in this study.

Surgical Technique—The procedures were not standardized but tailored to each patient's particular pathological findings. A lateral approach through a horizontal incision was used for 150 feet that were treated with in situ arthrodesis, and a posterolateral approach through a vertical incision was used for 34 feet that were treated with subtalar distraction arthrodesis.

Assessment of avascularity was performed intra operatively. Clinically important avascularity was arbitrarily defined as at least 2 mm of nonbleeding subchondral bone. The amount of avascular bone was measured from the level of superficial subchondral bone to the level of bleeding subchondral bone during preparation of the surfaces for the arthrodesis.

Results—The average ankle-hindfoot score according to the modified scale of the American Orthopaedic Foot and Ankle Society improved from 24 points preoperatively to 70 points at follow-up. The union rate was 84% overall and 86% after primary arthrodesis, and 71% after revision arthrodesis. The union rate was 92% for nonsmokers and 73% for smokers. Forty-two percent of the 184 feet had evidence of avascularity; all 30 nonunions occurred in this group. Excluding the subgroups of smokers, those with structural grafts, those with previous subtalar fusions, and those who had subtalar joint fusions with previous ankle fusions, the union rate improved to 96%.

Conclusions—The results suggest that the outcome following isolated subtalar arthrodesis is not as favorable as has been reported. The rate of union was significantly diminished by smoking, the presence of avascularity, and the failure of a previous subtalar arthrodesis. Other factors that may affect the union rate include the use of structural allograft and performing subtalar joint arthrodesis adjacent to the site of a previous ankle arthrodesis.—*O.T. Wang, D.P.M.*

♦ An isolated subtalar joint arthrodesis has been successfully used for treatment of many rearfoot problems. This current study shows a much lower union and higher complication rate than previously reported. Significant factors that lead to these results were smoking, presence of avascular bone, and a previous failure to fuse. To a lesser degree, the use of allograft and having a previous ankle arthrodesis were negative factors.

Therefore, it is imperative to require the patient to cease smoking before performing a subtalar joint or any other arthrodesis. It is the only factor that one can really control.—*S.H. Silvani, D.P.M.*

The Results of a Primary and Staged Pantalar Arthrodesis and Tibiotalocalcaneal Arthrodesis in Adult Patients

Acosta R, Ushiba J, Cracchiolo A (UCLA Medical Center, Los Angeles, CA)
Foot Ankle Int 21(3):182–194, 2000

Introduction—Arthrosis involving the ankle and rearfoot can cause pain, loss of motion, change in gait, and deformity. Arthrosis can be a secondary result of local arthritis, systemic arthritis, trauma, and infection.

Methods—Twenty-three patients with either a primary or staged pantalar fusion or a tibtalocalcaneal fusion were examined to determine their clinical situations. The main indication for surgery was severe pain and discomfort that did not respond to conservative therapy. Pantalar fusion is described as a combination of ankle joint, subtalar joint, calcaneocuboid, and talonavicular joint fusion. Fourteen feet had a pantalar fusion. Seven of these feet had either an ankle fusion of triple arthrodesis at an earlier time. The remaining seven feet had all joints fused feet had an ankle and subtalar joint fused during the same operation.

Results—All patients were followed for an average of 55 months from the time of their final fusion procedure. Overall, 23 of the 27 feet achieved a good fusion of all joints operated on. Four feet had a failure of fusion of only a single joint and all were in the pantalar group. The average time to radiographic fusion was 23 weeks and resulted in a plantigrade foot with an average tibia-floor angle of 87°. Complications occurred in 10 feet of which there were three deep infections: two ankle and one subtalar joint. These fusions resulted in marked relief of the patients' preoperative discomfort, which was the primary indication for surgery. Postoperatively, there was no pain in 11 feet, mild pain in 13 feet, and moderate pain only in three feet. Only five patients had an excellent clinical outcome. Nine were rated good, three rated fair, and six patients had a poor result.

Conclusion—These operations must be considered to be salvage operations. They are technically difficult to perform and major complications may occur. The combination of ankle and rearfoot fusions is a treatment option only in certain cases, and is the only alternative to amputation. If performed correctly, the operation can result in the relief of discomfort and correction of deformity which may result in some improvement in the patient's function.—*A. Ghamgosar*

♦ Major rearfoot arthrodesing operations are salvage procedures for severe arthritic and structurally deformed feet. They are intended to help reduce severe pain and do not improve function. The basic premise of any surgery is to direct the efforts towards the area that is affected and to do the least surgery that benefits the patient the most. Sometimes procedures are staged for symptom reasons, technical considerations, or poor local conditions. This study showed no significant outcome difference between staging or performing the procedure at one time.

Getting everything done at one time, if possible, affords the patient total correction with only one surgical exposure and hopefully fewer complications.—*S.H. Silvani, D.P.M.*

Peripheral Arterial Embolization: Doppler Ultrasound Scan Diagnosis

Nicholls SC, Smith W (University of Washington, Seatlle, WA)
J Vasc Surg 31(4):811–814, 2000

Introduction—Doppler ultrasound spectrum has been featured as a useful tool in detecting emboli in procedures such as carotid endarectomy. This use of Doppler ultrasound has been expanded to monitoring the ambulatory patients who are at risk for and/or show clinical signs of embolic activity. Such usefulness comes from the ability to monitor deep venous thrombosis, clinically silent lesions, and the progress of any anticoagulant therapy that is being done.

Case Report—The patient was 46-year-old male who initially underwent surgery for a short segment popliteal artery occlusion which continued on to various bypass grafts with limited success in achieving complete blood flow through the posterior tibial artery. Angiography revealed complete occlusion of the popliteal, peroneal, and anterior tibial arteries. The patient had no evidence of Buergers disease. On examination, the foot was cool to touch.

Using a 3-MHz Doppler probe, no embolic signals were noted proximal to the previously performed posterior tibial arteriotomy where duplex scanning had revealed normal flow. Distal to this site, however, there were multiple Doppler signals demonstrating emboli. Due to no clinical improvement, the patient was taken back to the operating room, revealing platelet thrombosis and emboli in areas of the arteriotomy that were consistent with the earlier Doppler embolic signals. Despite the use of urokinase and other antithrombotic measures, deterioration continued and a below-the-knee amputation ensued.

Conclusions—The incidence of embolism is clearly much higher than clinical presentation would suggest. Embolic showering is the culprit for many small vessel patencies such as stroke, "trash foot," and "blue toe." A delay in intervention of any of these may result in tissue loss. It has been shown that embolism monitoring with Doppler ultrasound in the high-risk patient gives the clinician a head start on any needed therapeutic measures such as antiplatelet therapy, thus reducing the incidence of stroke. Peripheral arterial embolization may occur after surgical procedures and being able to detect this phenomenon in the distal extremity will expand one's repertoire in the pursuit of efficient and effective patient care.—*S.B. Heninger*

♦ Doppler can now be used for detection of "embologenic" arterial lesions and to quantify the extent of embolic activity. This monitoring can detect clinically silent lesions and guide anticoagulant therapy. This practice, when it becomes widespread, will benefit all high-risk patients who undergo lower extremity surgery or casting.—*S.H. Silvani, D.P.M.*

Sinus Tarsi Approach with Trans-articular Fixation for Displaced Intra-articular Fractures of the Calcaneus

Ebraheim NA, Elgafy H, Sabry FF, Freih M, Abou-Chakra IS (Medical College of Ohio, Toledo, OH)
Foot Ankle Int 21:105–113, 2000

Introduction—The treatment of displaced intra-articular calcaneal fractures is a controversial topic. When operative intervention is preferred, various surgical approaches and several fixation options exist. The authors favor a limited exposure with minimal internal fixation to avoid additional damage to the lateral soft-tissue envelope.

Methods—The charts and radiographs of 99 patients with 106 intra-articular fractures of the calcaneus were retrospectively reviewed. All patients were treated with operative intervention by the same surgeon. Fractures were classified using the Sanders CT-based system.

Surgical exposure was achieved through an incision over the sinus tarsi. Reduction of the posterior facet was performed under direct visualization. The posterior tuberosity fragment was reduced indirectly under fluoroscopic guidance. The fracture was fixated with a threaded pin driven from the lateral process of the talus, across the subtalar joint, and into the reduced calcaneal fragment. In multiple fragment fractures, additional wires were inserted for fixation. The lateral calcaneal wall was then reduced with digital pressure. Postoperatively, patients were treated in a short leg cast for 6 weeks. Weightbearing was not allowed for 10 weeks. The threaded pin was removed after 6 weeks, and physical therapy was started.

Chart reviews and telephone interviews were performed on all patients. The American Orthopedic Foot and Ankle Society (AOFAS) Ankle-Hindfoot Score was used to grade clinical outcomes. Average follow-up duration was 29 months.

Results—According to the Sanders classification, 67% of fractures were type II, 23.6% were type III, and 9.4% were type IV. Postoperatively, 38.8% of fractures were rated as excellent, 36.7% were good, 13.2% were fair, and 11.3% were failures. The overall AOFAS Ankle-Hindfoot Score was 77.6. Mild to moderate limitation of subtalar joint motion was found in 85% of cases.

Discussion—The limited sinus tarsi approach with minimal transarticular fixation for the surgical repair of intra-articular calcaneal fractures offers adequate exposure to reduce the posterior facet and anterolateral calcaneus, while avoiding compromise to already damaged lateral soft tissues. The authors feel that this approach is a good option for management of calcaneal fractures.—*T.C. Melillo, D.P.M.*

♦ The treatment of calcaneal fractures is difficult at best, whether closed or open. Stiff, painful results commonly occur leading to subtalar joint arthrodesis. The extensile lateral approach, which I have been using for 11 years, offers a total view of the lateral body of the calcaneus, the cuboid articulation, and protects the sural nerve and the peroneal tendons. Direct visual reduction of all components of these complex fractures is provided by this approach. Various perimeter plates which hold the reduction without bone graft are easily applied. Even displaced sustentaculum fractures can be reduced by reaching through the fracture line across the body and grabbing the fragment. It is the secured by a compression screw through one of the plate holes.

This article advocates a limited sinus tarsi approach and transarticular pin fixation for severe calcaneal fractures. They reported fewer soft-tissue problems, excellent to good fracture scores, and some pin-tract infections. These results do not quite match those of large extensile approach series. Appropriate visualization of joint facets with anatomic reduction and rigid internal fixation allows early nonweightbearing range-of-motion exercises.

This study illustrates that different techniques work differently in each surgeon's hands. One must evaluate one's own skills and outcomes in reference to procedure selection and critically evaluate other surgeons' results. —*S.H. Silvani, D.P.M.*

9 The Diabetic Foot/ Wound Care

JOHN M. GIURINI, D.P.M.

Do Foot Examinations Reduce the Risk of Diabetic Amputation?
Mayfield JA, Reiber GE, Nelson RG, Greene T (Indiana University, Indianapolis, IN; Veterans affairs Puget Sound Health Care System, Seattle, WA; National Institute of Diabetes and Digestive and Kidney Disease, Phoenix, AZ; Cleveland Clinical Foundation, Cleveland, OH)
J Fam Pract 49(6):499–504, 2000

Background—The American Diabetes Association recommends "comprehensive vascular, neurological, musculoskeletal and skin and soft tissue evaluation should be done at least annually" in order to prevent lower extremity amputation. The efficacy of this recommendation has not been studied.

Methods—The Pima Indians from the Gila River Indian community in Arizona were the subjects of a population-based case-control study. The patients had type II diabetes with the case patients who had a first nontraumatic lower extremity amputation between January 1, 1985, and December 31, 1992 and the control group who had not had an amputation. A chart review was conducted determining the type of foot examinations, comorbid conditions, and foot risk factor present in the 36 months before the pivotal event, a preceding event that led to the amputation. The examinations that were for ulcer care were excluded. The types of exams where divided into three classifications: 1) foot scan—examined the skin for any sign of ulceration; 2) comprehensive foot exam—foot scan plus assessment of risk for ulceration, by noting bony prominences, neurological assessment, and vascular assessment; 3) therapeutic exam—debridement of callus, thick nails, prescription or dispensing of therapeutic footwear, or inspection of a previous ulcer site.

Results—Patients with 61 first nontraumatic amputations were compared to 183 patients who had no amputations. A total of 1166 preventive examinations occurred in the 36-month time interval. This study did not produce statistically significant results that proved a decreased risk for lower extremity amputation when foot examinations were performed.

Conclusion—Foot examinations in type II diabetes does help identify high-risk conditions that may lead to complications; however, there needs to be a better study with a larger patient population to support the American Diabetes Association's recommendations.—*T. Marshall*

♦ The purpose of this study was to determine the effect that regular foot examinations might have on the rate of diabetic amputations in a high-risk group, the Pima Indians of Arizona. During the 3-year study period, 1166 foot examinations were performed on 244 subjects. Case patients had seven foot examinations per year while control patients had three foot examinations per year.

The results of this study imply there was no statistically significant difference in the amputation rate between case patients who had more frequent foot examinations and control patients. This is a somewhat surprising conclusion.

Several factors can be extrapolated from the data of this study to explain this conclusion. The case patients as a whole were older, had diabetes longer, and had more comorbid conditions, including complications of diabetes such as neuropathy (43% vs. 14%), peripheral vascular disease (43% vs. 15%), underlying foot deformity (19% vs. 6%), and prior foot ulcer (33% vs. 8%). All these factors have been previously identified as risk factors for amputation. Additionally, the authors also identified nonadherence to recommendations as a major factor for lack of statistical significance. Forty-one percent of case patients failed to adhere to recommendations on footcare or shoegear modifications versus 23% of control patients.

The current study should be viewed not as pointing to the lack of importance of foot examinations, but rather the need for continued vigilance and education of the diabetic population. While this study was performed on a very select group of patients, the characteristics of this group match those of our more difficult patients.—*J.M. Giurini, D.P.M.*

The Prevelance of Multiple Diabetes-Related Complications

Morgan CL, Currie CJ, Stott NC, Smithers M, Butler CC, Peters JR (University Hospital of Wales, Wales, UK; University of Wales College of Medicine, Wales, UK; Glaxo Wellcome, Greenford, UK)
Diabet Med 17:146–151, 2000

Introduction—This study was conducted to determine the prevalence of diabetic complications. Patients with diabetes have an increased risk of coronary heart disease (CHD), cerebrovascular disease (CVD), nephropathy, retinopathy, and the neuropathic and vascular complications associated with the diabetic foot. The relationship between these complications and the age of the patient, age of onset of diabetes, and association with the other complications were studied.

Methods—The data were collected from two main sources, a general practice diabetes audit and a hospital-based record linkage-derived patient index. In addition, diabetic outpatients seen in ophthalmology were flagged for retinopathy and cataracts. The age of onset and duration of diabetes were also calculated. Patients who were diagnosed with diabetes at an age less than 35 were identified as having type I diabetes. Those who were diagnosed at the age of 35 or greater were said to have type II diabetes.

Results—A total of 10,287 patients with diabetes were identified. The data accumulated showed that 25.2% of the patients had CHD, 18.1% had complications of the diabetic foot, 16.5% had retinopathy, 9.6% had CVD, and 2% had nephropathy. If the outpatients from ophthalmology were included, then the rate for retinopathy increased to 28.9%. (The latter figure is probably more accurate.) Each of the macrovascular complications, CHD, CVD, and the diabetic foot, were shown to have a strong correlation with increase in age. The microvascular complications also had a correlation with age, but not as great as the macrovascular complications. Another factor that was studied was the percentage of patients with multiple complications. Of the diabetic patients studied, 52.1% had no complications, 30.2% had one, 12.7% had two, 4.1% had three, 0.8% had four, and only 0.1% had all five complications. The possibility of multiple complications increased with age. There was no correlation with gender.

It was also found that the prevalence of complications increased with the duration of the diabetes for both type I and type II. However, the onset of macrovascular complications occurred more rapidly with type II diabetics.

Conclusions—Almost half of the diabetic patients in this study were shown to have at least one coexisting morbidity, while almost one fifth had two or more. Even though the macrovascular complications have been shown to increase with age in the nondiabetic patient, diabetes accelerates the process even further. This was shown to be especially true for the type II diabetics. Resources should be directed for early identification and treatment towards those categories of patients with the greatest potential for morbidity.—*S. Patel*

◆ The authors of this study set out to determine the prevalence of complications of diabetes in a cohort of 10,709 patients identified as having diabetes. Information on macrovascular as well as microvascular complications was gathered.

The prevalence of coronary heart disease (CHD) was 25.2%, cerebrovascular disease (CVD) 9.6%, complications of the "diabetic foot" 18.1%, retinopathy 16.5%, and nephropathy 2.0%. Additional findings from this cohort of patients indicated that the macrovascular complications (CHD, CVD, and diabetic foot) were more advanced in type 2 diabetic patients at the time of diagnosis compared with type 1 patients. Additionally, all complications were clearly dependent on both age and duration of diabetes, but an association between microvascular complications (retinopathy and nephropathy) and duration of diabetes was more apparent. Another interesting finding was that while 52.1% of diabetic patients sampled had no comorbid conditions, nearly 20% had two or more complications of diabetes.

The current report quantifies and should serve to remind us of the multisystem nature of diabetes and the need to evaluate the entire person when examining the foot or contemplating foot surgery in patients with diabetes. It also should serve to remind us of the significance of duration of diabetes rather than chronological age in the development of many of these complications.—*J.M. Giurini, D.P.M.*

A Study of In-Shoe Plantar Shear in Patients with Diabetic Neuropathy

Lord M, Hosein R (King's College London, London, UK)
J Clin Biomech 15:278–283, 2000

Introduction—Diabetic patients with peripheral neuropathy are at an increased risk of plantar ulceration especially under major weightbearing structures like metatarsal heads (MTHs). One of the main causes of this is excessive mechanical stress, which consists of two different components: pressure, which is generated by ground reactive force pushing superiorly on the MTHs, and shear forces that act tangential to the plantar surface. Although increased pressure has long been accepted as a major risk factor, the role of shear forces has yet to be determined. This study was done to investigate the effects of plantar shear forces.

Methods—Six diabetic patients with a past history of plantar ulceration were given custom-molded shoes with a rocker bottom design. An F-scan system was used to measure peak plantar pressures throughout each patient's gait cycle. Bi-axial magnetic resistive transducers were then used to measure both longitudinal and transverse shearing forces at the same areas where the peak pressures were previously observed. All patients were observed with nylon hose on one foot.

Results—The highest area of shear force (longitudinal and transverse shear combined) was found under the first MTH in feet without hose and equally under the first and second MTHs in feet with hose. Also, the maximum shear in feet with hose was less at all measured sites. This correlates with the idea that socks may reduce friction. The maximum sites of pressure were observed under the second, first, and third MTHs, respectively.

Discussion—The general pattern of longitudinal shear was observed in a posterior direction under the heel and lateral MTHs throughout the first half of the gait cycle while the transverse shear was exhibited in a medial direction under these same areas. In the second half of the gait cycle, the longitudinal shear reversed into an anterior direction with the peak forces under the medial MTHs, while the transverse shear remained in a medial direction but also included the medial MTHs as well. When comparing this study with normal subjects, the diabetic group exhibited similar shear under the heal, less shear under the lateral MTHs, and more shear under the medial MTHs. This medial shift of shear forces in the diabetic population correlates with the most frequent area in which neuropathic ulcers occur.

Conclusion—Although increased pressure is a major factor in neuropathic ulceration, shear forces also exist with the peak incidence found under the medial MTHs during late stance phase of gait. These forces should be taken into consideration when managing the neuropathic patient.—*D. Carmack*

♦ It has long been felt there are two components to plantar pressures contributing to ulceration in the diabetic foot: dorsal-to-plantar peak pressures and shear pressures. Until recently, only dorsal-to-plantar pressures could be measured. The current study provides some insight into the magnitude and direction of shear forces during gait in patients with diabetes and may help explain the pattern of ulceration one sees in this patient population.

Although the current study is small in scope, it suggests there is an increased shear stress under the first/second metatarsal region in patients with diabetes versus an asymptomatic group where the highest magnitude of shear was localized under the third/fourth metatarsal regions. In patients who had a prior history of ulcerations, this region of maximum shear corresponded to eight of nine prior ulcer sites. A second interesting finding was that maximum shear was reduced at all sites when patients wore socks. This is not entirely unexpected as it is universally accepted that socks reduce friction.

The technology for measuring shear forces is relatively new and primitive. Already, however, data are emerging which appear to confirm the widely held belief that shear forces play a significant role in ulcer genesis. As the technology improves, it is expected that larger scale studies will provide even greater insight.—*J.M. Giurini, D.P.M.*

Efficacy of Injected Liquid Silicone in the Diabetic Foot to Reduce Risk Factors for Ulceration: A Randomized Double-Blind Placebo-Controlled Trial

Van Schie CHM, Whalley A, Vileikyte L, Wignall T, Hollis S, Boulton AJM
(Manchester Royal Infirmary, Manchester, UK; Withington Hospital, Manchester, UK; Lancaster University, Lancaster, UK)
Diabetes Care 23(5):634–638, 2000

Objective—The purpose of the study was to investigate the effectiveness of injecting liquid silicone into a diabetic foot to help reduce risk factors for ulceration.

Methods—In a randomized double-blind placebo-controlled trial, a total of 28 diabetic patients without peripheral vascular disease were administered 0.2 ml liquid silicone in the plantar surface of foot, or the same volume of saline in the placebo-controlled group. Areas of injection were chosen under metatarsal head sites with calluses or widened skin striae. After the initial injection, five subsequent injections were administered in 2-week intervals with a total of six injections given. Follow-up visits were scheduled at 3, 6, and 12 months after baseline to access efficacy.

Results—A total of 62 sites were chosen for injection, of which 34 sites were injected with silicone, and 28 were injected with saline. The median plantar tissue thickness had substantially increased from baseline with 1.8 mm, 2.0 mm, and 1.3 mm at 3, 6, and 12 months, respectively, in the silicone-treated group compared with no change in plantar thickness in the placebo group. A significant decrease in peak plantar pressure from baseline was measured in the silicone-treated group as compared to no change evident in the placebo group. No clinical evidence of any migration of injected silicone was observed throughout the study.

Conclusion—Injections of liquid silicone have been shown to be effective in increasing plantar tissue thickness and reducing plantar peak pressures. These results add a new treatment method to diabetic foot care with no clinical side effects reported in this study.—*Q. Solomon*

♦ This is a randomized double-blind placebo-controlled trial evaluating the efficacy of liquid silicone to reduce the risk of ulceration in patients with diabetes. Twenty-eight patients were randomized into two groups: one group of 14 patients who received injections of medical-grade liquid silicone in areas of callus formation and a second group who received an injection of equal volume of normal saline. While the podiatrist performing the injections was not blinded, the patients and investigators doing the evaluations were blinded. A total of six injections at 2-week intervals per site were given and one to five sites were selected for injections. Sites of previous ulceration were injected only if they had been healed for a minimum of 6 months. Therefore, no areas of open ulcerations were injected. Plantar peak pressures, callus formation and plantar tissue thickness were measured in both groups. Measurements were performed at 3-, 6-, and 12-month intervals.

The investigators discovered that liquid silicone did indeed reduce plantar peak pressures and plantar tissue thickness over injections of normal saline. However, there was not a statistically significant decrease in callus formation between the two groups. Further, six patients developed ulcerations at noninjected sites (three silicone-treated patients and three placebo), while one placebo-treated patient developed an ulceration at a site of injection. No other adverse reactions were noted.

Anecdotal reports encompassing thousands of injections exist concerning the efficacy of liquid silicone to prevent diabetic foot ulcerations. The present study, however, represents the first randomized, controlled trial on the use of liquid silicone for prevention of diabetic foot ulcerations. While this study quantifies the ability of liquid silicone to modify risk factors for ulcerations, it does not address the issue of reduction of rate of ulceration. As the authors state, further large-scale studies are needed to confirm their observations. Additional questions have also been raised by this study. For example, how many injections are optimal? Are booster injections needed? If so, how often and under what circumstances? The anecdotal data indicate that 50% of patients will require such booster injections. Additionally, one cannot ignore the public's concern over the use of silicone. This may be the primary limiting factor in the widespread use of injectable silicone. —*J.M. Giurini, D.P.M.*

Lack of Insulin-Like Growth Factor 1 (IGF1) in the Basal Keratinocyte Layer of Diabetic Skin and Diabetic Foot Ulcers

Blakytny R, Jude EB, Gibson JM, Boulton AJM, Ferguson MWJ (University of Manchester, Manchester, UK; Manchester Royal Infirmary, Manchester, UK)
Am J Pathol 190:589–594, 2000

Introduction—Wound healing is delayed in diabetes, resulting in chronic diabetic foot ulcers. The delay in re-epithelialization over the wound will increase the chance for infection at the wound or ulcer site. Studies link insulin-like growth factor (IGF) to increased keratinocyte production in vitro, thus, rapid re-epithelialization. Diabetic complications in mammalian studies are associated with decreased levels of IGF1 and IGF2, two isoforms of IGF, in basal keratinocytes of the epidermis. Therefore, this study uses monoclonal antibodies to assess wound healing with levels of IGF1 and IGF2 in diabetic skin, nondiabetic skin, and diabetic foot ulcers.

Methods—Full-thickness biopsies of human diabetic skin, diabetic foot ulcers, and nondiabetic skin were obtained from the lower limbs. Ulcer criteria required greater than 8 weeks in duration and no clinical signs of infection. Immunohistochemistry was used to evaluate levels of IGF1 and IGF2 in the epidermis of the three groups; furthermore, smooth muscle cells of the erector pili muscles and fibroblasts in the dermis were also immunolabeled for IGF1 and IGF2. The levels were scored by the immunostaining intensity.

Results—Intensity of staining for IGF1 in the basal layer of the epidermis and fibroblasts in the dermis was absent in sections from diabetic skin and diabetic ulcers. Normal skin sections revealed moderate levels of IGF1 in both the basal layer and fibroblasts. Moderate to strong intensity staining levels of IGF2 were found throughout the epidermis and fibroblasts in all three groups. Both IGF1 and IGF2 were found in smooth muscle cells from erector pili muscles in all three groups, but the IGF2 levels were more intense.

Conclusions—A major complication associated with diabetes is delayed re-epithelialization and wound healing, in which, absent levels of IGF1 in basal keratinocytes have been associated with this delay. IGF1 was not found in the basal cells of diabetic skin or at the ulcer edge, and IGF1 was also absent in fibroblasts from diabetic specimens. In contrast to mammalian studies, increased levels of IGF2 were found throughout the epidermis, including the basal layer, in all three groups. This lack of IGF1 with increased levels of IGF2 may be an important components of delayed wound healing with diabetes.—*M. Garrison*

♦ This study looks at the distribution of insulin-like growth factors 1 and 2 in the skin of diabetic and nondiabetic subjects. Additionally, the distribution of these factors in skin from diabetic foot ulcers was also assayed. The distribution of the two factors was similar in the skin of non-diabetic subjects being primarily localized in the epidermis and vascular endothelial cells of capillaries within the dermis. The immunolabeling profile of the two factors in the skin of diabetic patients showed significant differences. Insulin-like growth factor 2 (IGF2) was found throughout the epidermis while IGF1 was present only in the stratum granulosum and spinosum. Further, when diabetic foot ulcers were tested, IGF1 was found to be absent in the basal layer of the epidermis immediately adjacent to the ulcer, while IGF2 labeling was intense throughout all layers of the epidermis at the ulcer edge.

The significance of the findings of this study is not clear. IGF1 is known to induce chemotactic activity of several cell lines including proliferation and re-epithelialization. The lack of IGF1 in diabetic foot ulcers may lead to a decrease in the proliferative activity of keratinocytes and re-epithelialization, thereby resulting in slower wound healing. The high levels of IGF2 may serve as a compensatory mechanism for the lack of IGF1. Another function may be one of inhibition as IGF2 binds to the same receptors as TGFβ1, thereby blocking its activation and effect on wound healing.

While much is known about the activity of IGF1, much more needs to be discovered. This study should provide the impetus for further investigation into the effect this growth factor has on ulcer healing.—*J.M. Giurini, D.P.M.*

Neural and Endothelial Control of the Microcirculation in Diabetic Peripheral Neuropathy

Kilo S, Berghoff M, Hilz M, Freeman R (Beth Israel Deaconess Medical Center and Harvard Medical School, Boston, MA; University of Erlangen-Nuremberg, Germany)
Neurology 54:1246–1252, 2000

Introduction—The significant role that hyperglycemia plays in the causation of diabetic polyneuropathy is well-known, but the pathogenesis is poorly understood. The intention of this study was to evaluate endothelium-dependent and endothelium-independent vasodilation of the microcirculation and how it relates to neural microcirculatory control in type 1 and type 2 diabetic patients. Since the microcirculation is regulated by humoral, endothelial, and neural factors, there is a potential pathogenic vicious cycle in which microcirculatory dysfunction results in peripheral nerve dysfunction. This in turn results in dysregulation of the microcirculation, causing further nerve dysfunction.

Methods—Iontophoresis of acetylcholine and sodium nitroprusside in conjunction with laser Doppler provided data regarding endothelium-dependent, endothelium-independent, and C-fiber-mediated cutaneous microcirculatory function.

Results—Iontophoresis of acetylcholine increased cutaneous blood flow in diabetic and control subjects; however, the endothelium-dependent response of type 2 diabetics was significantly less than that of controls. Iontophoresis of sodium nitroprusside increased cutaneous blood flow quite evenly in all subject groups, suggesting that there is normal vascular smooth muscle function in the diabetic subjects. The C-fiber-mediated axon reflex increased cutaneous blood flow considerably in the control group and equally less so in both type 1 and type 2 diabetics. A noteworthy finding was that in the type 2 diabetics, the duration of diabetes was a significant predictor of the maximum endothelium-dependent response to acetylcholine.

Conclusion—The results suggest that the changes in cutaneous blood flow are characterized by neural and endothelial but not smooth muscle dysfunction. Moreover, notable C-fiber impairment in both diabetic groups and the greater dysfunction in endothelium-dependent vasodilation in type 2 diabetics suggest that endothelial function and nitroprusside play a greater role in the pathogenesis of type 2 diabetic peripheral neuropathy. The results imply that the pathogenesis of diabetic neuropathy may be different in type 1 and type 2 diabetic patients and should receive greater attention in future studies.—*J.M. Dawson*

♦ Peripheral sensory neuropathy remains the primary risk for diabetic foot ulceration. Yet, the precise pathogenesis of this complication remains poorly understood. Vascular and metabolic mechanisms have been proposed as possible causes. Recently, neural control of the microcirculation of the endothelium has been studied in hopes of unraveling the pathogenic mechanism. The current report is one such study.

The investigators examined endothelial vasodilatory response in three groups of subjects under various stimuli. Cutaneous blood flow was measured in type 1 diabetic patients, type 2 diabetic patients, and controls following iontopheresis with acetylcholine (endothelium dependent) and sodium nitroprusside (endothelium independent). Measurements were made with use of the laser Doppler. While cutaneous vasodilation was impaired in both diabetic groups, type 2 patients showed a greater impairment than type 1 patients. The endothelium-independent vasodilation response was normal in both diabetic groups, suggesting that vascular smooth muscle function was normal in this group of diabetic patients. Therefore, it may be presumed that reduced nerve blood flow is one mechanism for the pathogenesis of diabetic neuropathy and that this abnormality plays a greater role in type 2 diabetic patients than in type 1.

The current study gives physiologic support to the concept that endoneurial ischemia resulting from impaired synthesis and release of nitrous oxide is a cause of peripheral neuropathy in diabetic patients. Additional studies using laser Doppler assessment are currently underway which will provide an even greater understanding of the pathogenesis of peripheral neuropathy and the individual contributions of vascular and neural factors.—*J.M. Giurini, D.P.M.*

Results of Decompression of Peripheral Nerves in Diabetics: A Prospective, Blinded Study

Aszmann OC, Kress KM, Dellon AL (University of Vienna, Vienna, Austria; The Johns Hopkins University School of Medicine, Baltimore, MD)
Plast Reconstr Surg 106(4):816–822, 2000

Introduction—Diabetic neuropathy is traditionally thought of as a progressive and irreversible condition. It is usually treated by controlling the hyperglycemia and prophylactic care of soft tissue at risk for sensory loss. It has been proposed that the pathophysiology of diabetic neuropathy can be explained by the increased susceptibility to compression of the diabetic nerve. If this were true, then decompression of the nerves should be a viable option to alleviate some of the symptoms of neuropathy. This study was conducted to measure the sensory recovery in patients with diabetic neuropathy after surgical decompression of the peripheral nerve.

Methods—A total of 20 patients, 14 insulin-dependent and six non-insulin-dependent, with diabetic neuropathy were evaluated. A total of 31 nerves were decompressed. A numerical grading scale based on two-point discrimination was used to determine the preoperative and postoperative measurements. These measurements were performed by a therapist blinded to the surgical procedure. The decompression procedure was performed on the median nerve, ulnar nerve, and the posterior tibial nerve. The surgical procedure was performed on only one limb, while the contralateral limb was not treated. The extremity chosen was the one the patient felt to have the worst symptoms. The nerve chosen had to have a positive Tinel sign, which indicated regenerative potential. Assessment of the nerves postoperatively was done on an average of 23 months.

Results—The surgically decompressed nerves showed improvement in sensation in 79% of the cases. When comparing the upper and lower extremities, 88% of the upper extremity cases showed improvement and 69%

of the lower extremity cases improved. The numerical grading system showed that the lower extremity nerves treated had worse scores than the upper extremity. None of the decompressed nerves decreased in sensation based on the grading scale, whereas 32% of the nontreated nerves worsened.

Conclusion—The study demonstrated that surgical decompression is an effective treatment option in patients with peripheral neuropathy. There was improvement in 88% of the upper extremity cases and 69% of the lower extremity cases. The discrepancy in these results is probably based on the more advanced neuropathy in the lower extremity cases. The most appropriate situation in which to consider surgical decompression would be when the patient presents with abnormal two-point discrimination (>4 mm in the fingertip and >8 mm in the big toe) and a positive Tinel sign at the site of anatomic narrowing (i.e., the tarsal tunnel). This may serve as a cost-effective method for preventing the sequelae of diabetic neuropathy which include ulceration, infection, and amputation.—*S. Patel*

♦ This current paper presents the results of tarsal tunnel releases in diabetic patients with presumed neuropathy. The basic premise of this study, as in other similar studies by the senior author, is that diabetic neuropathy results from an entrapment of the posterior tibial nerve and therefore may be reversible. This has been a controversial subject in the past. The current article does little to settle this controversy.

Twenty diabetic patients underwent decompression of the posterior tibial, medial plantar calcaneal, and lateral plantar calcaneal nerves. A total of 16 lower extremity nerves were decompressed. In order to be included in the study, all patients had to have a positive Tinel's sign. Sixty-nine percent of these lower extremity nerves showed improvement in sensory testing versus 88% of upper extremity nerves.

What remains unclear is what the authors are treating. The presence of a Tinel's sign suggests a true compression neuropathy. Therefore, the authors are operating on a very select group of diabetic patients. Even in this group, the results were less than universal and significantly less than upper extremity nerves (69% vs. 88%). It is presumed that the lack of comparable results may be related to the metabolic effect of hyperglycemia on peripheral nerves of the lower extremity. For this reason, one must proceed with great caution in performing tarsal tunnel release in diabetic patients with clinical evidence of peripheral neuropathy.—*J.M. Giurini, D.P.M.*

Treatment of Diabetic Neuropathy by Decompression of the Posterior Tibial Nerve

Caffe HH (University of Florida College of Medicine, Gainesville, FL)
Plast Reconstr Surg 106(4):813–815, 2000

Objective—Nerve deterioration is believed to be a cause of diabetic neuropathy. Procedures to treat this have not proved to be promising. A newly proposed theory about endoneural edema claims that swelling makes the nerve prone to compression. By this theory, nerve decompression should reverse the pathologic events. The purpose of this study is to evaluate the effect of posterior tibial (PT) nerve decompression on diabetic peripheral neuropathy.

Patient Profile—Thirty-six patients had a total of 58 PT nerve decompression surgeries performed. Twenty-two had bilateral surgery and 14 had unilateral procedures done. Of the 14 unilateral procedures, six had a previous contralateral amputation. Eleven patients presented with foot ulcers, 28 presented with painful paresthesia, and all 36 patients had decreased sensation measured by Semmes-Weinstein monofilament. Patients with ischemia were excluded from the study.

Surgical Technique—The procedures were performed with the patients in supine positions, general or spinal anesthesia, and tourniquets. Incisions were made from above the medial malleolus to the medial aspect of the foot. The tarsal tunnel was opened so that the PT nerve could be visualized. The fascia underlying the abductor hallucis muscle and septum was freed so that the medial plantar nerve, lateral plantar nerve, and calcaneal branch could be identified for about 1 cm. The tourniquets were removed and hemostasis was maintained with bipolar coagulation. Single-layer skin sutures and soft compression dressings were used. Only the patients with ulcers were required to stay longer than the 1st preoperative day. Restrictive ambulation was advised for up to 10 days.

Results—All in all, the surgical candidates tolerated the bilateral surgery well. Seven of the 36 patients had delayed wound healing. One patient developed a wound infection on the 5th postoperative day but recovered following IV antibiotic treatment. All other patients recovered without complications. Only four patients did not have relief from pain postoperatively. However, two of these four had improved pressure sensation. No one claimed to have increased pain. Of the eight insensate patients, four claimed to have improved sensory perception, one had burning sensation, and one denied sensory perception but was able to feel the Semmes-Weinstein monofilament.

Discussion—Metabolic and vascular components have been implicated in diabetic peripheral neuropathy. This study was designed to eliminate patients whose neuropathy could be related to vascular issues. However, nerve constriction at the tarsal tunnel could cause localized ischemia. Since previous studies have shown clinical improvement of nerve pain with nerve decompression, the goal of this study was to see if decompression of the PT nerve could alleviate symptomatic diabetic peripheral neuropathy. Based on the results of this study, it appears that PT nerve decompression is a valuable procedure for symptomatic diabetic neuropathy and of minimal risk. Clearly, if nerve decompression can restore protective sensation, it may prevent the formation of neuropathic ulcers. In addition, being able to relieve the burning sensation postoperatively is an obvious reward for patients who cannot even sleep due to the discomfort. Perhaps earlier surgical intervention may have yielded better results. These results would prove to be more conclusive had the study included a placebo effect and more formal sensory measurement. In summary, this procedure appears to be a safe and effective treatment option for diabetic peripheral neuropathy.—*G.H. Jhala*

◆ This paper represents a single investigator's experience with tarsal tunnel release for the treatment of diabetic neuropathy. The author performed 58 procedures on 36 patients over a 9-year period. The primary presenting symptoms were either pain (28 patients) or foot ulcerations (11 patients). Surgical decompression consisted of release of the posterior tibial nerve as well as the medial and lateral plantar nerves at the porta pedis.

Of the 28 patients who underwent the procedure for relief of painful neuropathy, 24 experienced some relief, while four experienced no relief or minimal improvement. Of the eight patients who presented with loss of sensation (five patients) reported a feeling of increased sensation in, although this could not be demonstrated objectively.

There are several problems with this study. First, it is a retrospective study. Therefore, objective preoperative testing for neuropathy or nerve compression is lacking. Second, objective postoperative evaluation is likewise inconsistent and is mostly subjective. Third, there is a lack of control. It is possible that much of the patients' perceived improvement can be attributed to a placebo effect. Fourth, the author suggests that the procedure was safe with minimal complications. However, not including those patients who received no benefit from the surgery, seven patients demonstrated slow healing and one patient developed a postoperative wound infection requiring hospitalization. This is a 28% complication rate. No surgeon should accept this complication rate as being insignificant.

What is most notable, however, is that this report suggests there may be some efficacy in treating recalcitrant painful neuropathy with nerve decompression, but that restoring impaired sensation to the neuropathic foot is less predictable. This once again points to the need to understand what is being treated and what the expected goals of the surgery should be. That tarsal tunnel syndrome may serve as an etiology of neuropathic pain should not come as a surprise. Clearly, there is much we do not know about diabetic neuropathy. However, to expect to reverse years of metabolic hyperglycemic damage to nerves by decompression of the posterior tibial nerve may not be a realistic expectation as demonstrated by this report.—*J.M. Giurini, D.P.M.*

Prospective Study of Transcutaneous Oxygen Tension (TcPO$_2$) Measurement in the Testing Period of Spinal Cord Stimulation in Diabetic Patients with Critical Lower Limb Ischaemia

Petrakis E, Sciacca V (University of Rome, Rome Italy)
Int Angiol 19(1):18–25, 2000

Introduction—Spinal cord stimulation has successfully been used in improving microcirculatory blood flow, and relief of pain due to neuropathy and ischemia. Spinal cord stimulation has also been shown to reduce the healing time for trophic ulcers and has reduced the rate of amputation in the arterial compromised patient. In this prospective study, Petrakis and Sciacca set out to assess the possibility of using transcutaneous oxygen tension (TcPO$_2$) measurements to decide if a given diabetic patient with peripheral arterial occlusion is a candidate for permanent device implantation.

Methods—Thirty-nine men and 21 women (age range 46–75) with peripheral vascular disease, who failed conservative or surgical treatment, were implanted with a temporary spinal cord electric generator. The clinical status was classified as Fontaine's stage III and IV with the main pathology being diabetic vascular disease. Doppler toe pressures were recorded at 2 weeks before and 4 weeks after implantation as were the TcPO$_2$ measurements assessed at the dorsum of the foot and ankle. The patients were followed postoperatively for 18 months.

Results—Out of the 60 patients, 35 experienced 75% pain relief with limb salvage of greater than 6 months, which was considered a success. Partial success, defined as pain relief of 50% and a limb salvage of up to 6 months, was obtained in 12 patients. In 13 patients, spinal cord stimulation failed and the affected limbs were amputated.

Within 2 weeks after implantation, TcPO$_2$ had shown increases among those considered as successes (from 21.4 to 31.5 in patients with rest pain, $p = .03$; from 15.1 to 22.0 mmHg, $p = .03$, in those patients with trophic lesions under 3 cm^2 in size; from 12.1 to 17.9 mmHg, $p = .025$, in those patients with trophic lesions over 3 cm^2). These increases, however, were unrelated to the stage of the disease and the initial TcPO$_2$. Ankle brachial indices and toe pressures did not change under the spinal cord stimulation, and TcPO$_2$ changes were related to the feelings of paraesthesia and warmth in place of pain during the trial period.

Conclusion—When considering spinal cord stimulation for treatment of peripheral arterial occlusive disease in diabetic patients, a 2-week trial period should be done before permanent implantation is contemplated. As noted by Petrakis and Sciacca, only diabetic patients with significant increase in TcPO$_2$ and clinical improvement, during the test period, should be considered for permanent implantation and not merely all patients with pain relief. Furthermore, because limb salvage was achieved only in those with significant TcPO$_2$ increases within 2 weeks of temporary implantation, this could be a reasonable way of predicting the success of permanent spinal cord stimulation therapy in individual patients.—*S.B. Heninger*

♦ The current study looks at the predictive value of TcPO$_2$ measurements in diabetic patients treated with spinal cord stimulation in the presence of nonreconstructible peripheral arterial occlusive disease. Of the 60 patients studied, 27 had failed bypass procedures. Another 24 had exploration of their distal vessels but were not submitted to bypass due to advanced atherosclerotic disease. Twenty patients had trophic lesions smaller than 3 cm^2 and 20 had trophic lesions greater than 3 cm^2. Twenty patients suffered from rest pain. All patients had implantation of a spinal cord stimulator to improve microcirculatory blood flow and had TcPO$_2$ measured to document improvement of flow.

This study suggests that TcPO$_2$ was a useful tool to select patients who might respond to spinal cord stimulation. An increase in TcPO$_2$ implied that a patient's pain was due more to ischemia than neuropathy, while little to no increase in TcPO$_2$ implied peripheral neuropathy as the primary cause of lower leg pain. In this case, spinal cord stimulation should be terminated for lack of effect on peripheral circulation.

This study suggests that an increase in TcPO$_2$ warrants permanent implantation of a spinal cord device. However, the long-term results fail to support this conclusion. Thirty-five of 60 patients (58%) achieved limb salvage for 6 months, while 25 patients (42%) underwent lower extremity amputation by 6 months. What is not clear is what happened to the 35 patients beyond 6 months. In fact, clinical improvement diminished over the ensuing 12 months. The current paper is reminiscent of the use of sympathectomy for the treatment of peripheral vascular disease. Over the past 10 years this surgical procedure has rightfully fallen out of favor as being ineffective. The current study does little to make one reconsider this mode of surgical intervention.—*J.M. Giurini, D.P.M.*

Popliteal-to-Distal Bypass Grafts for Critical Leg Ischaemia

Biancari F, Kantonen I, Alback A, Ihlberg L, Lehtola A, Lepantalo M
(Helsinki University Central Hospital, Helsinki, Finland)
J Cardiovasc Surg 41(2):281–286, 2000

Introduction—Atherosclerosis is a prevalent disease in the lower extremity that not only affects the femoropopliteal segment but also the crural and pedal arteries distally. The incidence is higher among diabetics. A 7-year study was done to further investigate the efficacy of popliteal-to-distal bypass grafts in the management of isolated severe crural and pedal atherosclerotic disease.

Materials and Methods—Hundreds of bypass procedures were reviewed and 81 bypass grafts using the popliteal artery as the inflow source were chosen. Of those, 66 popliteal-to-distal bypass grafts performed in 61 patients with critical leg ischemia (CLI) were focused on. The criteria for CLI was a ankle systolic pressure of ≤50 mmHg or a toe systolic pressure of ≤30 mmHg which was corroborated by low ankle/brachial indices, ankle pulse volume recording amplitudes below 5 mm, and by clinical signs and symptoms. All patients underwent angiography to evaluate the extent of the disease and choose the appropriate inflow and outflow vessels. There were 12 surgeons participating, all with varying degrees of experience. The patency of the bypass was assessed every 3 months during the first year and every 6 months thereafter by using clinical pulse examination, ABI, duplex Doppler, and angiography (if failure was suspected). The mean follow-up period was 15.2 months and all data were analyzed with multiple statistical protocols. The main measurements analyzed were bypass graft patency, leg salvage, survival, and success.

Results—Four patients died during the immediate postoperative period. Nine patients had another operation for the management of surgical complications. At 1-month, 1-year, and 2-year follow-up, the primary patency rates were 87%, 58%, and 55%, corrected patency rates were 89%, 59%, and 56%, secondary patency rates were 95%, 70%, and 67%, leg salvage rates were 97%, 88%, and 88%, while 88%, 70%, and 66% of patients were alive with legs at the same intervals. No statistical significance was found between popliteocrural and popliteopedal bypass grafts, while there was a statistical difference between above-knee grafts versus below-knee grafts, the former being better. The reconstruction material did not show any impact on the patency rates. Multivariate analysis showed ages above 80 years have a higher risk of graft occlusion. Further analysis showed diabetes had an impact on both survival rate with leg salvage. Uremia and coronary artery disease had significant impact on survival rates. There was no correlation between the level of inflow source and the angiographic runoff status.

Discussion—The data confirmed that the popliteal artery is a good inflow source for bypass surgery to crural and pedal arteries in severe, isolated infrapopliteal atherosclerotic disease. Although successful, above-knee grafts still maintain to have better patency rates. The preoperative angiographic runoff data were not predictive of patency, leg salvage, and survival outcome. This may be due to the severity of the occlusion. Diabetics and uremic patients did show to have short-term survival after popliteal-to-distal bypass surgery.—*F. Nejad*

◆ The authors of this study report on their experience of distal bypass surgery in diabetic patients with critical leg ischemia. Primary patency rates of 87%, 58%, and 55% were achieved at 1-month, 1-year, and 2-year follow-up. Secondary patency rates of 95%, 70%, and 67% and limb salvage rates of 97%, 88%, and 88% were also reported.

The above patency rates are comparable to well-established vascular services performing large numbers of these procedures in the United States on comparable patients. The authors conclude that above-knee popliteal-to-distal bypass grafts are well tolerated among diabetic patients and worthwhile for the treatment of severe lower leg ischemia. This should establish this procedure as the standard of care for the treatment of nonhealing ischemic ulcers in diabetic patients worldwide.—*M. Giurini, D.P.M.*

Lower Extremity Revascularization in Diabetes: Late Observations

Akbari CM, Pomposelli FB, Gibbons GW, Campbell DR, Pulling MC, Mydlarz D, LoGerfo FW (Harvard Medical School, Boston, MA)
Arch Surg 135:452–456, 2000

Introduction—Many studies report success with distal arterial reconstruction on diabetic patients, but long-term function and survival rates have been poorly defined. This may play a role with less aggressive approaches to managing diabetic patients with peripheral arterial disease, often resulting in amputation and mortality. Therefore, late function and survival are assessed, at a minimum 5-year follow-up, from diabetic and nondiabetic patients undergoing revascularization procedures to the lower extremity.

Methods—Data on all consecutive patients who underwent infrainguinal arterial bypass with vein graft from 1990 through 1993 were reviewed. At the time of surgery, patient demographics and indication for operation were recorded. Initial follow-up visits occurred at 1 month, then every 3 months for the first year, and subsequent visits continued every 6–12 months. The results were recorded following each visit. Statistical analysis concerning primary and secondary patency, limb salvage, and survival rates were performed.

Results—Nine hundred Sixty-two vein grafts were performed on 843 patients, in which, 795 grafts were performed on diabetic patients. Demographic data revealed diabetic patients were younger as compared to the nondiabetic group. Diabetic patients experienced lower in-hospital perioperative mortality rates versus nondiabetic patients. Moreover, indication for operation data revealed tissue loss, defined as gangrene or ulcer, as the main indication in both groups. No difference was found among the two groups between primary and secondary patency, limb salvage, and 5-year survival rates.

Conclusion—Long-term graft patency, limb salvage, and 5-year survival rates show no difference between diabetic and nondiabetic patients who have undergone lower extremity revascularization procedures. This shows diabetic patients should have equal opportunity to aggressive attempts of limb salvage.—*M. Garrison*

◆ This study comes from a tertiary referral center with the largest experience in lower extremity revascularization in patients with diabetes in the United States. In a 3-year period, 843 total infrainguinal arterial bypass procedures were performed using vein graft. Seven hundred ninety-five (82.6%) were in patients with diabetes mellitus (DM) and 167 (17.4%) in patients without diabetes (NDM). The results of this study showed there was no statistically significant difference in primary graft patency between DM and NDM patients (75.6% vs. 71.9%), secondary graft patency (77.0%

vs. 73.6%), and overall limb salvage rate (87.3% vs. 85.4%). Five-year survival was also similar between the two groups (DM group, 58.2%; NDM group 58.0%). Of note, the perioperative mortality between the groups did show a statistically significant difference with the DM patients faring better than NDM patients (0.9% vs. 4.2%).

The current study concludes that diabetic patients are at no greater risk than nondiabetic patients when requiring lower extremity revascularization. They fare as well if not better in various measures than the nondiabetic patient. This may in part be due to recognition of the comorbid conditions of the diabetic patient and vigilance to perioperative monitoring. It also demonstrates the importance of close communication between the vascular surgeon, anesthesiologist, primary care physician, and cardiologist.

The overall conclusion by these very experienced authors is that no diabetic patient should be denied a potentially limb-saving bypass procedure simply because they have diabetes. This now sets the standard of care for the ischemic extremity.—*J.M. Giurini, D.P.M.*

Arthrodesis as an Early Alternative to Nonoperative Management of Charcot Arthropathy of the Diabetic Foot

Simon SR, Tejwani SG, Wilson, DL, Santner TJ, Denniston NL (Beth Israel Medical Center, New York, NY; University of California at Los Angeles School of Medicine, Los Angeles, CA; Grant Medical Center, Columbus, OH; Ohio State University College of Medicine, Columbus, OH)
J Bone Joint Surg 82-A(7):939–950, 2000

Background—The current standard treatment of Eichenholtz stage I Charcot arthropathy is the application of a nonweightbearing (NWB) total-contact cast. Although largely effective, such conservative management may fail to restore normal anatomy, malunion or nonunion may occur, and resulting deformities may produce ulceration of the foot that require operative treatment. This study evaluates the efficacy of tarso-metatarsal arthrodesis for treatment of stage I Charcot arthropathy in diabetic patients by assessing clinical results, financial impact, gait pattern, and abnormal foot pressures.

Methods—Between 1991 and 1996, 43 diabetic patients presented with clinical and radiographic evidence of Eichenholtz stage I Charcot arthropathy: 29 were managed with total-contact cast immobilization; 14 requested operative intervention because of potential sequela from foot deformation that may result from conservative treatment, after much discussion of the risks involved. The subjects had diabetic neuropathy, adequate blood supply, and stage I disease confirmed by histopathology. Secondary diabetic complications or medications were not deemed contraindications to surgery. The operative technique was identical for all patients, consisting of debridement, autologous bone graft, stabilizing the medial and medial-to-lateral tarso-metatarsal column with plate and/or screws by AO technique, and fluoroscopic imaging to confirm adequate reduction. Patients were immobilized in a NWB cast for a 6-week minimum and evaluated clinically and by serial radiographs until complete healing was evident. The final follow-up visit at 41 months (mean) consisted of gait analysis with plantar pressure measurement. These data were compared with similar data from two groups of 14 patients with diabetic neuropathy: one with below-knee amputation, and one without history of plantar ulceration. Retrospective review assessed comorbidity in each group and financial charges in the operative treatment groups.

Results—All arthrodesis procedures were successful, with no clinical evidence of immediate or long-term postoperative complications and no patient reports of ulceration. Assisted weightbearing took place by 10 ± 3.3 weeks (mean), unassisted weightbearing by 15 ± 8.8 weeks (mean), and return to regular shoes by 27 ± 14.4 weeks (mean). Comorbidity was lowest in the nonulcerative group, mildly higher in the arthrodesis group, and slightly higher in the amputation group. The mean charge for arthodesis was $11,579 less than the mean expense for the amputees. All arthrodesis patients regained preoperative walking ability, and confidence interval analysis demonstrated no differences between this group and the two comparison groups with regard to joint range of motion and gait patterns. Plantar peak pressures were highest at the first metatarsal, hallux, and heel, with little difference amidst the groups.

Discussion—Deformity increases local mechanical stresses and pressures, with peak plantar pressures higher in patients with a history of neuropathic ulceration, and especially high forefoot pressures in acute Charcot arthropathy patients. There is no evidence that exostectomy or late-stage arthrodesis reduces forefoot peak pressures, and could alter plantar pressure distribution that may predispose to ulceration. All 14 patients undergoing stage I arthrodesis had anatomical reduction, clinical union, and stability without increased risk of complications. Healing time was not lengthened and plantar pressures were restored to values similar to those in neuropathic patients 2 years after operative treatment. Given the importance of avoiding lower limb complications, early arthrodesis should be a consideration in diabetic patients with stage I Charcot arthropathy.—*D. Collman*

♦ This paper provides a review of Charcot neuroarthropathy in patients with diabetes. The authors subsequently present their experience with primary arthrodesis for the treatment of Eichenholtz stage I neuroarthropathy. In a 5-year period, the authors performed 14 primary arthrodesis of the tarso-metatarsal region (Lisfranc's joint). In all cases, primary fusion was achieved. Assisted weightbearing occurred in 10 ± 3.3 weeks, while return to regular shoegear occurred at 27 ± 14.4 weeks. Furthermore, no patient developed an ulceration following arthrodesis.

This study represents the first known report of surgical intervention in Eichenholtz stage I Charcot joint disease as an alternative to nonoperative management. The results are quite impressive and go against the old principle of not to operate on Charcot joint during the acute phase. The examples given by the authors represent neuropathic disease with little bony fragmentation. It would appear that if caught at this early stage where there is little fragmentation and disruption, the surgical technique would be quite straightforward. Clearly, the natural history of the disease process is known. Early surgical intervention in most cases provides a more stable foot, resistant to foot ulceration. However, this study does not answer the question of what to do in those cases of acute Charcot characterized by severe fragmentation and joint disruption. It is this author's opinion that little is lost by treating these cases conservatively until Eichenholtz stage II Charcot joint disease is reached.—*J.M. Giurini, D.P.M.*

10   Biomaterials—New Devices for Management of Conditions

Vincent J. Hetherington, D.P.M.

Osteoinductive Applications of Regional Gene Therapy: Ex Vivo Gene Transfer
Oakes DA, Lieberman JR (UCLA School of Medicine, Los Angeles, CA)
Clin Orthop 379S:S101–S112, 2000

Background—Problems with bony repair can sometimes be a formidable task for surgeons dealing with the likes of fracture nonunion, revisional total arthroplasty, tumor resection, and spinal fusion. Surgeons have found no satisfactory options to current methods. With autogenous bone grafts, tissue is of limited supply and donor site morbidity is common. Prosthetic implants, too, have significant limitations, and although allograft provides an osteoconductive scaffold, it lacks osteoinductivity.

Such limitations compel consideration of alternative measures like recombinant growth factors. Transforming growth factor-β (TGF-β), platelet-derived growth factor, fibroblast growth factor, and insulin-like growth factor all have osteoinductive properties but need to be in supraphysiologic concentrations and need well vascularized bone and sufficient soft tissue. Most nonunions, however, lack this optimal healing environment.

Gene therapy stands as a new frontier in medical science; manipulation of the body's endogenous cells can generate osteoinductive proteins. Transduction is the process by which the chosen gene is introduced into the target cell. Vectors enhance entrance of the DNA into the cells' nucleus where it can utilize the necessary machinery. Next, carriers enhance the delivery system to the bone and function to diminish diffusion and provide an osteoconductive scaffold.

Two approaches target the gene to the bone. With the ex vivo process, target cells are harvested, expanded in culture, transduced with the desired

163

gene, and reimplanted into the anatomic site. No viral particles are directly injected into the patient, cells to be transduced are selected, and a high cell transduction efficiency is achieved. The in vivo approach transduces target cells without removing them from the body; the gene is introduced directly into the body. It is a simple process with no harvesting step and is lower in cost, but transduction of the target is inefficient due to both diffusion of the vector from the treatment site and the immune response against the foreign proteins.

To maximize target efficiency, the ex vivo method is used and appropriate cells are harvested; mesenchymal stem cells differentiate into osteoblasts, chondroblasts, and fibroblasts and serve as a good transducing medium. Cells are expanded by 300 times physiologic levels, then transduced. These transduced pleuripotent stem cells secrete growth factors that attract and stimulate other stem cells. In the senior author's lab, bone marrow cells transduced with bone morphogenetic protein via an adenorival vector (adBMP) secretes BMP which not only induces mesenchymal cells to differentiate into osteoblasts, but also drives themselves into an osteogenic lineage.

Methods—The senior author's lab studied methods for filling an 8-mm rat femoral defect. Autologous marrow cells were harvested, transduced with adBMP, mixed with a bone matrix carrier, and implanted into the defect; 22 of 24 healed by developing a coarse, dense trabeculation with a large amount of bone per unit area. This was compared with a pharmacologic dose of recombinant BMP which healed all 16 defects with equal torsional strength, but developed a thin, lacelike trabecular bone.

In another lab, an in vivo approach was tested with adenovirus containing either BMP or TGF-β. The BMP treatment group showed bony union at 13 weeks, and TGF-β at 16 weeks, highlighting their osteogenic potential.

Success was seen in other labs using in vivo regional gene therapy with a collagen sponge as a carrier for naked DNA. Successful DNA transfer within a femoral gap was quantified and shown to remain there for 6 months, and the higher the concentration of plasmid within the matrix, it was shown, the more complete the healing process. It is thought that the gene-activated matrix holds the plasmid in place until endogenous fibroblasts arrive and undergo transduction, now able to function as bioreactors generating osteoinductive signals.

Success was seen with ex vivo regional gene therapy for induction of spinal fusion in rats. A transcription factor was transduced into bone marrow cells with a plasmid vector and a liposome solution which were introduced into a demineralized bone matrix carrier and placed into the level of fusion. All treatment groups healed, and no controls healed, again showing the potential of ex vivo techniques, this time with a transcription factor.

Discussion—Gene therapy offers surgeons an opportunity to enhance their bone healing capacity by manipulating the potential of endogenous cells.

Future application of this treatment will represent a continuum based on specifics of each case. Small defects with good vascularity may only require recombinant growth factors while bone loss associated with a compromised tissue bed or large segmental defect may respond to regional gene therapy. Even osteoporosis may be amenable to such treatment. Animal models have shown their efficacy; human trials are the next step to utilizing this promising clinical tool.—*C. Jacka*

◆ Research in biotechnology for enhancing bone healing and other musculoskeletal problems, such as arthritis, is advancing treatment options at a rapid pace. Gene therapy may also hold promise for tissue regeneration and wound repair. An understanding of what gene therapy is and the advantages over current techniques and technology will be important for podiatric practice in the new millennium. The use of osteoinductive gene therapy in treatment of delayed union of bone, genetic abnormalities of bone, joint resurfacing, and perhaps Charcot joint reconstruction, is just around the corner. Knowledge of the basic science of gene therapy and clinical applications should be included in all aspects of postgraduate training. Progressive podiatrists need to be conversant in the processes of transduction, vectors, transcription, translation, and expression on a relevant clinical basis. The use of regional gene therapy as described experimentally in this article has direct application to podiatric medicine following refinement of the technology and technique.— *V.J. Hetherington, D.P.M.*

Biodegradable Implants in Sports Medicine: The Biological Base

Weiler A, Hoffmann RFG, Stahelin AC, Helling H-J, Sudkamp NP
(Humboldt University of Berlin, Berlin, Germany; Basel, Switzerland; University of Cologne, Cologne, Germany)
Arthroscopy 16(3):305–321, 2000

Introduction—The realm of biodegradable implants within the operative field of sports medicine offers secure internal fixation strength while allowing degradation and replacement by the host tissue. The implants consist of different polymeric raw materials. Unfortunately, these biodegradable polymers differ significantly in terms of material characteristics, tissue response, and biocompatibility. In addition, the degradation process varies from slow degrading polymers to fast-degrading materials. Degradation starts when the implant begins to fragment into smaller pieces. Macrophages and polymorphonuclear leukocytes then phagocytose the particles to further the process of degradation. Soft-tissue reactions can be directly correlated with the clearing capacity of the tissue, represented by macrophages and polymorphonuclear cells.

Method—Based on clinical experiences and previous investigations, a standardized classification system has been developed in order to divide the foreign-body reactions from these biodegradable implants into osseous, extra-articular, and intra-articular synovial inflammatory soft-tissue responses. The purpose of this scheme is to standardize the information on the incidence and severity of tissue reactions in relation to the choice of implant design, specific polymer, and/or anatomic location.

Results—

- *Osteolysis*—Bone resorption is the first reaction at the implant site to occur. Plain radiographs and computed tomography (CT) scans show radiolucencies that may vary from mild osteolytic changes at the implant site to cystic-like extended resorption cavities. If the osteolytic changes are mild, fracture healing, soft-tissue fixation, or the static properties of bone probably are not affected. Interference with fracture healing or graft fixation occurs if the osteolytic changes exceed a certain level.

- *Extra-articular Soft-Tissue Reactions*—Application of material extra-articularly in soft tissue or in cancellous bone of the metaphysis can create debris at the implant site, which accumulates during degradation. The debris can then be expelled into the surrounding tissue to result in an inflammatory response.

- *Intra-articular Synovial Reactions*—Due to the fact that most of these implants are used intra-articularly, this area of biocompatibility is of special interest. In addition to the final stage of degradation, the inflammatory response can also be associated with loosened fragments or wear debris released before implant degradation. Osteolytic changes are also seen.

Discussion—As a result of the degradation process, accumulation of implant fragments results in soft-tissue reactions, which correlate with the clearing capacity of the tissue. Therefore, most of the soft-tissue reactions seen are associated with fast-degrading implants. Moreover, research and in vivo long-term studies need to be focused on testing biodegradable implants in terms of intraosseous, soft-tissue, and intra-articular biocompatibility with a standardized classification system.—*A. Duckworth*

◆ This article presents an excellent overview of biodegradable (absorbable) fixation including a review of materials and complications. It contrasts the different materials properties and associated tissue reactions. The author documents the evolution of the earlier devices made of polyglycholic acid (PGA) to the devices made of polylactic acid (PLLA) and combinations of PLLA, and PGA. They point out that as the change of materials occurred from PGA to PLLA, the number of material complications declined. Current PLLA and PLLA-copolymers are not without problems, but the incidence is less. Osteolysis can occur as a result of the use of absorbable devices and delay the replacement of the device by bone. In general, this reaction appears to have no effect on bone healing, but potential structural weakness may be a concern.—*V.J. Hetherington, D.P.M.*

Response of Articular Cartilage and Subchondral Bone to Internal Fixation Devices Made of Poly-L-Lactide: A Histomorphometric and Microradiographic Study on Rabbits

Böstman O, Viljanen J, Salminen S, Pihlajamäki H (Helsinki University Hospital, Helsinki, Finland)
Biomaterials 21:2553–2560, 2000

Introduction—With the increased use of absorbable internal fixation in the orthopedic community, the desire to find a biologically ideal material that has the capability to achieve intra-articular fixation without disruption of joint function has also grown. One of the main concerns with biodegradable polymers has been the fact that the chemical composition of the materials used in the past, such as polyglycolide, is triggering inflammatory foreign-body reactions. As a result, other materials like polylactide are being utilized, leaving the question of their total effectiveness. This particular study investigates the tissue (polylactide)–implant interface and the effect of the implant on the adjacent articular cartilage and subchondral bone.

Materials and Methods—Implants used were sterile poly-L-lactide screws and pins, with a self-reinforced composite manufacturing structure. Screw measurements were 4.5 mm thread diameter, 1.8 mm thread pitch, and 30 mm in length. Cylindrical pins were 4.5 in diameter and 50 mm in length. Twenty-four mature rabbits were used, and 10 pins and 14 screws were individually placed through the intercondylar portion of the patellofemoral joint directed through the distal femur into the intramedullary canal of the bone, while the contralateral limb was left intact for a control. Particular attention was made to leave the implants flush with the articular surface.

At 38 and 48 weeks, the rabbits were injected with oxytetracycline (50 mg/kg) to mark newly formed bone. As the femurs were harvested and fixed with 50% ethanol, they were embedded in methylmethacrylate. Five-micrometer thick. thick sections of each specimen were cut longitudinally with implant in place; one side was then stained by the Masson-Goldner trichome method to visualize trabecular bone and the adjacent section was stained with toluidine blue to visualize the Articular cartilage. Under histomorphometric analysis, the "nature of the reparative tissue covering the articular-surface defect" and "the total volume of subchondral bone trabeculae including the subchondral bone plate, and the fractional osteoid formation surface of the trabeculae" were determined, during which the contralateral limbs were analyzed for comparison. A scoring system was used to characterize the reparative and pre-existing cartilage, and under statistical evaluation correlations were made between the implanted samples and the intact controls.

Results—

- Articular cartilage:
  - Reparative tissue over the implant was composed of undifferentiated mesenchymal tissue and was quantitatively less when compared to the existing articular cartilage.
  - Only two specimens showed near normal matrix histologically.
  - No inflammatory cells were seen within the bone.
  - Degenerative chondrocytes were observed within the pre-existing articular cartilage with a zone of 400 μm around the tissue–implant boundary.
  - There were no qualitative or quantitative differences of the reparative tissue between pin and screw.
  - The reparative tissue only covered the entrance of the implant channel without any signs of erosion or degradation to the implant.

- Tissue–implant interface and subchondral bone:
  - The average thickness of new bone formation at the tissue–implant interface was 220 μm. There was a walling-off type response that seemed to subside between 36 and 48 weeks.
  - There was a significant increase in osteoid formation surface of the trabeculae with the screw implants when compared to the control side at 36 weeks, and at 48 weeks the osteoid formation did not differ from that of the intact bone of the control side.
  - There was no surface erosion of the implant or osteolytic change in the trabecular bone surrounding the implant.

Discussion—It is obvious that an inflammatory response to poly-L-lactide pins and screws is not any concern, but the zone of degenerative chondrocytes of the existing cartilage is troubling. Due to the slow processes of degradation (5 years or greater) of poly-L-lactide, the osteoclastic and new-bone response is minuet when compared to polyglycolide. This also makes it hard to accept conclusions of good biocompatibilty for poly-L-lactide implants in studies that have only followed a few weeks of progress. Screws tend to induce more osteoid activity than pins, but the increase in surface area of the screw can be attributed to this.

Furthermore, it has been well documented that pre-existing cartilage is not necessary for healing of a cartilage defect. It is thought, however, that "proper new subchondral-bone formation and restoration of the trabecular bone architecture at the level of the original chondro-osseous junction seems to be a prerequisite for the regeneration of normal or near-normal articular cartilage," which in the case of poly-L-lactide materials could take up to 6 or 7 years. "Meanwhile, the articular-surface defect [that persists] may result in even more extensive degenerative changes in the vicinity of the implant channel...," as was evident in this study. It must be acknowledged, however, that the large size of the implant in relation to the recipient bone sections does warrant conclusive limitations.

It is clear that in the quest to find fixation that is truly biocompatible, it must be a biodegradable polymer that has a shorter degradation time than that of poly-L-lactide, without the inflammatory foreign-body reactions that occur with the faster degrading polyglycolide.—*S.B. Heninger*

♦ This article suggests, following an in vivo animal trial, that absorbable polymers with long degradation time may not be suitable for repairs involving the placement of absorbable devices through cartilage. The polymer (poly-L-lactide) evaluated revealed no inflammatory response. However, peri-implant cartilage revealed evidence of degeneration and the prolonged degradation time of poly-L-lactide devices may have adversely affected the repair of the cartilaginous surface. The authors suggest use of a polymer with a fast or intermediate degradation time. Polyglycholic acid may not be suitable because of reactions associated with that polymer thought to be a result of rapid device degradation. Poly-*p*-dioxanone or copolymers of polylactic and polyglycholic acids may be suitable in this application, but would need to be evaluated. It is interesting to note that several surgeons fixate Austin osteotomies by placement of an absorbable pin through the articular cartilage of the first metatarsal head with reports of good results and few, if any, complications. Long-term follow-up of these patients may reveal if fixation delivered through joint cartilage is of concern clinically.—*V.J. Hetherington, D.P.M.*

Long-Term Follow-up of Patients with Osteochondral Allografts: A Correlation Between Immunologic Responses and Clinical Outcome

Friedlaender GE, Strong DM, Tomford WW, Mankin HJ (Puget Sound Blood Center and Northwest Tissue Center, Seattle, WA; Yale University School of Medicine, New Haven, CT; Massachusetts General Hospital, Harvard Medical School, Boston, MA)
Orthop Clin North Am 30(4):583–588, 1999

Introduction—Animal models predict that allogeneic bone grafts are highly immunogenic due to their histocompatibilty cell surface antigens. In fact, research suggests that immunologic response in animal models is highly predictive of the viability of the bone graft. In addition to cryopreservation of allogeneic grafts, immunosuppression has decreased the rejection rates of allograft incorporation. Human-derived data are scarce at best; thus it is common that evidence is extrapolated from the parallel alloreactivity response in animal models.

Materials and methods—A single surgeon utilizing a large osteochonbdral allograft reconstructed 33 patients who sustained major bony deficits due to tumor excision or trauma. Two patients received amputations of the affected limb and two others died of malignant causes, leaving a remaining total of 29 patients. The Orthopedic Oncology Unit of Massachusetts General Hospital applied a functional grading system to all patients in long-term evaluation. Serum samples were collected from each patient for 4 years and were tested for presentization to class I and II HLA antigens.

Results—Seventy-nine percent of the 29 patients in long-term follow-up achieved excellent clinical results; 15 patients had complications, with four patients having more than one complication. Eighty percent of patients with class I responders and 63% of class II responders to surgical reconstruction with frozen allografts were judged to have a satisfactory clinical outcome.

Discussion—These data support the hypothesis that patients who have a match of class II histocompatibility antigens in both donor and recipients of allografts have improved long-term clinical outcome. Information is scarce and confirms the parallel nature of human and animal bone allograft immuno-genicity. Studies show that freeze-dried bone specimens profoundly reduce the immunologic response of the host. There is also improved bone allograft incorporation in the presence of immunosuppressive treatment.

Summary—As found in the animal models, matching histocompatibility to class II antigens improves clinical outcome and viability of implantation of massive bone allograft in humans. In this study, 79% of the patients had a good-to-excellent outcome, thereby indicating that prior sensitization do not preclude a satisfactory outcome. However, these data and clinical correlation does not directly assess the presence of recipient immunologic responses against donor-specific cells. Reactivity to a representative panel of cells determined the immunogenicity of these subjects, which suggest that more definitive research must be undertaken to provide concrete evidence of the human model and its histocompatibility antigens.—*K.E. Van Voris*

♦ Various methods have been used to surgically treat arthritis and osteocartilaginous defects of the foot and ankle. In podiatric medicine emphasis has been placed primarily on the ankle and first metatarsophalangeal joint, and to a lesser extent the subtalar joint. This article discusses alternatives to stimulate cartilage growth and repair by using such techniques as bone marrow stimulation, microfracture, and autologous chondrocyte implantation versus osteochondral grafts, such as mosaicplasty of joint defects. The authors accurately point out how animal research cannot completely represent human disease to allow for direct application clinically. This article's importance is in stressing the need for clinical outcome studies of procedures to restore viable joint articular surfaces which measure multiple factors, including clinical function, patient satisfaction, and quality of repaired tissue.—*V.J. Hetherington, D.P.M.*

Use of Hydroxyapatite to Fill Cavities After Excision of Benign Bone Tumors: Clinical Results

Yamamoto T, Onga T, Marui T, Mizuno K (Kobe University School of Medicine, Kobe, Japan)
J Bone Joint Surg 82-B(8):1117–1120, 2000

Introduction—The purpose of this study was to evaluate the clinical use of hydroxyapatite to bone defects after curettage of bone tumors. Previous studies have revealed that calcium hydroxyapatite has excellent osteoconductive properties and is safe to use as a bone-graft substitute. However, there is a scarcity of research concerning its use after bone tumor curettage.

Methods—Seventy-five patients with benign bone tumors were used as subjects for the study. Of these 75 patients, there were 28 women and 47 men. The mean age was 27.7 years and the ages ranged from 3 to 80 years. There were a wide variety of bone tumors in a variety of bones but all were treated by curettage and then filling the defects with a hydroxyapatite compound. The compound consisted of 70% hydroxyapatite and 30% tricalcium phosphate. External stabilization with splints or slings was used postoperatively for patients at risk of pathological fracture. The mean follow-up time was 41.3 months.

Results—

- Overall, the results supported the use of hydroxyapatite for the purpose of filling in the defect left by curettage of a bone tumor.
- Histopathological study showed removal of the hydroxyapatite by histiocytes and multinucleated giant cells and the formation of appositional, thick lamellar bone.
- Radiographic evaluation showed the implanted hydroxyapatite to be well incorporated into the surrounding host bone within a mean period of 4.2 months. In the specific cases where the hydroxyapatite implantation was just below the subchondral bone of an articular joint, no degenerative changes were observed in the joints.
- No patient developed a postoperative infection.
- Two patients suffered fractures in the postoperative period; however; these were due to either trauma or noncompliance with postoperative instructions.

- Two patients, both of which had echondromas of the fingers, complained of pain. This pain was attributed to particles of hydroxyapatite in the soft tissues and this diminished within six months. At the final follow-up, no patient complained of local pain.
- Local recurrence of tumor was seen in three cases; however, the authors stated that this is similar to the recurrence rate for such tumors without the implantation of hydroxyapatite and reflects the biological nature of the tumor.

Conclusion—The authors concluded that hydroxyapatite is an excellent bone-graft substitute in surgery for benign bone tumors since it has minimal complications and can be used safely near the joints.—*B. Hoffman*

♦ Bone graft substitutes are alternatives to autogenous and allogenic bone grafts. These substitutes must provide long term biological and mechanical compatibility. The authors in a variety of applications demonstrated the incorporation of calcium hydroxyapatite (HA) as a viable bone-graft alternative. Included in the study were the small bones of the hand and fingers as well as the tibia, fibula, and calcaneus. In addition to manufactured HA products, porous coraline ceramics also provide an alternative to bone grafts and demonstrate osteoconductive potential. Other material to provide an osteoconductive surface for bone repair includes collagen (biological) and absorbable polymers (nonbiological) plus calcium phosphate derivatives (plaster of Paris), tricalcium phosphate or calcium sulfate. The addition of specific bone-stimulating proteins and growth factors such as bone morphogenic protein to these osteoconductive biomaterials will add an osteoinductive component with the potential of enhancing bone healing.—*V.J. Hetherington, D.P.M.*

Evaluating Methods of Restoring Cartilaginous Articular Surfaces

Buckwalter JA (University of Iowa College of Medicine, Iowa City, IA)
Clin Orthop 367S:S224–S238, 1999

Introduction—Physicians and scientists have been seeking ways to restore cartilaginous surfaces. This has come about as the development of artificial materials approaches but never duplicates the adaptability, durability, and functionality of real cartilage. Many methods have been sought to restore cartilaginous surfaces. These include two primary categories: stimulating repair and regeneration, and transplanting of articular surfaces. In spite of the large volume of research toward these ends, there is still uncertainty as to the value of individual techniques and procedures. Critical evaluation of research should include consideration for the limits of experimental models, specifically in terms of their applicability to clinical disorders and appropriate outcome measures.

Experimental Models and Clinical Disorders—

1. *Defect type*—This is broken down into two types: focal defects in an otherwise normal joint and degenerative defects. Loading forces produce focal defects. Local osteochondral defects mostly occur in young adults, whereas older adults have mostly chondral defects from the same forces. Degenerative defects have less well defined margins and generally occur over longer durations. Most are not evident until middle age. Cartilage fibrillation and degeneration occur in most people, but not all cases of cartilage fibrillation have clinical osteoarthritis. Osteoarthritis presents with attempted remodeling as evidenced by radiographic subchondral sclerosis, and cystic changes. There are also soft-tissue differences in osteoarthritic joints compared with joints with cartilage fibrillations. Several animal experiments have attempted to isolate mechanisms predictive of osteoarthritis with little clear success.

2. *Age*—Cartilage changes with increasing age in ways that increase its vulnerability to degeneration and inability to repair itself. Molecular changes include decreased aggrecan size, decrease in proteoglycan aggregation, water content, and increases in collagen cross-linking and accumulations of degraded molecules. It is therefore important to consider the age of the subjects in experimental trials before drawing clinical correlations.

3. *Species differences*—Animal experiments are useful starting points in transplant and other research. It must be interpreted with caution because of differences between species exist in joint structure, loading forces, and molecular and cellular components. Animal studies can, by themselves, be considered at best a limited clinical trial.

Measuring Outcomes—Many studies measure outcomes by evaluating the structure and composition of new or transplanted tissue. This is not enough information to make clinical inferences and recommendations. Outcomes need to consider the following factors: general physical function and quality of life, joint function, joint structure, and chondral repair tissue structure (including structure, composition, and mechanical properties).—*D. Clement*

♦ Immunologic reaction to frozen bone allografts can complicate bone reconstruction. These immunologic responses are due to reactions to class I and II histocompatability antigens. Allografts also raise the concern of transmission of disease. Allografts are indicated for long bone replacement under weightbearing conditions. This article focuses on the use of large grafts for which alternatives may not be available or advisable. Alternate methods of preparation reduce the antigenicity but may compromise biologic or mechanical properties of the bone.

Bone-graft substitutes may be more accessible and carry less risk because of the small amount of graft needed in foot surgery. — *V.J. Hetherington, D.P.M.*

Grafton® Demineralized Bone Matrix: Performance Consistency, Utility, and Value
Russell JL (Osteo Tech, Eatontown, NJ)
Tissue Eng 6(4):435–440, 2000

Background—Treatment of some orthopedic pathology necessitates a bone graft, and allografts are proving to be a viable option to autologous bone. Bone allograft products have been shown to be safe with adequate inactivation of viruses such as HIV and hepatitis B and C viruses, and, as shown here, produce equivalent, superior even in some cases, results when used to support bone healing and regeneration.

Methods—The various forms of Grafton® demineralized bone matrix (DBM) (gel, flex, and putty) all show comparable degrees of osteoinduction across a spectrum of donor ages and between genders. Demineralized bone powder was harvested from human tissue and 40-mg quantities were histologically studied for signs of endochondral ossification. Using a numerical score to evaluate bone formation at 28 days, no statistical differences were noted between the osteoinductive capacity of samples from the different ages and sexes of the donor.

Using a rabbit spine procedure, Grafton products proved comparable to autograft. Lumbar intertransverse process arthrodesis with iliac crest autograft showed 70% successful fusion. Using a 50/50 mix of autograft and Grafton gel revealed equal success. When used without autograft, putty and flex displayed comparable results to autograft alone. Moreover, putty and flex maintained a roughly one-third fusion rate with guanidine extraction which removes all autologous forms of osteoinductive properties, indicating the superior osteoinductive potential of putty and flex.

Grafton products proved useful in human fusion procedures addressing a number of spinal disorders. A control group of 54 patients received iliac crest bone grafts, and 36 patients got a composite of Grafton Gel with autografts from either iliac crest, posterior parts of the spine near the operative site, or both. Groups were matched based on age, gender, and level of fusion; and a radiologist, blinded to treatment groups, measured radiographic evidence of fusion at 2 years postoperatively. The radiologist also scored mineralization with a four-point scale conveying no statistical difference between groups. Although those needing a three- and four-level fusion tended to have the composite graft because of lack of autologous graft, use of Grafton Gel made iliac crest harvest unnecessary.

A second study used two groups matched to age and gender and a radiologist blinded to the groups. Fifty-six patients were given a mix of gel plus autologous graft from the local laminectomy, and a group of 52 received graft from their iliac crest alone. The radiologist noted no difference between the mineralization values, and by 2 years 60% of Grafton and only 56% of autografts were judged to be fused.

A mix of bone marrow and DBM putty was studied on rabbits and used as a model to study the treatment for trauma necessitating bone graft. Twelve consecutive subjects presented with high-impact injuries requiring fixation where bone grafting was deemed appropriate. Bone marrow was aspirated from the iliac crest and one part marrow was combined to three parts Grafton putty. All fractures were treated with this graft mixture and nine were followed for up to 12 months with blinded radiographic analysis looking for successful trabeculation. Each patient succeeded in healing, with structural union and bone formation without any graft-related complications of aspirate site pain. This illustrates the usefulness of Grafton/marrow composites: achieving a satisfactory fracture healing, here obviating an iliac crest bone harvest altogether.

Grafton Gel was finally shown to provide a superior alternative to current treatment of osteonecrosis of the femoral head. One group of 90 hips with confirmed osteonecrosis got the traditional core decompression, and 28 hips got core decompression plus Grafton Gel. The Grafton was used without autologous bone this time and inserted into the core defect. Sixty-seven percent of hips with moderate osteonecrosis survived (i.e., did not need replacement) compared to the 83% survival rate for decompression plus gel. The addition of Grafton Gel proved to be a significant improvement for severe osteonecrosis with a 69% survival rate with Grafton compared to only 28% with decompression alone.

Conclusion—Grafton products meet the requirements of safe and effective material for bone grafting across a wide range of orthopedic indications. When mixed with marrow, Grafton allows for adequate bone formation to advance. Quite importantly, this allogenic bone graft eliminates, or at least reduces, the need for additional surgical sites for bone harvest, thus reducing the cost of procedures and lowering patient morbidity.—*C. Jacka*

♦ Grafton is an allogenic bone morphogenic protein (demineralized bone matrix) that is supplied in three forms, dependent upon the carrier. The method of preparation reduces the antigenicity and eliminates the potential for transfer of viral disease. This is an example of biologic engineering currently available to podiatric surgeons to manage problem bone healing. Bone morphogenic proteins may be used in conjunction with osteoconductive materials or as an extender of an autogenous bone graft. The combination demineralized bone matrix with demineralized cortical bone cubes provides for osteoconduction as well as osteoinduction. — *V.J. Hetherington, D.P.M.*

Use of Small Cannulated Screws for Fixation in Foot Surgery

Burns AE (California College of Podiatric Medicine, San Francisco, CA)
J Am Podiatr Med Assoc 90(5):240–246, 2000

Introduction—Bone screws, the most commonly used orthopedic implants, are the primary fixation device of the Swiss Association for the Study of Internal Fixation (ASIF) technique. In order to achieve ASIF fracture treatment recommendations, the lag technique is followed, which generates compression between two opposing ends of bone while inducing primary vascular bone formation. In addition, this method of fixation allows for mobilization of the affected limb. Due to the stability of the bone ends, pain is not created from the movement of free nerve endings. Failure of screw compression is evidenced by perceived patient pain and periosteal callus formation on radiograph.

Cortical screws, which have a narrow pitch, can purchase dense and compact cortical bone better than cancellous screws, which are designed to purchase cancellous bone due to their wider pitch. While both screws are available in partially or fully threaded varieties, the use of the lag screw technique requires partial threading. Full threading is required, however, if bone plate fixation is indicated.

Methods—A prospective study was engineered using the Mini Lag Screw System produced by Alphatec Manufacturing, Inc (Palm Desert, CA), available in 2.7, 3.5, and 4.0 mm sizes. All screws were titanium alloy, self-tapping, and partially threaded, with low-profile heads. Cannulated screws were used as the exclusive means of fixation in 70 procedures that were performed on 49 patients between January 1992 and October 1993. The procedures consisted of 61 osteotomies and 9 fusions, and all patients were followed for 2 years. Postoperative evaluation parameters were comprised of fixation failure, implant fracture, and periosteal callus formation.

Results—There was no incidence of fracture among the 70 implants used in the study. However, there were six patients who developed periosteal callus formation and seven patients with implant-fixation failure that was attributed to surgeon error or patient noncompliance.

Conclusion—The use of the cannulated screw system in fixating osteotomies and fusions of the foot is effective and reliable. Advantages of cannulated bone screws include a reduction in possible sources of error in angulation and three-dimensional placement, thus decreasing surgical time and producing more precise screw placement.—*E. Zarutsky*

♦ Cannulated bone screws have streamlined the technique for internal fixation as compared with noncannulated screw systems. This is especially true for self-tapping systems. Cannulation of smaller screws does not seem to compromise the strength of the screws needed for clinical application. Cannulated absorbable fixation screws are available but due to inherent material properties cannot be self-tapping or reaming at present. As the author points out, cost is a significant factor when comparing standard screws to cannulated systems creating use and availability problems in a managed care environment.—*V.J. Hetherington, D.P.M.*

Emerging Strategies of Bone and Joint Repair

Schultz O, Sittinger M, Haeupl T, Burmester GR (Humbolt University of Berlin, Berlin, Germany)
Arthritis Res 2:433–436, 2000

Introduction—Biomedical tissue engineering has provided today's physician with many alternatives to treating the patient who suffers from failure of vital structures, such as chronic inflammation and degeneration.

Cell Transplantation—Studies in cartilage repair have proven transplantation of differentiated autologous cells taken from biopsy of similar tissue has three disadvantages: 1) limited availability of these cells, 2) donor site morbidity, and 3) unpredictable viability and subsequent differentiation of the transplant. Current studies focus on in situ mobilization of mesenchymal precursor stem cells. Supplementing the local tissue repair process with controlled release of regulatory bioactive molecules such as growth factors, cytokines, cell adhesion molecules, and chemokines is under current study.

Morphogenic Factors—With increasing age there is a declining number of progenitor cells in the reservoir for tissue rejuvenation. It is known that bone morphogenic proteins (BMP 2, 4, and 7) and growth factors (GDF 5 and 6) are integral to the osteochondrogenic morphogenesis as well as tissue homeostasis. Studies have shown that the incorporation of BMPs with carrier molecules result in faster revitalization of cartilage and bone defects.

Bioartificial Tissues—Resorbable polymer scaffolds combined with hydrogels might achieve the embryo-like state required to provide biocompatibility of implants and/or transplants. Encapsulation of the bioartificial tissue by semipermeable membrane is a key factor in both protecting it from immune response and maintaining the integrity of the tissue. New "smart" polymers will incorporate functional groups, side chains, matrix proteins, and cell adhesion molecules to provide a more dynamic structure capable of adaptation, promoting differentiation, and matrix formation.

Clinical Aspects—The use of "smart" polymers and growth factor gradient release systems broadens the spectrum of clinical applications. The regenerative potential of mesenchymal stem and progenitor cells has been shown with sufficient osseous bridging and bone formation in clinical trials. However, due to the increase in the amount of joint injuries sustained by the clinical population, studies are currently being conducted to assess the viability of cartilage transplants. The two determinant factors in the viability of replacement joint cartilage are the pressure resistance and transplant fixation. Alternatives to present procedures for replacement of joint cartilage consist of 1) osteochondral transplants which consist of artificial cartilage tissue cultured directly on porous calcium carbonate and 2) the transplantation of fibroblast-seeded scaffolds cultured under specific tensile strengths with concomitant administration of growth factors.

Genetic Engineering—The possibility of transferring genes of the BMPs or their receptors will give regenerative and anti-inflammatory properties to the transplant. Gene therapy itself lends us the advantage of a genetically modified population of cells in which the optimal differentiation and protection can be controlled. Systemic delivery of stem cells with "homing" sites for various regions of the body presents future opportunities for treatment of systemic disease.

Conclusion—Bioregenerative medicine has been able to predict cell destiny and dramatically improve the possibility of treating chronic disease and hard-to-resolve tissue deficit with advanced biomaterials, bioactive molecules, and gene therapy.—*K.E. Van Voris*

♦ As reported in other reviews in this chapter the field of biomaterials is evolving to ultimately include genetically engineered materials and products such as growth factors, engineered cells and gene therapy. This advance signals the move from the field of replacement to what the author's of this article refer to as bioregenerative medicine (Fig. 1). This article deals with the advances in biomaterials discussing

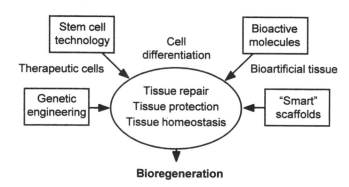

FIGURE 1. Tools for tissue engineering. (Reproduced, with permission, from Schultz et al., *Arthritis Res* 2:433–436, 2000. Copyright © 2000 by Current Science Ltd.)

combinations of static biomaterial with active cells and inductive proteins combining to form bioartifical tissues. We need to educate our profession to rapidly move with these changes.—*V.J. Hetherington, D.P.M.*

Hallux Rigidus Treated by Carbon Fibre Arthroplasty of the Proximal Phalanx

Minns RJ, Muckle DS, Nabhani F (Dryburn Hospital, Durham, UK; Middlesborough, General Hospital, Middlesborough, UK; University of Teesside, Middlesborough, UK)
Foot Ankle Surg 5:245–250, 1999

Introduction—Hallux rigidus is a painfully restricted first metatarsophalangeal joint, which can be treated both conservatively and surgically. Many of the current surgical options shorten the metatarsal or phalanx, thus increasing range of motion but leaving a "floppy toe" sequelae. The joint replacement options, including the Silastic implants, have not afforded good results either, resulting in removal of the implant. Although total joint replacements of larger joints have been successful, smaller joints are under greater biomechanical stress and require more precise placement of the implant to prevent failure. After animal trials with a small carbon fiber pad implant, humans with diagnosed hallux rigidus secondary to osteoarthritis were considered for the interpositional hemiarthroplasty.

Materials and Methods—The carbon fiber pads are porous nonwoven layers of Polyacrylonitrile, which is flexible and easy to cut. After the initial incision, the capsule is then opened and a Rose bur of 3 mm diameter is used on the base of the proximal phalanx to make a concavity with peripheral undermining. Lyofoam is used to produce the final shape of the implant. Then the implant is inserted and both the capsule and the skin are closed, separately. Seventy-three patients were operated on; 48 were available for follow-up.

Results—Radiographs show successful positioning of the implant without any degradation of the implant. Osteosclerotic borders indicate new bone formation. Histologically there was evidence of a pseudo-fibrocartilaginous weightbearing surface. The new bone formed grew into the deeper layer of the implant, thus anchoring it. The joint space was maintained for as long as 17 years and pain in the joint was much lower postoperatively.

Discussion—Failure of the Silastic implants is mainly from "pistoning" effects during loading, but this is not the case with carbon fiber pad due to the tissue ingrowth. With this implant, the joint space is preserved, the implant is fixed in place, and a fibrocartilaginous surface is formed which can later create an articular cartilage matrix, which is all pain free and fully functional.—*F. Nejad*

♦ Carbon as a biomaterial has proven to be generally well tolerated in animal and human implantations. The study reported a mean follow-up of 9.2 years. The implant was well tolerated and provided significant pain relief. The nonbiodegradable implant provides a scaffold for reparative tissue ingrowth and analysis retrieved cases provides for a suitable articulation surface. The scaffolding matrix with resultant soft-tissue ingrowth may provide for a more biomechanically compatible articulation than metal hemiarthroplasty by more closely mimicking normal articular cartilage and bone.—*V.J. Hetherington, D.P.M.*

Replacement Arthroplasty for Hallux Rigidus: 21 Patients with a 2-Year Follow-up

Olms K, Dietz A (Agnes Karll Hospital, Bod Schwartau, Germany; Rikshospitalet, Oslo, Norway)
Int Orthop 23:240–243, 1999

Introduction—Patients with severe degenerative changes to the first metatarsophalangeal joint (MPJ) require joint destructive procedures such as Keller-Brandes procedures, fusion of the first MPJ, or implant arthroplasty. This paper reviews outcomes 2 years after insertion of a two-component implant of the first MPJ.

Methods—Twenty-one patients underwent total first MPJ replacement with follow-ups greater than 24 months. Sixteen patients with stage III and stage IV hallux rigidus had primary reconstruction. Five patients had revision surgery with this implant. Data were collected from clinical and radiographic evaluation as well as from a patient questionnaire.

The implant (Bio-Action Great Toe Implant, MicroAire Surgical Instruments, Charlottesville, VA) was introduced in 1991, and is a nonconstrained two-component system designed to reproduce the function of the first MPJ. The phalangeal component has a polyethylene articular surface and is made from titanium. The metatarsal head component has an ionated surface to reduce polyethylene wear and is made from chrome-cobalt.

Surgical Procedure—The joint is exposed through a dorso-medial incision and a T-capsulotomy is made at the medial capsule. Bony hypertrophy is removed from the head of the metatarsal and the base of the proximal phalanx. More bone is resected from the base of the proximal phalanx than the head of the metatarsal to prevent shortening of the first ray and prevent metatarsalgia. The implants are press-fit without cement.

Results—There were no cases of infection or revision surgeries. There was good cosmetic closure and no signs of synovitis or swelling at follow-up. Five patients had lack of toe purchase. Four had metatarsalgia relieved with orthotics. First MPJ dorsiflexion increased from 0°–10° to an average of 50° at follow-up. Thirteen patients had pain anytime preoperatively versus four patients postoperatively. Six patients had pain in shoes preoperatively while only four patients had pain after surgery. Thirteen patients had pain and stiffness prior to surgery as compared to three after surgery. Of the 21 patients, 17 had less or no pain and 17 had the same or greater activity level.

Discussion—The Bio-Action Great Toe Implant increased dorsiflexion from 10° to an average of 50°, which allowed for greater movement and better function. There was no narrowing of the joint space, as seen on X-ray. The implant did not cause synovitis like the Silastic implants. In the 2-year review, no infections or implant complications occurred and no implants were subsequently removed. The patients who had lack of toe purchase and metatarsalgia were successfully treated with orthotics.—*O.T. Wang, D.P.M.*

♦ Few studies have been reporting on two-component first MPJ replacement with a follow-up of 2 years. The results presented are encouraging but several questions remained unanswered. How was toe purchase measured? Did the toe function in gait with toe purchase or just passively dorsiflex? Was the lack of toe purchase associated with metatatarsalgia in the same patients? Did 11 of 21 patients continue to have pain or were multiple pain complaints received individually from patients (e.g., pain with shoes, pain and stiffness). What accounted for the cosmetic complaints? Was stiffness associated with periarticular ossification? Did preservation of the plantar shelf maintain toe function and purchase?

The authors present results consistent with good patient satisfaction, pain relief, and activity. Further study with this implant will be needed to answer functional concerns or if the implant is functioning as a spacer. — *V.J. Hetherington, D.P.M.*

11 Biomechanics of the Lower Extremity

RONALD L. VALMASSY, D.P.M.

In Vivo Strain Measurements to Evaluate the Strengthening Potential of Exercises on the Tibial Bone
Milgrom C, Finestone A, Simkin A, Ekenman I, Mendelson S, Millgram M, Nyska M, Larsson E, Burr D (Hadassah University Hospital, Jerusalem, Israel)
J Bone Joint Surg 82-B(4):591–594, 2000

Introduction—The increasing concern about osteoporosis has provided the impetus to find an exercise activity to best stimulate an increase in bone strength. It is thought that mechanical loading during physical activity produces forces (strains) within bones which act as a stimulus for the structural adaptation of bone. The goal of this study was a first step toward defining the dose-response relationship of physical loading and mechanical strengthening of bone. The study involved measuring the tibial bone strains and strain rates in vivo during common fitness exercises and comparing them with those during walking, an activity which is considered to have little effect on bone mass.

Methods—Tibial strains and rates of strain were measured in vivo in six mature adults during running, stationary bicycling, leg presses, and stepping and were compared to those of walking. The six subjects included four men aged 37, 39, 45, and 52 years and two women aged 27 and 33. All of the subjects were healthy with no previous history of medical problems. Into each patient's right leg, three strain-gauged staples were inserted percutaneously in a rosette pattern in the medial aspect of the midshaft of the tibia. The gauges were hooked up to amplifiers and the signals were recorded on cassette recorders. All of the patients wore the same type of shoe gear as they participated in the following activities: running, walking, exercise bicycle, stepmaster, and leg presses. The following measurements and calculations were made: peak principal compression, tension, and shear strains and the strain rates.

183

Results—

1. *Strain:*
   - There was no statistical difference in the principal tension, compression, and shear strains between walking, leg presses, or stepmaster.
   - Principal tension, compression, and shear strains were significantly higher during running than those during walking.
   - Principal tension and shear strains were significantly lower in stationary bicycling than in walking.

2. *Strain Rates:*
   - The maximum tension strain rates during walking were significantly higher when performing leg presses, using the stepmaster, or stationary bicycling.
   - There was no statistically significant difference between tension strain rates during walking and running.
   - The maximum compression and shear strain rates during walking were significantly higher than those while performing stationary bicycling and leg presses. Running had higher compression and shear strain rates than the other exercises.

*Conclusion—*The authors believe that if bone strains and/or strain rates higher than walking are needed for bone strengthening, then of the exercises measured in this study, only running can influence the adaptive remodeling response in bone so that it can be considered an effective strengthening exercise for the tibia.—*B. Hoffman*

♦ This study is noteworthy in that it recruited individuals who allowed transducers to be implanted into a tibia to assess impact forces through this segment. The salient features of this study indicate that running has a higher potential than walking to influence adaptive remodeling to strengthen the midshaft of the tibia. This certainly has long-term ramifications for decreasing the likelihood of osteoporosis in our older patient populations. My only derogatory comment with regard to this study is that there was no evaluation of foot function among the study participants, thereby eliminating the possibility of obtaining additional useful information regarding increased shock to the tibia relative to foot function.—*R.L. Valmassy, D.P.M.*

Effect of Immobilization on Ankle Dorsiflexion Strength

Geboers JFM, van Tuijl JH, Seelen HAM, Drost MR (iRv, Hoensbrock; SRL/Hoensbroek; University Maastricht, The Netherlands)
Scand J Rehab Med 32:66–71, 2000

---

*Introduction—*Currently two opposing thoughts are presented in the literature in regards to ankle-foot orthoses (AFOs). Ankle-foot orthosis are prescribed to patients with paresis of the dorsiflexors of the foot. One of the thoughts is that AFOs help the person to stimulate synergistic muscles to aid in walking. The other is that the AFO restricts ankle movement with in turn causes disuse atrophy in the remaining dorsiflexors of the ankle. If the later thought were true, it would be harmful to prescribe an AFO.

In addition there have been many different studies to evaluate disuse atrophy by looking at ankle torque measurements; unfortunately the studies have shown significant differences. This is partly due to different test protocols. The studies have all shown that the tendency of muscles to weakness depends of muscle type, position, and length of duration. This study wanted to establish a reproducible way to determine ankle torque range and then to apply it to patients who have been immobilized in order to decide whether an AFO is the best treatment.

Methods—Seventy-two healthy volunteers were used to gather reference values for ankle torque. The volunteers were between the ages of 18 and 80 years old, had no incidence of fracture, trauma, or contractures of the lower limbs, and had no history of musculoskeletal, rheumatological, neurological, or orthopedic lower extremity problems. Isometric torque was measured. The patients were in a supine position with the knee in extension with the leg fixed to the table to ensure only ankle forces were being measured. A horizontal rod was at the level of the metatarsophalangeal joint dorsally. A Tedea-Huntleigh model 601 load cell was used to measure the torque after 5 minutes of warm-up and then patients were instructed to pull against the beam for 5-second intervals for 10 times; a 30-second break was given to ensure fatigue was not a factor. This was done with the foot in 0° of plantarflexion and 30° of plantarflexion.

The immobilization group consisted of 15 people who were immobilized in a weightbearing below-the-knee cast for 40 days. The first ankle torque measurements, as described above, were taken immediately after the removal of the cast and the second were taken 43 days later. The injury that these 15 sustained required no internal fixation, and they were capable of holding the foot in 0° and 30° of plantarflexion without risk of re-injury.

Results—The same differences in gender, age, and ankle position again showed differences in the range study. In the study to establish reproducible ankle torque, the average of both ankles at 0° of plantarflexion was 41.8 Nm for males 20–49 years old, 27.2 Nm for males 50–80 years old, 31.2 Nm for females 20–49 years old and 22.3 Nm for females 50–80 years old. The average of both ankles at 30° of plantar flexion was 54.4 Nm, for males 20–49 years old, 44.8 Nm for males 50–80 years old, 38.9 Nm for females 20–49 years old, 32.1 Nm for females 50–80 years old. In the immobilized group the ankle torque in the average of the first measurement was 24.6 Nm and the second measurement was 33.3 Nm at 0° of plantarflexion. The ankle torque average at 30° of plantarflexion was 29.7 Nm in the first measurement and 41.9 Nm in the second measurement.

Discussion—The reproducible ankle torque measurements were in agreement with other studies with some minor differences, once again attributed to different testing and had a mean coefficient of variation of 4.2% (SD = 3.6). The findings of the effect of immobilization showed 28% strength loss in the initial measurement. Because of this decrease in strength, the use of an AFO may prove to cause some weakness. Immobilization, however, did not seem to affect the optimal length of the dorsiflexors when casted in the neutral position because of the very small difference in the 0° of plantarflexion and 30° of plantarflexion. Recovery took 6 weeks.—*T. Marshall*

♦ This article attempted to determine whether or not protracted immobilization of an ankle following injury resulted in any significant weakness. I was quite surprised to note that the study, which overall was conducted in a most appropriate fashion, concluded that normal strength of the ankle took place within 6 weeks following immobilization without any specific treatment. This is certainly at odds with my personal experience which indicates that there are a host of patients who fare very poorly with their immobilization treatment regimens. My experience is that an essential portion of the treatment of any lower extremity injury is that a period of immobilization should always be followed by quite vigorous and consistent muscle strengthening exercises. I have often seen individuals re-injure their foot and/or ankle due to the fact that they have not completely rehabilitated their lower extremity strength following a period of immobilization. There have been multiple instances of chronic foot and ankle pain for 1 or more years following a period of injury or immobilization if specific strengthening exercises have not been recommended. It is for this reason that I feel that the appropriate treatment following any period of lower extremity immobilization calls for rigorous range-of-motion exercises and strengthening of the involved intrinsic and extrinsic foot muscles.—*R.L. Valmassy, D.P.M.*

Relationship Between Calf Muscle Size and Strength After Achilles Rupture Repair

Leppilahti J, Lähde S, Forsman K, Kangas J, Kauranen K, Orava S (Oulu University Hospital, Oulu, Finland)
Foot Ankle Int 21(4):330–335, 2000

Introduction—Studies in the past have shown that muscle strength and/or size decreases in immobilized limbs. The purpose of the study was to investigate the recovery of calf muscle size and strength after surgical repair of an Achilles tendon rupture. Past studies show that muscle strength is recovered more easily than muscle size.

Methods—This study consisted of 85 athletes, 75 men and 12 women, who underwent Achilles tendon rupture surgical repair via Lindholm's plasty (65) or Silfverskiöid's plasty (20). Surgical technique included suture repair and reinforcement with one or two gastrocnemius aponeurosis flaps. Patients were casted for 6 weeks postoperatively; first 3 weeks in plantarflexion followed by 3 weeks at 90° to the leg (neutral). After immobilization, rehabilitation was conducted in four phases, starting with range of motion leading to strength and endurance training. At 6 weeks, jogging was permitted, and at 9 months, there was no limit to activity.

Results—Calf muscle size (cross-sectional area) was normal in 30%, mildly atrophic in 40%, moderately atrophic in 20%, and severely atrophic in 4% of patients. Isokinetic strength was good to excellent in 73%, fair in 19%, and poor in 18% of the patients.

Discussion—The study found that the average plantarflexion strength per unit cross-sectional area was greater on the injured side than the noninjured side at an average of 3 years after surgical repair. While 73% regained good-excellent calf muscle strength, only 30% regained calf muscle size. It is concluded that recovery of strength is obtained more readily than size. Rehabilitation plays a role in the recovery of size and strength. Exercise with high loads (80–100% max) will induce muscle strength, while repetitive lower loads (60–80% max) will induce muscular hypertrophy (size). Rehabilitation technique may help in the recovery of calf muscle size.—*K. Carriero*

♦ I found this to be a clinically relevant article and quite useful for anyone dealing with a large number of athletic patients. We certainly all have had the opportunity to treat patients with ruptured Achilles tendons and have noted that although patients generally will recapture their muscle strength, they will always demonstrate some asymmetry in overall calf size. This study indicates that calf muscle size was normal in only 30% of the patient population evaluated in this study. The reasoning for this is that the type of exercises performed to regain strength—few repetitions of increased weights—typically will not build up muscle size. Conversely, multiple repetitions of lesser weights will build up muscle size, but will have little effect on the overall strength. Needless to say, regaining one's strength following a ruptured Achilles tendon is more important to normal biomechanical function than is the overall size of the calf muscle.—*R.L. Valmassy, D.P.M.*

Reliability of Measurements of Pressures Applied on the Foot During Walking by a Computerized Insole Sensor System

Randolph AL, Nelson M, Akkapeddi S, Levin A, Alexandrescu R (New York Medical College, Valhalla, NY)

Acad Phys Med Rehabi 81:573–578, 2000

Introduction—Patients with diabetes mellitus, peripheral vascular disease, leprosy, and other conditions associated with reduced sensibility of the foot frequently suffer plantar foot ulceration, which often results in disability and occasionally amputation. Ulceration is most common at areas of high pressure, and it has been shown that diabetics with reduced sensibility have even higher foot pressures. In the prevention of foot ulcer development, the ability to measure accurately the pressures on the foot during ambulation is largely important. This information can be used to create devices to redistribute the weightbearing forces on the foot, reducing the pressures to a safer level. This study reports the reliability of the insoles used with the F-scan device, which was developed for this purpose.

Methods—Foot pressures were recorded on 10 subjects who each walked three 6-second periods using four different pairs of insoles in their own shoes. Data were interpreted for the hindfoot, midfoot, and forefoot of the patients.

Results—The mean standard deviation peak pressure was about 11.1 psi at the hindfoot, 3.5 psi at the midfoot, and 11.3 psi at the forefoot. The intrasubject mean difference was 0.2 psi at the hindfoot, 0.4 psi at the midfoot, and 0.3 psi at the forefoot. There were no statistically significant differences observed among the groups. The data suggest that information obtained using this system is sufficiently reliable to compare data among various subjects and insoles.

Discussion—There are many techniques for measuring the pressures on the sole of the foot, but they all have their shortcomings. Direct visualization from beneath a transparent surface hinders positioning and quantifying pressures. Evaluation of imprints limits accuracy and precision. Strain gauges measure force through deformation of a conducting material; however, this system permits only a single determination. Pressure pads and other insole measuring devices that are taped under bare feet present difficulties in proper instrument placement, preventing the device from shifting after placement, and receiving accurate data when the bulk of the device artificially alters it. The results indicate that the F-scan system can reflect the pressures on the foot during ambulation in shoes more accurately than other methods or devices. The disadvantages of this system are its cost, as well as the insole cost ($25 each), a lengthy data analyzation time, the necessary training to use the system, and the lack of recognition of this as a reimbursable service by health insurers. In conclusion, the pressure data derived from the F-scan system are sufficiently reliable to be used for the prevention of ulcer formation, particularly in the diabetic patient with reduced sensibility of the foot.—*J.M. Dawson*

♦ This is another article in a long series of studies demonstrating the effectiveness of various modalities to evaluate plantar foot pressure. This study demonstrates the reliability of the F-scan insole in being able to reliably demonstrate abnormal pressures on the plantar aspect of the foot. The practitioner should be aware of the various types of pressure-measuring systems in order that they might direct their at-risk patients for this type of diagnostic testing. Although this type of system may not be appropriate for all practitioners' offices, one should possess the knowledge of where such systems exist in their respective communities in order to assist with their patients' lower extremity problems.—*R.L. Valmassy, D.P.M.*

Do the Hamstrings and Adductors Contribute to Excessive Internal Rotation of the Hip in Persons with Cerebral Palsy?

Arnold AS, Asakawa DJ, Delp SL (Stanford University, Stanford, CA; Northwestern University, Evanston, IL; Rehabilitation Institute of Chicago, Chicago, IL)
Gait Posture 11:181–190, 2000

Introduction—It is common to find excessive internal rotation of the hip causing gait abnormalities in people with cerebral palsy. It is thought that spastic medial hamstrings or the adductors play a role in the excessive internal rotation. Patients with cerebral palsy often have excessive anteversion of the femur and frequently walk with exaggerated flexion of the hips and knees. The purpose of this study was to determine the rotational moment arms of the medial hamstrings and the adductors during gait, and to see if any of these muscles contributed to excessive internal rotation.

Methods—Graphic models were created for three subjects with cerebral palsy and excessive internally rotated hips. The limb that showed the greatest degree of hip internal rotation was selected. These models were developed based on MRI. The accuracy of the methods to create the models was tested. The rotational moment arms of the muscles were calculated based on the limb positions corresponding to each subject's internally rotated gait.

Results—All three of the patients showed that the semimembranosus, semitendinosus, and the gracilis have external rotation moment arms throughout the gait cycle. The adductor brevis and adductor longus had internal rotation moment arms in subject 2. The adductor longus also had an internal rotation moment arm in subject 3. However, in both subjects, the internal moment arms of the muscles were small. This suggests that neither the medial hamstrings nor the adductor muscles contribute substantially to the excessive internal rotation of the hip.

Conclusions—Based on previous models, the medial hamstring, adductor brevis, and adductor longus have the ability to internally rotate the hip in a normal upright, standing position. However, this study showed that the medial hamstrings and the adductor muscles have no influence on internal rotation of the hips in children with cerebral palsy. Therefore, surgical procedures done to lengthen the hamstrings and the adductors in cerebral palsy patients with excessive internal hip rotation may be inappropriate.—*S. Patel*

♦ Overall, I found this to be a quite interesting and informative presentation on a very commonly held precept regarding spastic gait disorders in pediatric patients. Years ago I learned and subsequently taught that tight hamstrings and adductors are involved in the overall gait anomalies evidenced in patients with cerebral palsy. This paper represents an excellent research model which attempts to determine what the overall net effect is when the aforementioned muscles are contracted in involved children. The overall net conclusion of this study is that the medial hamstrings and adductors do not contribute to excessive internal rotation of the hip in individuals with cerebral palsy who walk with a crouched, internally rotated gait pattern. This information is of significant importance in that surgical lengthening of these structures was commonly performed and continues to be performed to this day in an attempt to reduce excessive intoeing in this patient population. Certainly the information presented in this paper would cause one to reconsider recommending surgical procedures for the involved structures.—*R.L. Valmassy, D.P.M.*

Biomechanics of the First Ray. Part II: Metatarsus Primus Varus as a Cause of Hypermobility. A Three-Dimensional Kinematic Analysis in a Cadaver Model

Rush SM, Christensen JC, Johnson CH (Northwest Surgical Biomechanics Research Laboratory, Providence Seattle Medical Center, Seattle, WA)
J Foot Ankle Surg 39(2):68–77, 2000

Introduction—Pathological manifestations of first ray mechanics such as hypermobility and hallux abductovalgus (HAV) are not well understood. Abnormal function and consequent progressive deformity can occur from an imbalance of the structures responsible for the stability of the first ray. The role of these components, the plantar ligaments, plantar aponeurosis, and extrinsic muscles inserting on the first ray, is to inhibit dorsal translation occurring at the metatarsocuneiform joint. This study was designed to address the role of the plantar aponeurosis in stabilizing the first ray through the windlass mechanism.

Methods—Six fresh frozen cadaver specimens with intact feet and ankles and pre-existing metatarsus primus varus (MPV) and HAV deformity were evaluated radiographically using a loading frame to simulate weightbearing. This analysis allowed for classification of foot type and measurement of absolute intermetatarsal angle and sesamoid position. Specimens with any metatarsal valgus rotation were excluded and care was taken to preserve capsuloligamentous integrity during dissection. Following the precise removal of a 15-mm section of diaphyseal bone, a two-component titanium alloy metatarsal jig was secured onto the first metatarsal using Kirschner wires. The specimens were then loaded into a custom acrylic load frame and had 100 N dorsally directed forces passed through them with varying hallux positions and intermetatarsal angles. Three-dimensional tracking was attained by fastening positional receiving radio signal transducers to the medial cuneiform, second metatarsal, and the head and base of the first metatarsal.

Results—An increased ability to plantarflex the first ray and engage the windlass mechanism was achieved with re-establishment of first ray alignment as compared to presence of MPV or HAV deformity. This increase was detected in metatarsal head, base, and cuneiform sagittal motion.

Discussion—The results of this study suggest that functional stability is lost with the development of first ray deformity. There was a noticeable increase in first ray drift with HAV deformity, signifying the inability of the first ray to stabilize itself through the windlass mechanism. Functional stability of the first ray, and thus medial column stability, is decreased with "damping" of the windlass mechanism or compromise of the sesamoid articulations. A 26% increase in closed kinetic chain plantarflexion was observed following first ray deformity correction. This indicates that a component of measured first ray hypermobility is reversible. Therefore, first ray motion is largely dependent on first ray alignment, and correction of MPV and HAV deformity markedly reduces first ray hypermobility.—*E. Zarutsky*

◆ This is an excellent study that demonstrates the various factors involved with a hypermobile first ray. The most salient feature of this article demonstrates what we have understood from a clinical perspective for a number of years, that is, that increased first ray stability may be gained with a reduction in the intermetatarsal angle. I feel that a review of this article by podiatric surgeons will allow them to better appreciate the results that are achieved with various osteotomy procedures of the first metatarsal. Additionally, I continue to feel that the best long-term results for bunion surgery in individuals with excessive abnormal pronation is the postoperative use of functional foot orthoses. — *R.L. Valmassy, D.P.M.*

The Influence of Orthotic Devices and Vastus Medialis Strength and Timing on Patellofemoral Loads During Running

Neptune RR, Wright IC, van den Bogert AJ (The University of Calgary, Calgary, Canada; The Cleveland Clinic Foundation, Cleveland, OH)
Clin Biomech 15:611–618, 2000

Introduction—Patellofemoral pain (PFP) represents 26% of all running injuries. PFP includes all disorders associated with discomfort in the anterior knee joint. The most common conservative treatments of PFP are prescription orthotics and exercise programs directed at vastus medialis obligue (VMO) strengthening.

Objective—There is disagreement in the scientific community as to what causes PFP and which treatment is most effective. The study is conducted via the use of musculoskeletal models to determine the cause and the most appropriate treatment in regards to VMO strengthening versus prescription orthotics.

Methods—A forward dynamic musculoskeletal model was used to produce simulations of heel-toe running. Experiments were performed on nine healthy subjects to examine the influence of VMO strength, VMO timing, and orthotics on patellofemoral loads during running. To access the treatment, a two-way mixed factor was used to measure the peak lateral joint constraint and impact forces.

Results—Based on the lateral impact peak, it was found that the impact peak force was never lowered with the use of orthotics and only slightly decreased by VMO activation timing. The statistical analysis showed that VMO strength was the only treatment to significantly reduce the peak lateral constraint force.

Conclusion—The study is limited in that the musculoskeletal model was not customized to the anatomy of individual subjects, and the orthotics used in the study did not change the shape of the foot–ground interface, but only increased support in the arch area. The experiments showed that increased VMO strength had the greatest effect on decreasing both peak and lateral constraint force. The effect of VMO activation timing did reduce joint loading, although the ability to selectively activate VMO while running is a highly debated, complex issue. Orthotic treatment had a beneficial effective in some subjects and had no effect in other subjects. However, an adverse effect was never observed. VMO strength had the most consistent results across subjects, yet selective VMO strengthening is also a difficult task. The study suggests that techniques that selectively strengthen VMO, combined with effective orthotic treatment, might be the best way to help patients with patellofemoral pain.—*K. Carriero*

♦ This article is certainly interesting in that it attempts to determine if strengthening of the vastus medialis obliques or an orthotic device would be more beneficial in treating chronic patellofemoral dysfunction problems. I have some issues with the article in that the authors did not utilize prescription foot orthoses, nor did they fully evaluate the biomechanical function of their subjects' feet. My clinical perspective on this is that chronic patellofemoral dysfunction responds exceptionally well to a combination of specific quadriceps and vastus medialis obliques strengthening activities and an appropriately designed orthotic device that is capable of reducing all abnormal subtalar joint pronation. Treatment with only muscle strengthening or orthotic devices alone often proves ineffective in treating our patient population for this disorder.—*R.L. Valmassy, D.P.M.*

Effects of Lateral-Wedged Insoles on Kinetics at the Knee

Crenshaw SJ, Pollo FE, Caltron EF (Baylor University Medical Center, Dallas, TX)
Clin Orthop 375:185–192, 2000

Background—Patients with osteoarthritis of the knee experience it in the medial compartment 10 times more often than in the lateral, probably due to higher loads during gait. While ambulating, a varus moment about the knee takes place throughout the majority of stance. Both the higher loads and varus moment are thought to be partly responsible for the greater incidence of osteoarthritis in this compartment. Articular cartilage degeneration narrows the medial joint space, which results in a shift in alignment towards varus. This increases the moment of the ground reactive force and results in an even higher varus moment. Past studies have shown that lateral-wedged insoles placed the entire limb in a more upright position, changed the angle of force through the joint, and reduced lateral thrust, lessening the load on the medial compartment.

Methods—Gait and medial knee compartment loads were analyzed to determine the effects of 5° lateral-wedged insoles.

Results—Lateral-wedged insoles generally reduced both the external varus moment about the knee and the calculated medial compartment load. The lateral-wedged insoles had no significant effect on velocity, cadence, stride length, swing and stance ratios, or kinematics about the hip, knee, or ankle. Though not tested in this analysis, past studies have shown an increase in the valgus position of the subtalar joint.

Discussion—In osteoarthritis, the articular cartilage degenerates, leading to collapse of the affected compartment and an increase in coronal plane angulation and moments. This increased compartmental load can be reduced by the lateral-wedged insole, slowing the progression of this disease.—*J.M. Dawson*

◆ I found this to be a very straightforward and informative article dealing with the mechanics of the foot and knee and how they relate to each other. Clearly, in our practices we encounter numerous patients with marked degenerative changes associated with the medial joint line of the knee. Unfortunately, many of these patients present to our offices with a chief complaint of foot or ankle discomfort. In that our immediate reaction often involves the reduction of abnormal pronation, we find that, in many cases, we have exacerbated a mild knee problem or precipitated the onset of what might prove to be chronic knee problems. Excessive correction of abnormal foot function is likely to precipitate medial knee pain. If, in fact, the patient does present with a chief complaint of medial knee pain which can be delineated at the level of the medial jointline, then an orthotic device that pronates the foot at heel contact and in midstance proves quite effective. One of the orthotic modifications that I have found to be quite effective in treating these patients is the initiation of a reverse Kirby scive along the lateral heel cup. This will flatten the orthotic device along the lateral margin of the calcaneus and evert the heel at heel contact. In addition, a 3°–5° extrinsic forefoot valgus post is also capable of everting the foot and reducing the varus thrust to the medial knee jointline.—*R.L. Valmassy, D.P.M.*

Influence of Ankle Support on Joint Range of Motion Before and After Exercise: A Meta-Analysis

Cordova ML, Ingersoll CD, LeBlanc MJ (Indiana State University, Terre Haute, IN; State University of New York, Oswego, NY)
J Orthop Sports Phys Ther 30(4):170–182, 2000

Introduction—Ankle sprains are the most common injury occurring during sports activities. Ankle support studies have had inconsistent results partly due to varied measurement of range of motion, different applications of adhesive tape, and different styles of commercial lace-up braces and semi-rigid orthoses. This article combines the data available in literature in a meta-analysis to provide greater understanding of the role of ankle supports on joint range of motion before and after exercise. A meta-analysis is a statistical procedure that combines the results of related studies in a systematic and comprehensive manner.

Methods—It has been shown that ankle bracing and taping are effective in reducing ankle injuries in sports. These devices function best to restrict frontal plane (inversion/eversion) movement of the subtalar joint. The devices include ankle taping, lace-up braces, and semi-rigid orthoses (i.e., Air Cast stirrup).

This analysis examined a total of 253 cases from 19 studies. The treatment variables were ankle support (tape, lace-up, and semi-rigid) and time (before and after exercise). Range of motion was then examined (inversion, eversion, dorsiflexion, plantarflexion) before and after exercise using the three modalities.

Results—The semi-rigid device demonstrated greater restriction of inversion and eversion before and after exercise as compared to the tape and lace-up modalities. No difference was noted between the tape and lace-up devices. The lace-up brace was able to provide greater reduction in eversion than taping.

As far as ankle dorsiflexion and plantarflexion are concerned, only the tape and lace-up conditions were analyzed. When looking at dorsiflexion, the tape condition was more restrictive than the lace-up brace prior to and after exercise. There was no difference between the two modalities for plantarflexion. Overall, there was less restriction of plantarflexion after exercise for both modalities.

Conclusion—Ankle supports mainly function to restrict frontal plane motion, specifically, inversion sprains. The semi-rigid condition has greater restriction of this motion due to the stronger material used to restrict this motion. Even more important, the semi-rigid device maintained its support throughout and after exercise.

The data suggest that both lace-up braces and adhesive tape support are equally effective and should be adequate for prophylactic use in uninjured ankles. These supports offer a good compromise between restriction and mobility. However, since semi-rigid braces offer the greatest support before and after exercise, they should be used in athletes who have a history of ankle injuries or have chronic ankle sprains.—*O.T. Wang, D.P.M.*

♦ This article is interesting to me in that I was unfamiliar with the term "meta-analysis." This study reviewed *all* existing studies regarding ankle supports and ankle braces and was able to quantitate the information from all of the various studies into one body of information. Overall, the results were not contrary to anything already realized. The studies reviewed supported the fact that semi-rigid braces are certainly more appropriate to restrict ankle range of motion than tape or lace-up restrictive devices. The most salient clinical features of this article relate to the fact that taping loses its restrictive properties within 10 minutes after exercise and that both taping and lace-up braces are adequate prophylactic treatments, while a more rigid type of brace is advocated for the athlete with a history of ankle injuries or chronic lateral ankle instability.—*R.L. Valmassy, D.P.M.*

The Efficacy of Tone-Reducing Features in Orthotics on the Gait of Children with Spastic Diplegic Cerebral Palsy

Crenshaw S, Herzog R, Castagno P, Richards J, Miller F, Michaloski G, Moran E (Baylor University Medical Center, Dallas, TX; Alfred I. duPont Hospital for Children, Wilmington, DE; University of Delaware, Newark, DE)
J Pediatr Orthop 20(2):210–216, 2000

Objective—The objective of this study was to compare the effects of orthotics with and without tone-reducing features and with and without plantarflexion limitation using objective clinical measures of ambulation.

Methods—Three types of orthotics were used in this study: a standard articulating ankle–foot orthotic (AFO) molded to the heel but having a flat sole plate that extended to the tips of the toes, a modified standard articulating AFO with tone-reducing features (TRAFO), and a supramalleolar orthotic (SMO). Eight children (three girls and five boys) diagnosed with spastic diplegic cerebral palsy volunteered for this study. To qualify for the study, the children had to be able to walk independently with no assistive devices for 12 m. Each had to exhibit neutral (0°) dorsiflexion bilaterally with hindfoot and forefoot in maximum varus and 15° of inversion and eversion bilaterally.

Gait analysis was performed using a high-resolution video analysis system with 25 body markers located on the trunk, arms, pelvis, and lower extremities. A standard gait analysis was performed on each individual, and in each of the three different orthotic types, and in a baseline shoes-only condition. A 4-week accommodation period was allotted for each of the three devices.

Results—The most significant differences in this study were found in the kinematics at the ankle, which is the joint affected directly by the orthotics. For the maximal plantarflexion moment for the ankles, the AFO and the TRAFO conditions produced higher values than the SMO and the shoes-only conditions. Since both of the AFO devices limit plantarflexion, these values were expected. These differences support the concept that the benefit of the orthotic is limited to the direct mechanical effect of the orthotic on the joint it covers.

At the conclusion of the study, the parents and children were asked which orthotic they liked best. Three chose the standard AFO, four liked the TRAFO, and two preferred the SMO.

Conclusion—There were no clinically significant differences between the shoes-only and the SMO conditions and no clinical or statistical differences between the AFO and the TRAFO conditions. Based on the results of this study, the tone-reducing features of an AFO do not alter the gait appreciably when compared with the gait of the standard AFO.—*Q. Solomon*

◆ I found this article to be quite informative and useful with regard to this patient population. Numerous practitioners have attempted to utilize a variety of devices for children with cerebral palsy. At one time, it was quite acceptable to utilize AFOs with various tone-reducing features built into them in order to improve the overall gait pattern and stability of a child with cerebral palsy. The results of this article indicate that the various tone-reducing changes incorporated into an AFO do not increase the overall stability and function of a child with cerebral palsy. In fact, the traditional AFO seems to be efficient due to the fact that it clearly is capable of limiting plantarflexory range of motion during gait. This study indicates that it is this specific feature of an AFO more than all the tone-reducing modifications that allow a youngster to be more stable in gait. I would like to add that in cases of lesser degrees of involvement, functional foot orthoses of the UCBL type or Blake inverted variety seem to work especially well in reducing significant degrees of pes planus deformity with these children. Specifically, with an inverted device, the use of a 55° inverted orthosis with a 6-mm medial scive and the addition of a medial flange seems to work exceptionally well in improving the gait of this patient population.—*R.L. Valmassy, D.P.M.*

The Influence of Foot Positioning on Ankle Sprains

Wright IC, Neptune RR, van den Bogert AJ, Nigg BM (University of Calgary, Calgary, Canada; Cleveland Clinic Foundation, Cleveland, OH)
J Biomech 33:513–519, 2000

Introduction—Ankle sprains are one of the most common causes of sports injury. Previously injured ankles are more prone to spraining their ankles. There are many factors which may contribute to excessive supination that cause inversion sprains. One of these factors is the position of the foot as it initially makes contact with the ground. The purpose of this study was to test the hypothesis that inappropriate foot positioning at touchdown increases the likelihood of ankle sprains.

Methods—Computer simulations of 10 subjects performing side-shuffle movements were analyzed. The landing surface, subtalar joint angle, and the talocural joint angle were each varied to allow for a multitude of various conditions. A sprain was considered to have happened if the torque about the subtalar joint or the angular displacement at the subtalar joint exceeded a respective given value. These threshold values were varied.

Results—When the initial supination angle was increased, there was a small increase in the occurrence of sprains. When there was a decrease in the initial supination angle, there was a small decrease in the occurrence of sprains. This was only true when the supination torque threshold or the supination angle threshold was low. There was very little influence on initial supination angle when the thresholds were relatively high.

When the thresholds for the angular displacement at the subtalar joint and the torque about the subtalar joint were large, dorsiflexion and plantarflexion influenced the occurrence of sprains. There was an increase in the occurrence of sprains when the initial plantarflexion angle was increased, while the opposite was true for when there was an increase in the initial dorsiflexion angle. These effects were not observed when the threshold values were low.

Conclusions—To get an accurate result, only the data collected when the threshold was large should be analyzed. In this scenario, the initial supination angle had little effect on sprain occurrence. On the other hand, initial plantarflexion had a high influence on the occurrence of ankle sprains when the thresholds were set high. This agrees with earlier data showing that the anterior talofibular ligament is the most commonly sprained ligament. This ligament is sprained when the foot is in a supinated, plantarflexed position. This study showed that an initial plantarflexion had a greater influence on the occurrence of sprains than an initial supination. The use of an ankle brace or taping of the ankle may help reposition the unloaded foot, and help keep it from landing in a plantarflexed position.—*S. Patel*

♦ I found this to be a quite interesting, informative, and useful article regarding the mechanics involved with inversion ankle sprains. The information presented that was most salient concerns the fact that a more plantarflexed foot in touch-down would increase the likelihood of that individual sustaining an inversion sprain. The results of the information presented in this article suggest that an increased plantarflexed position of the foot at touch-down increases not only the sprain susceptibility, but also the severity of the sprain. The authors' conclusion is that external techniques such as bracing and taping reduce the overall range of motion of the ankle joint and decrease the ability of the foot to be maintained in a plantarflexed attitude. If this is the case, then certainly there would be a decreased likelihood of an individual spraining an ankle. The information presented in this article also should make one consider the appropriate use of range-of-motion and strengthening exercises following any type of inversion sprain. In our clinic population, we find that the most likely individuals to sustain recurrent injuries are those who have not been properly rehabilitated. Again, I must stress the importance of muscle strengthening exercises following this type of athletic injury in order to decrease the likelihood of subsequent episodes of involvement.—*R.L. Valmassy, D.P.M.*

The Effectiveness of Gait Plates in Controlling In-toeing Symptoms in Young Children

Redmond AC (University of Western Sydney–Macarthur, New South Wales, Australia)
J Am Podiatr Med Assoc 90(2):70–76, 2000

Introduction—Although in-toeing is a common pathology found in young children, many parents find it disconcerting to see their child walk this way. The most common complaints these parents have are abnormal shoe wear, increased fatigue with walking, and recurrent tripping. This study evaluated the parents' satisfaction following gait plate therapy for controlling in-toed gait.

Materials and Methods—A rigid plastic plate, which covered the sole of the foot up to the metatarsals and extended onto the fifth toe with the medial side cut at a 45° angle, was used as a gait plate on 18 children with in-toed feet. The children selected for the study were between 18 months and 5 years, had only postural abnormalities, experienced symptoms associated with in-toeing, and had an in-toeing angle greater than −3°. The plates were contoured, not posted to neutral, and worn with flexible, lightweight canvas athletic shoes. Questionnaires were given to the parents prior to the children wearing the devices and then 1 month after the intervention. The parents were asked about the frequency of tripping, the extent of injury following tripping, the preferred sleeping position for the child, and how concerned the parent was versus how concerned the child was about the in-toeing. Since the data collected from the parents was subjective, the questions were written so that they could be cross-referenced. Associations between the answers were studies with the use of the Spearman rank correlations. Overall, there appeared to be a high degree of consistency in the responses.

Results—There was a 6° improvement in the foot placement angle with gait plates in situ. After 1 month of wearing the gait plate, only one parent denied improvement in the frequency of tripping. Only one parent stated that the gait plate was not a worthwhile treatment option. In general, the parents' responses to the questionnaire revealed that they were pleased with the outcome of the treatment.

Discussion—Long-term effects of using the gait plate are still doubtful. Also, the relationship between sleeping patterns and in-toeing is still questionable. This study may have been skewed since the responses were confidential but not anonymous and there may have been a positive placebo effect. In the author's opinion, these results show that further evaluation of gait plate treatment for in-toed gait should be done. —*G.H. Jhala*

♦ I found this to be a quite informative and well written paper regarding the use of gait plates. Over the years, I have experienced varying results with the use of gait plates in my patient population. However, I must agree with the author who states that there certainly is a reduction in the tripping and falling element of an adducted gait pattern. I feel that the use of gait plates does often improve overall stability in gait and may, in fact, introduce some minor element of cosmetic improvement as well. One specific point of utilizing gait plates that I feel is clinically significant is that they seem to function best when utilized in a child's flexible shoe. Typically we find that a stiffer soled, rigid shoe works better with a functional foot orthosis to decrease abnormal pronation. However, in the use of a gait plate, the shoe should be more flexible in order to allow for some abduction and pronation to occur. Finally, I have found that a gait plate does not last as long as a functional foot orthosis. I typically advise parents that a functional foot orthosis will last from 2 to 3 years for their children. When I have prescribed a gait plate, I have found that the device will typically last between 18 and 24 months due to the fact that the distal-lateral margin of the orthotic becomes a source of irritation as the child's foot grows. —*R.L. Valmassy, D.P.M.*

12 Anatomy of the Lower Leg and Foot

STACEY A. PAUKOVITZ, D.P.M.

Management of Ischemic Heel Ulceration and Gangrene: An Evaluation of Factors Associated with Successful Healing
Treiman GS, Oderich GSC, Ashrafi A, Schneider PA (University of Utah School of Medicine, Salt Lake City, UT; Hawaii Permanente Medical Group, Honolulu, HI)
J Vasc Surg 31(6):1110–1118, 2000

Introduction—Development of wounds over the heel is a frequent problem in bed-bound patients. Ulceration of the ischemic heel is difficult to treat and often leads to gangrene or foot amputation. Difficulty is generally seen as multifactorial. This study seeks to identify factors associated with increased healing rates.

Methods—Charts were reviewed of all patients with heel ulcers and documented arterial insufficiency treated at four different institutions from 1994 to 1999. Revascularization was performed at the discretion of attending vascular surgeons. Debilitated patients, where revascularization was not an option, were not included in the data analysis. Most patients with occlusive lesions proximal to the ankle received bypass. Most bypasses were to the posterior tibial artery. Demography, cardiovascular risk factors, details of the operative procedure, and clinical course were statistically analyzed. Graft patency and foot salvage were determined by the life table method.

Results—Ninety-one patients had interventional treatment. Cardiovascular risk factors included diabetes, hypertension, impaired renal function, tobacco use, existing heart disease, and hyperlipidemia. Average duration of nonhealing was 6 months. Overall treatments consisted of topical wound care and one or more other modalities, including operative debridement, nonweightbearing, tissue transfer, limited amputation, bypass grafting, and below-knee amputation (BKA). Of grafts, primary patency was 87%, while secondary patency was 91%. After grafting, 90% had at least one patent tibial artery to the ankle. Ankle-brachial index (ABI) improved from 0.40 to 0.91. Seventy-three percent of ulcers healed, 16% remained unhealed, and 11% went on to BKA.

Limb salvage was 86% at 3 years. All patients with wound healing had one or more patent tibial arteries. After revascularization, statistically significant factors for healing included normal renal function, cigarette smoking, absence of hyperlipidemia, palpable pulses, patent posterior tibial artery, and one or more patent tibial arteries.

Discussion—Based on the results of this study, the greatest likelihood for success of healing ischemic heel ulcers is achieved when a patient has a patent posterior tibial artery and good renal function. This study confirms the fact that renal failure, in spite of patent arteries, is an inhibitor to wound healing. However, there were enough patients with diabetes and renal failure who were successful in healing to argue for offering vascular reconstruction to these patients. One limitation of this study is the absence of off-loading devices as a treatment modality factor. Also, the presence of smoking as a positive factor is perhaps an indication of a small population sample leading to a type II statistical error.—*D. Clement*

◆ This article reiterates what those experienced in wound care already know—ischemic heel ulcers are quite challenging. It is well known that diabetes mellitus, ESRD, malnutrition, peripheral vascular disease, and systemic infection impair wound healing. Unfortunately, this is the patient population often requiring limb-salvage procedures.

In this particular study, the factors associated with wound healing were inconsistent, making it difficult to predict a successful outcome. Patients with palpable pedal pulses often resulted in amputation and cigarette smokers had better success rates than nonsmokers. Such results seem unlikely, and may be due to statistical error and low patient population.

It has been my experience that two major factors influencing success are 1) patency of the posterior tibial artery (which maximizes regional perfusion to the heel), and 2) whether the patient has end-stage renal disease. This study confirms that patients with renal insufficiency or renal failure are at significantly increased risk for limb loss, even with intact arterial circulation to the foot. However, this should not exclude these patients from attempts at revascularization and limb salvage. Increasing perfusion and aggressive wound debridement by a multidisciplinary team approach yields the best results, but with no guarantees.—*S.A. Paukovitz, D.P.M.*

Result of Arthrodesis of the Hallux Metatarsophalangeal Joint Using Bone Graft for Restoration of Length

Myerson MS, Schon L, McGuigan FX, Oznur A (The Union Memorial Hospital, Baltimore, MD)
Foot Ankle Int 21(4):297–306, 2000

Introduction—Arthrodesis of the hallux metatarsophalangeal (MTP) joint is often performed for patients who suffer from arthritis, hallux rigiditus, and complications that arise from hallux valgus surgery. Maintaining the length of the first metatarsal and hallux is important to ensure a favorable outcome and eliminate the sequela of a short first ray. Unfortunately, there are cases in which avascular necrosis, infection, congenital a condition, or a previous surgery has caused the first metatarsal or hallux to be short. In this patient population one must consider using a bone graft in order to achieve the desired length. Arthrodesis with cancellous bone graft is associated with shortening. This study looks at an alternative way to restore the length of the metatarsal using an interpositional structural bone graft.

Methods—Twenty-four patients (18 women, six men) with an average age of 45.4 years old were treated using a bone graft for the restoration of the length of the first ray. Patients had previous surgeries that had shortened the first ray. In addition, seven patients had deep bone infection preoperatively, one patient had septic arthritis, and nine had avascular necrosis, although none of them had diabetes or were immunocompromised. Fifteen patients had concomitant callosities and metarsalgia of the lesser digits. Those with infections had staged arthrodesis using antibiotic-impregnated bone cement, then had an arthrodesis 4–6 weeks later. All patients had either a structural autograft or structural allograft. The allograft was harvested from the femoral head and either unicortical or bicortical in eight of the patients, the autograft was from the iliac crest and tricortical (15 patients) or distal medial tibia (one patient). To fill any defects in the metatarsal or base of the proximal phalanx, cancellous bone was harvested either from the iliac crest or from additional allograft. Fixation that was used was determined by assessing the quality and shape of the metatarsal and proximal phalanx. The following were all used: beaded Steinmann pins (two patients), beaded Steinmann pins and screws (one patient), screws (three patients), dorsal plates and screws (seven patients), screws and beaded Kirschner wires (four patients), dorsal plates screws and Kirschner wires (two patients), and Kirschner wires (one patient). Patients were placed in a posterior plaster splint until sutures were removed, then they were placed in a short leg cast for 5 weeks, and then a rigid wooden shoe until arthrodesis was achieved clinically and radiographically. At the final evaluation (mean 63 months after surgery), all patients were required to complete the American Orthopedic Foot and Ankle Society's (AOFAS) score; clinically the range of motion of the interphalangeal joint and the metatarsalcuneiform joint was assessed and the calluses were appreciated.

Results—

- *AOFAS scores*: Because the nature of the arthrodesis procedure, the total amount of points attainable was 95 due to the loss of range of motion of the hallux MTP joint. The mean score preoperative was 40 points with a range of 22–60 points. The mean score postoperatively was 79 points with a range of 66–90.

- *Calluses/metatarsalgia*: Preoperatively 15 patients had calluses that with metatarsalgia. Postoperatively the conditions improved although the study did not use quantitative methods to assess. Four patients had mild metatarsalgia, but no calluses, and all reported improvement from the preoperative status.

- *Graft size/first ray length*: The average length of the graft inserted into the first MTP joint was 22 mm with a range of 11–35. The actual lengthening of the first ray was assessed using the lateral radiograph from the end of the proximal phalanx to the base of the first metatarsal. The mean was 13 mm, with a range of 0–29 mm.

- *Fusion*: At 13 weeks 79% of patients had fusion of the hallux MTP joint. The range of time to achieve fusion was 11–16 weeks. Nonunion occurred in 21% of the patients. These patients had the iliac crest autograft. Three patients had fixation with dorsal plate and screws and two had screws combined with threaded K-wires. Two patients had initially treated with a silastic arthroplasty and a total joint replacement and had osteomyelitis. The other three had previously undergone silastic arthroplasty. Two of these nonfusions were asymptomatic, the other three underwent subsequent procedures.

Conclusion—This procedure proved to help obtain fusion and restoration of length of the first ray.—*T. Marshall*

♦ First MTP joint arthrodesis has gained recent popularity over other joint destructive procedures such as the Keller bunionectomy or implant arthroplasty. It is also used as a secondary salvage procedure from failed MTP joint surgery. This article was a good compilation of the authors' experience utilizing bone graft for first MTP joint fusions. Grafting was necessary due to bone loss from unsuccessful metatarsal osteotomies, implant arthroplasties, Keller resections, and total joint replacements. Interpositional structural bone graft must be considered to restore length of the first ray and weightbearing function in order to eliminate an existing metatarsalgia.

Interestingly, the nonunions that occurred in this study were associated with iliac crest autograph. It is well documented that interpositional bone graft has a higher rate of nonunion than an in situ arthrodesis. It is also known that in revisional procedures, autograph is superior to allograph. Autogenous grafts have the advantage of viable cell transfer and immunologic compatibility. They are ideal for areas that require osteogenesis and where vascularity is a concern. The authors attribute their failures to possible choice of fixation, methods of exposure, and initial poor bone quality.

The authors compare their work to a study using an in situ arthrodesis that had a higher arthrodesis rate (94%). In addition to the first MTP joint procedure, resection of the lesser metatarsal heads was necessary to preserve weightbearing function. The authors feel this procedure is ablative, therefore, a poor choice. Lesser MTP joint function should be preserved whenever possible.—*S.A. Paukovitz, D.P.M.*

Optimisation of the Non-invasive Assessment of Critical Limb Ischaemia Requiring Invasive Treatment

Ubbink DTh, Tulevski II, de Graaff JC, Legemate DA, Jacobs MJHM
(Academic Medical Centre, Amsterdam, The Netherlands)
Eur J Vasc Endovasc Surg 19:131–137, 2000

Introduction—As arterial insufficiency threatens the viability of the leg, the surgeon must make a decision when to act. This judgment is largely based on objective findings from peripheral blood pressures. The European Consensus Document (ECD) utilizes the Fontaine staging criteria for the diagnosis of "critical limb ischaemia" (CLI), but there are no treatment algorithms that follow these criteria. The current study seeks to determine the "optimal cut-off values of toe blood pressures and transcutaneous oxygen pressure ($TcpO_2$)" to aid in the detection of CLI.

Patients and Methods—Patients with Fontaine stages III and IV were examined. A total of 49 patients, (65 legs) were studied. Gold standard of CLI was determined to be invasive treatment required within 6 weeks of diagnosis. Validity of this gold standard was also ascertained.

Surgeons were blinded to $TcpO_2$ and toe blood pressures taken. "Ankle pressure" was defined as the highest pressure value of the two ankle arteries. "Toe pressure" was defined as the highest pressure obtained from both the hallux and second digit. $TcpO_2$ was taken from the dorsum of the foot.

The noninvasive results were examined with the therapeutic action taken to determine the best cut-off criteria used for the determination of CLI. Receiver-operator characteristic (ROC) curves were established for the measurements taken. Statistical analysis was performed.

Results—Of the 65 legs included in the study, 38 (58%) required invasive treatment. Four amputations were performed in this group. Those in this group also showed a significant increase in systolic pressures postinvasive treatment.

Toe pressure showed a linear relationship between the sitting and supine positions. The $TcpO_2$ showed a more logarithmic curve. Toe pressure and $TcpO_2$ measured in the supine or sitting position are equally diagnostic. In the sitting position, all patients with a toe pressure of ≤ 70 and $TcpO_2$ of ≤ 40 mmHg were ruled to have CLI.

Discussion—CLI, when defined using the Fontaine staging criteria and ankle blood pressure, does not imply the need for invasive treatment. Additional measurements such as $TcpO_2$ below 25 mmHg and toe pressure below 30 mmHg measured in the supine position, when used in combination, increase the pretest probability to 12.4.

Conclusion—A definition of CLI is needed to guide the clinical treatment of patients and design effective algorithms. Measurements taken in the sitting position are not more effective in the diagnosis.

For the patient with severe leg ischemia, toe rather than ankle pressure measurements may be more predictive of the need for invasive treatment. Transcutaneous oxygen pressure values may also aid in the definitive diagnosis of severe leg ischemia.—*G. Grant*

♦ This study defines critical limb ischemia (CLI) as severe leg ischemia requiring invasive treatment within 6 weeks, including primary amputation. It attempts to establish optimal cut-off values to detect CLI requiring invasive therapy.

Evaluation of a single test is often misleading—for example, ankle-brachial indexes (ABIs) are often falsely elevated from calcified vessels; TcpO^2 values may be influenced by cellulitis and edema; and digital temperatures influence Toe Pressures.

CLI defined by ABIs alone had low (58%) pretest probability. With the addition of toe pressures and TcpO^2 measurements, predictive values increased considerably. Evaluation of a single parameter alone is of little use, but collectively, noninvasive testing plays an important role in decision-making. Obviously, we should never treat values alone, and correlating these with the clinical picture is crucial. Unfortunately, application of toe and oxygen pressures is not standard practice. Using an experienced center that performs a comprehensive exam is important.—*S.A. Paukovitz, D.P.M.*

Congenital Tarsal Coalition: Multimodality Evaluation with Emphasis on CT and MR Imaging

Newman J, Newberg AH (New England Baptist Bone and Joint Institute, New England Baptist Hospital, Boston, MA)
RadioGraphics 20(2):321–332, 2000

Introduction—Tarsal coalition, a frequent source of foot and ankle pain, is defined as abnormal fusion between two tarsal bones. Approximately 90% involve the talocalcaneal (TC) or calcaneonavicular (CN) joints. Tarsal coalitions can be subclassified as fibrous, cartilaginous, or osseous. Initial presentation is rearfoot or tarsal pain or stiffness, exacerbated with weight gain, increased athletic activity, or after antecedent trauma. It is a common etiology of peroneal spastic or rigid flatfoot conditions. Physical examination reveals a decrease in rearfoot motion with concomitant pes planus and calcaneal valgus deformity.

Radiography of Tarsal Coalitions—Initial evaluation of suspected tarsal coalition requires three views of the foot: anteroposterior, 45° internal oblique, and lateral. Most talonavicular (TN) and CN coalitions can be diagnosed by conventional radiography alone. CN coalitions are best seen on the 45° internal oblique view. Furthermore, the lateral view may demonstrate the "anteater's sign," an elongated anterior dorsal calcaneus. The middle facet at the level of the sustentaculum tali is most commonly involved in TC coalition. Secondary radiographic signs of this subtype include talar beaking, posterior subtalar joint (STJ) narrowing, rounding of the lateral process of the talus, and an obscured middle facet on lateral radiographs.

Computed Tomography (CT) of Tarsal Coalitions—CT of the rearfoot and ankle should be performed in the coronal and axial planes, with 3-mm section thickness and both feet imaged simultaneously. The advantages of CT imaging over conventional radiographs are in the precise evaluation of the extent of coalition, involvement at the STJ, and associated degenerative changes. CN coalitions display a broadening of the medial aspect of the anterior and dorsal calcaneus as it lies in apposition to the navicular, and are best visualized with cross-sectional imaging. TC coalitions are best viewed with coronal scans. The orientation of the sustentaculum tail and middle facet of the STJ are crucial to the identification of this pathology. In a normal foot, the sustentaculum tali slopes upward medially. However, in TC coalition, it slopes downward or the articular surface is oriented in the transverse plane.

Magnetic Resonance (MR) Imaging of Tarsal Coalitions—Axial or oblique axial, coronal, and sagittal plane images should be obtained of the rearfoot and ankle. T1- and T2-weighted fast spin-echo images are adequate for evaluation purposes; however, the use of at least one fat-suppressed sequence in the coronal or sagittal plane is recommended to assist in identifying bone marrow and soft-tissue edema or inflammatory changes. CN coalitions are best pictured with sagittal and axial MR views, while TC coalitions are best assessed with coronal plane images. Bone marrow contiguity across the fused articulation is observed in osseous coalitions, while joint space narrowing is seen in nonosseous coalitions. In addition, cartilaginous coalitions may evidence an area of joint space signal intensity similar to that of fluid or cartilage.

Treatment—Conservative treatment includes orthotics, casting, nonsteroid anti-inflammatory drugs, steroid injections, or physical therapy. Operative treatment is indicated if this regimen is not successful in alleviating symptoms. CN coalitions may be resected, and regrowth of the bony bridge may be precluded with interposition of the extensor digitorum brevis muscle. Similarly, TC coalitions may be treated with middle facet resection and fat interposition. Significant degenerative TN joint disease or excision failures lend themselves to eventual triple arthrodesis.—*E. Zarutsky*

♦ When a patient presents with rearfoot pain, stiffness, and decreased range of motion, a tarsal coalition should be high on the list of differential diagnoses. Standard radiographs (AP, lateral, and oblique) taken in the office may identify the coalition, but in many cases, further imaging is needed.

This article is a good review of clinical findings and imaging features (radiographs, CT, and MR Imaging) of congenital tarsal coalition. CT and MR imaging are also useful for surgical planning to depict joint involvement and secondary degenerative features.

CT scanning is the "gold standard" in identifying coalitions, but this is conclusive only if the union is osseous. MR imaging is needed to identify fibrous or cartilaginous coalitions, and should be used for children who have not yet reached osseous maturity. — *S.A. Paukovitz, D.P.M.*

Saving the Diabetic Foot

Smith RJ (Memphis, TN)
J Natl Med Assoc 92(8):405–410, 2000

Introduction—Approximately 16 million Americans suffer from diabetes, and of those, 15% will eventually develop a foot ulcer at some point in their life. Typically, the diabetic ulcer is a result of vascular and muscle changes, which often lead to necrosis and tissue loss, unfortunately before appropriate therapy is implemented. The diabetic situation is further complicated by neuropathy, for it affects all the nerves in the foot: motor, sensory, and autonomic. Consequently, approximately 50% of major leg amputations occur in diabetic patients as a result of an infected foot ulcer.

Methods—Early infections can be treated on an outpatient basis if the level of blood glucose is monitored closely, proper care of the feet and skin is taken, and a broad-spectrum antibiotic is administered. Bed rest is advised for these patients for 1–2 weeks and, if needed, crutches may be used. The patient is to return to the clinic in 1 week. If the infection has not improved after this week, hospitalization is recommended. In order to decrease further tissue loss, drainage and debridement of the specific compartment involved should occur during the 1 or 2 day of admission. Follow-up therapy can be instituted on an outpatient basis and includes a whirlpool, weekly visits, and local debridement.

Case I—A 50-year-old woman presented with hyperglycemia, marked sepsis, and a gangrenous right foot. Hydration and antibiotics were administered and she was then taken to surgery, where all four compartments were drained. Whirlpool therapy, intravenous antibiotics, and bed rest in a skilled nursing facility for 6 weeks constituted her therapy. The wound healed without amputation of the foot.

Case II—A 59-year-old man with type 2 diabetes (insulin dependent) presented with a 2-week history of infection and swelling of the left foot. He proved to have significant vascular occlusive disease and the fifth toe and lateral compartment showed signs of wet gangrene. On May 17, 1995, the patient underwent surgery where Ray amputation of the fifth toe occurred and drainage of the lateral compartment allowed the open wound to be packed. Whirlpool therapy and weekly local debridements were implemented. A follow-up in 1998 showed both feet in good condition and a continuance of the patient's control over his disease.

Case III—A 60-year-old woman with diabetes presented with an ulcer measuring 3.5 cm on the sole that had been present for several months. Her foot was warm and enlarged, pulses were good, and both the transverse and longitudinal arches were absent. Upon review of her X-rays, Charcot osteoarthropathy of the midfoot with a rocker bottom deformity was discovered. Furthermore, a needle was found imbedded deep within the foot, even though the patient gave no history of this occurring. Treatment began with frequent debridement and control of hyperglycemia, in addition to the use of an insole. After 5 months, the ulcer showed signs of improvement and eventually healed completely.

Discussion—It is imperative that therapy for the severely infected diabetic foot includes evaluation of the vascular supply to the foot and anatomical location of the infection in the foot, wide debridement, drainage, and appropriate antibiotics. Ulcers should be treated promptly and aggressively. Patients need to be educated in foot care, most importantly on how to control hyperglycemia and skin care.—*A. Duckworth*

♦ This article provides a very basic overview of the diabetic foot, and adds very little new information to the current literature. In fact, it barely skims the surface of ulcer management.

Our profession understands the diabetic foot better than any other medical specialty. The key is prevention and patient education, but unfortunately, it is usually not that simple. Quite often we initially see the patient with deep ulcers and limb-threatening infections already present. In these instances, aggressive measures must be initiated.

A large percentage of my practice involves diabetic management and limb salvage. The key to success has been because of our close affiliation with the vascular surgeons. Peripheral vascular disease occurs earlier and more frequently in the diabetic patient, but does not necessarily adversely influence the outcome of arterial reconstruction. Many times revascularization must be performed prior to any foot surgery. Foot debridement only takes precedence in emergent cases involving gas gangrene, sepsis, or plantar space infections that need immediate incise and drainage.—*S.A. Paukovitz, D.P.M.*

MR Imaging of Disorders of the Posterior Tibialis Tendon

Schweitzer ME, Karasick D (Thomas Jefferson University Hospital, Philadelphia, PA)
AJR 175:627–635, 2000

Introduction—Posterior tibial tendon dysfunction (PTTD) is best thought of as a continuum of disorders. Because most of these disorders are not clinically painful, patients seek medical attention relatively late. Therefore, later stages of the disorder are frequently seen on imaging.

The posterior tibialis tendon forms in the distal third of the leg, courses behind the medial malleolus, and inserts into the medial navicular and the plantar aspects of the cuneiforms and the bases of the second through fourth metatarsals. Blood supply to the tendon is most tenuous at its midportion; additionally, the mesotendon is absent distally.

Most PTTD is caused by a combination of impingement and ischemia. Important systemic risk factors are hypertension, obesity, lupus, gout, rheumatoid arthritis, and Reiter's syndrome.

MR Imaging—The axial plane is optimal when obtaining MR images for evaluation of the posterior tibialis tendon; controversy exists whether the images should be captured perpendicular to the long axis of the tendon or perpendicular to the long axis of the leg and foot. Sagittal imaging is the secondary plane. Contrast material is indicated in cases of suspected synovitis, infection, and inflammatory arthritis, and for insertional tendonitis.

On MR imaging, tendon is typically black, without any internal signal intensity. In a healthy person, the posterior tibialis tendon is roughly twice the size of the two adjacent tendons. A small amount of fluid in the synovial sheath of the posterior tibialis tendon is normal; this fluid measures 1–2 mm, and is almost never circumferential. Because there is no normal sheath distally, fluid observed at the distal aspect of the tendon is abnormal.

Staging of PTTD—Clinically, the first presenting stage of PTTD is paratendonitis or synovitis. MR images reveal partially circumferential high signal intensity located distally. At this stage, the tendon itself is normal.

The next stage of PTTD is tendonosis. Pathologically, there is intratendinous degeneration of collagen, local necrosis, calcification, and hypocellularity. If visible on MR imaging, there is subtle focal high signal intensity in the tendon.

Microscopic tears eventually become macroscopic tendon fiber tears. Tears can scar over and lead to tendon thickening, retract and lead to thinning, or severely weaken the tendon and result in a gap.

Secondary signs of PTTD can include talonavicular fault, uncovering of the talus, focal spurring of the distal tibia, and heel valgus. PTTD can also cause focal marrow edema, typically seen underneath the course of the tendon in the tibia, the talus, or the navicular.—*T.C. Melillo, D.P.M.*

♦ Over the course of the last decade, posterior tibial tendon dysfunction has been recognized as a common cause of unilateral flatfoot, and disabling rearfoot pain. Its diagnosis can be made clinically, and a careful physical exam is essential. Standard radiographs may demonstrate secondary signs associated with this disorder, including heel valgus, talonavicular fault, forefoot abduction, and collapse of the longitudinal arch. Further studies, such as MR imaging, help to accurately diagnose and stage the deformity. Conti et al developed a classification scheme of tears of the PTT based on MR imaging specifically for this purpose.

Some controversy exists over the exact role of MR imaging in the treatment plan of PTTD. Some feel it is used too frequently in clinical practice, and not necessary to make a diagnosis. Others find it necessary in staging the dysfunction and formulating an appropriate treatment plan. MR imaging has provided clear detail of abnormalities of the PTT and should be correlated with clinical findings. It is a useful tool in staging the deformity, managing, and planning surgical intervention. This article is a good review of finding on MR imaging associated with this common disorder.—*S.A. Paukovitz, D.P.M.*

Ankle Arthrodesis: Indications and Techniques

Abidi NA, Gruen GS, Conti SF (Jefferson Medical College, Thomas Jefferson University, and Rothman Institute, Philadelphia, PA; University of Pittsburgh Medical Center, Pittsburgh, PA)
J Am Acad Orthop Surg 8(3):200–209, 2000

Introduction—When conservative treatment modalities for arthritic and associated pain or deformity experienced only at the ankle joint fail, ankle arthrodesis is indicated. Several options of surgical technique are available with the ankle arthrodesis. As a general rule, patients with significant osteopenia or septic ankle joint require external fixation; the arthroscopic arthrodesis is utilized in patients with mild deformity, while the open arthrodesis is utilized during severe malalignment and deformity of the foot and ankle. Many complications can be associated with ankle arthrodesis; studies reveal nonunion is the most encountered complication.

Methods—The authors reviewed three surgical techniques, including external fixation, arthroscopic arthrodesis, and open arthrodesis, while comparing results from scoring systems measuring ankle functionability before and after operative treatment. Furthermore, several risk factors for nonunion were reviewed.

Results—Scoring systems and various studies have demonstrated success with and indications for ankle arthrodesis. The most successful technique combines an open approach with compression and internal fixation. Risk factors associated with nonunion, noted in one study, include severity of the fracture, open injury, local infection, osteonecrosis of the talus, and smoking.

Conclusion—Surgical techniques utilized in ankle arthrodesis are determined by the underlying disorder, but the open approach using internal fixation appears to have greater success postoperatively. Preoperative examination of other lower extremity joints, limb alignment, and the relationship of the hind-foot to the forefoot, as well as gait appraisal should be performed. The major complication is nonunion, which is associated with risk factors that include smoking and osteonecrosis of the talus. Furthermore, regardless of the appropriate surgical procedure selected, the talus should be posteriorly displaced, the ankle externally rotated 5°–10°, and the rearfoot placed in valgus by 5°–7°. Studies reveal ankle arthrodesis as a successful treatment modality for ankle arthritis, deformity, and pain with appropriate surgical technique and proper candidate screening.—*M. Garrison*

♦ This article was a good review of the indications for ankle arthrodesis as well as the methods of fixation available. Ankle arthrodesis is an end-stage salvage procedure to provide relief of long-term pain and functional disability. It is associated with multiple complications, including nonunion rates in as high as 40% of patients. Prior to considering ankle fusion, all nonoperative measures should be fully exhausted and patients should be screened carefully for identifiable risk factors.

With advances in surgical techniques and fixation devices, success rates have increased. It is a technically demanding procedure, and should be performed by the experienced surgeon. Arthroscopic ankle fusions have gained popularity and shown joint fusion almost 6 weeks earlier than conventional internal fixation. However, this is indicated for minimal deformities not requiring aggressive bone resection. There is a high learning curve associated with external fixation application, but it offers many advantages over other techniques. With proper planning, choice of fixation, operative techniques, and the experienced surgeon, ankle arthrodesis can be a reliable procedure.—*S.A. Paukovitz, D.P.M.*

The Role of Bone Scanning in Severe Frostbite of the Extremities: A Retrospective Study of 88 Cases

Cauchy E, Chetaille E, Lefevre M, Kerelou E, Marsigny B (Chamonix Hospital, Chamonix, France; Bonneville Hospital, France)
Eur J Nucl Med 27(5):497–502, 2000

Objective—The objective is to perform a retrospective study of the results of two-phase technetium-99 m hydroxymethylene diphosphonate bone scans in 88 patients with severe frostbite of the extremities.

Methods—This study analyzed the bone scans performed on 88 patients with frostbite at the Chamonix Hospital in France. Of the 88 patients, six were women and 82 were men, with an average age of 32.1 years. The inclusion criteria were based on the topography and features of the lesions, including the insensitive area and the presence of cyanosis extending proximally beyond the distal phalanx of at least one finger or toe. All patients were evaluated within 48 hours after rewarming and all underwent a first bone scan (BS1) within 5 days after rewarming. In the BS1, the radiotracer used was sodium hydroxymethylene diphosphonate coupled to technetium-99 m. The bone scans were completed in two phases: an early tissue phase 2–3 minutes after intravenous administration of the tracer and a bone phase taken approximately 180 minutes later. A second bone scan (BS2) was performed in 36 patients more than 5 days after rewarming when low tracer uptake or absence of uptake had been observed in one or more phalanges.

Results—The bone scans of 88 patients included 53 scans of the hands, 48 of the feet, and 13 of both hands and feet. An excellent correlation was found between low tracer uptake, or absence, in the phalanges and later amputation. This correlation was especially strong during the bone phase of the scans. Normal or high uptake of the tracer in the phalanges was a reliable indicator of ultimate healing. The sensitivity of the examination was enhanced even more by the addition of a second bone scan which was performed on 36 of the 88 patients due to low uptake of the tracer. A comparative analysis of BS1 and BS2 demonstrated that some of the lesions were still evolving between day 2 and day 8. In the case of severe sepsis, the results of BS1 can serve as an indication for an emergency amputation.

Conclusion—On the basis of the findings, it is recommended that bone scans be performed close to day 2 after rewarming in all patients who present with lesions extending proximally to include the entirety of one or more phalanges. BS2 should be performed close to day 8 if there is an area of low or absence of tracer uptake. This is an excellent means by which to access frostbite to the extremities. As early as day 2 after injury, bone scanning can indicate whether amputation is necessary.—*Q. Solomon*

◆ Bone scanning has been shown to be an invaluable tool in the management of severe frostbite. It helps to predict tissue viability and level of later amputation. However, surgical intervention should only take place after complete demarcation. Depending on the severity of the frostbite, this may take up to 8 weeks. Until that time, local wound care is performed. Immediate amputation may be necessary in cases of severe sepsis, hypothermia, and gas in the soft tissues.

This study recommends an initial bone scan between days 2 and 4, and a second between days 7 and 10. Nonviable tissue appears as a defect in perfusion—the viable tissue is hyperemic and shows increased uptake. Limitations to this study included the presence of blisters, subjectivity of reading the scans, and improved bone scan quality during the course of the study.—*S.A. Paukovitz, D.P.M.*

Giant Cell Tumor of the Bones of the Hand and Foot

Biscaglia R, Bacchini P, Bertoni F (University of Verona, Verona, Italy; Rizzoli Orthopedic Institute, Bologna, Italy)
Cancer 88(9):2022–2031, 2000

Introduction—Giant cell tumors (GCT), although rarely seen in the bones of the hand and foot, share many radiographic and histological features with other giant cell lesions such as aneurismal bone cyst (ABC), giant cell reparative granuloma (GCRG), and giant cell osteogenic sarcoma. Therefore, it is important that GCT still be included in the differential diagnosis when dealing with nonspecific bone lesions of the hand and foot.

Methods—The Rizzoli Orthopedic Institute in Italy has studied hundreds of cases of GCTs over the past 50 years. Of these, only eight GCTs were found in the small bones of the hand, while 21 were found in the small bones of the foot. All 29 cases were followed and studied with emphasis put on clinical presentation, radiographic findings, histological analysis, and surgical outcomes.

Results—Nineteen lesions were found in females and 10 in males with the average age of diagnosis being 27.4 years. Foot lesions were predominantly found in the tarsal bones (most commonly the talus), while hand lesions were solely found in the metacarpals. No lesions were found in the phalanges. GCTs demonstrated a predilection for the epimetaphyseal region of bone and were exclusively found in skeletally mature patients in which the physes were closed. The most common presenting symptoms were pain, edema, and pathological fractures. Radiographically, the lesions were purely lytic and expansive in nature showing areas of cortical destruction with poorly defined borders. No periosteal reaction was observed. Histologically, all tumors demonstrated multinucleated giant cells mixed with oval-round mononuclear cells. One third of the tumors involved the surrounding soft tissue; however, vessel involvement was rare.

Conclusion—Although radiographic findings are very supportive, other lesions can mimic GCT on X-ray. Therefore, histological analysis is necessary in confirming the diagnosis of GCT. Even then, GCT can be confused with other giant cell rich lesions which can further complicate the matter. Fortunately, no patients in this study died from the disease and none reported metastasis. Nonetheless, GCTs of the hand and foot typically demonstrate a more violent nature than other giant cell lesions and therefore must be treated aggressively with thorough curettage, utilizing phenol, or resection with a bone graft.—*D. Carmack*

♦ Radiographic presentation of bone tumors is nonspecific. Therefore, we rely on histological findings for appropriate diagnosis. This article specifically reviews giant cell tumors (GCT), and shows that even the histological features may overlap with other giant cell rich lesions. This was often found with insufficient intraoperative specimens.

Various treatment options were also reviewed in this paper. GCT is a very aggressive bone tumor, and its recurrence is common. The best outcomes were with thorough curettage followed by phenolization or a resection.

A few points should be made about bone tumors. First, they are relatively uncommon in the foot. Second, recurrence rates are high and aggressive measures are necessary, being careful to preserve function. Lastly, an important diagnostic key of bone tumors is location. Giant cell tumors in the foot are commonly "tarsal" with a significant concentration in the talus. Most are found in the epiphysis or metaepiphysis. Erratic location for giant cell rich lesions should alert the physician to a possible sarcoma. — *S.A. Paukovitz, D.P.M.*

Local Flaps

Paragas L, Attinger C, Blume PA (Yale University; VA Healthcare System, New Haven, CT; Georgetown University, Washington, DC; Yale School of Medicine, New Haven, CT)
Clin Podiatr Med Surg 17(2):267–318, 2000

Background—A local cutaneous skin flap is a mass or tongue of tissue for transplantation with an intrinsic blood supply by a pedicle or stem. Local flaps are comprised of the epidermis, dermis, and subcutaneous tissue, and may include underlying fascia and/or muscle. They should be employed for closure of foot defects because of their versatility, reproducibility, and long-term functional outcomes, and they are the ideal choice for covering defects with insufficient vascularity to support a skin graft. This paper presents local flaps according to movement and provides a thorough investigation of their applications.

Discussion—Numerous perioperative concerns are paramount for local flap survival. Patient health factors, including disease, age, medication, nutrition, and smoking, must be addressed. Noninvasive vascular studies and the elimination of infection are important requisites to tissue reconstruction. Blood from cutaneous, musculocutaneous perforating, and fasciocutaneous arteries form angiosomes that supply composite blocks of skin. The artery at the flap base determines flap success, not the ratio of flap length to width. Pedal flaps must be positioned to maximize local blood supply; large plantar rotation flaps should be based medially. Donor site selection is based on tissue mobility and elasticity, skin composition, avoidance of bony prominences, and proximity to perforator arteries.

Safe flap design advocates axis placement along the lines of maximum extensibility (LME), indicating the direction of desired movement and determined by the pinch test. Incision lines should be parallel to the relaxed skin tension lines (RTSL) which run perpendicular to the LME. Flap dissection and transposition requires atraumatic technique, meticulous hemostasis, mild tissue undermining, and the elimination of dead space. Lying or standing cones (dog-ears) may result from flap angle closure and should be corrected by excess tissue excision via Bürow's triangles. After closure, flaps must be evaluated for adequate vascularity and excessive tension, ideally 15 minutes after suturing to allow for skin relaxation. Flap ischemia can be reduced with topical applications of 60% dimethylsulfoxide (DMSO) solution. Flap bandages should be well padded but loose, with patients restricted to limb nonweightbearing and nondependency for 1–2 weeks. Flap viability may be evaluated by stab wound bleeding. Complications can result from patient risk factors and noncompliance, poor flap design and surgical technique, infection, excessive tension, and intrinsic metabolic, hemodynamic, or neurologic changes.

Advancement flaps move in one direction, allow for primary closure of donor and recipient sites, are best suited for areas with good tissue laxity and elasticity, rely on direct cutaneous perforators, and should be placed perpendicular to the RSTL and advance parallel to the LME. They include single or double advancement, M- and T-plasty (ellipse excision alternatives), V-to-Y, double V-to-Y (for defects >2 cm), crescentic (for triangular defects), and oblique sigmoid island flaps (for small circular defects). Their use in the foot is limited by mobility restrictions and they fail to redistribute tension.

Rotation flaps pivot around a point and move through an arc, provide tension redistribution and redirection from the primary defect to the donor site, may be axial or random, and are often used in areas of convexity or curved tension lines. They include single rotation (for triangular/circular defects), double rotation (for circular defects as ellipse alternative), and the Satterfield-Jolly (for painful plantar forefoot lesions). They may be elevated from nonweightbearing to weightbearing surfaces, are often used to correct heel defects, and are a useful adjunct for Charcot foot reconstruction.

Transposition flaps move adjacent skin to close a defect by the redistribution of tension via rotation and advancement. The flap must extend beyond the defect to ensure adequate length. These flaps include the single lobe (for circular/oval/semicircular large defects) and bi-lobed flap (large tissue recruitment for defects 1–3 cm), Z-plasty and double-Z rhomboid (for scar contractures and cosmetic enhancement), double-opposing Z-plasty, four-flap Z-plasty (for maximal scar lengthening), double opposing semicircles (for large circular defects 2–5 cm), W-plasty (for scar modification), rhomboid or Limberg flap (versatile for pedal wound closure), flap of Dufourmentel (for other rhombic defects), 30° transposition flap, double and triple rhomboid flaps (for large rectangular/circular defects), and the note flap (for circular defects

<2 cm). These flaps represent a wide range of geometric constructs for skin defect closure.—*D. Collman*

♦ The authors present an excellent, comprehensive review of local flaps that are commonly utilized in podiatric surgery. The article provides information on the principles, indications, and techniques associated with advancement, rotational, and transposition flaps. These flaps allow repair of tissue defects with minimal patient morbidity.

The most challenging aspect of soft-tissue coverage is choosing the appropriate flap. Knowledge of the detailed anatomy of the foot is the basis for flap design and survival. A thorough understanding of current plastic surgical techniques is paramount for success. Other nonvariable factors must be considered in the preoperative planning, such as the patient's general health. A history of diabetes mellitus, renal disease, peripheral vascular disease, local infection, peripheral neuropathy, nutritional status, and anemia may contribute to graft failure.

When simple excision with primary closure is not possible, local flaps are an excellent alternative that avoids sacrificing healthy tissue. Appropriate design, planning, and surgical technique will determine flap viability and avoid potential complications.—*S.A. Paukovitz, D.P.M.*

Anterior Tarsal Tunnel Syndrome

Akyüz G, Us Ö, Türan B, Kayhan Ö, Canbulat N, Tomi Yilmar I (Marmara University Institute of Neurological Sciences, Istanbul, Trukey; Marmara University Medical School, Istanbul, Turkey)
Electromyogr Clin Neurophysiol 40:123–128, 2000

Background—Namaz is an Islamic faith prayer form that is performed five times a day, which may take between 5 and 25 minutes each time. Namaz consists of a series of body movements, which includes standing up, bending forward, sitting down with knees together, and prostration with head and arm movements. In Namaz, foot positioning during sitting and prostration faces Kiblah (Mecca) but differs between men and women. For men, the right foot should be perpendicular to the floor and the left foot should be parallel to the floor. For women, their feet should be parallel to the floor but are directed to the right.

Introduction—Anterior tarsal tunnel syndrome (TTS) can manifest clinically as motor weakness of the extensor digitorum brevis muscle(EDB), paresthesias between the first and second toes, and blunt undefined pain to the dorsum of the foot, and/or anterolateral leg. Common causes of anterior TTS include compressive trauma from tight shoe gear, compression from osteophytes/bony structures, ganglions, chronic stretching of the nerve, and systemic causes such as diabetes and uremia. Nerve conduction studies of the deep peroneal nerve and electromyography of the EDB of diagnosed patients with anterior TTS who improperly practice Namaz suggests that this may cause anterior TTS.

Methods—Three hundred twenty Muslim patients, who had been practicing Namaz ranging between 10 and 53 years, were diagnosed with anterior tarsal tunnel syndrome. None had anterior TTS predisposing factors except for practicing Namaz. All patients have been placing their feet perpendicular to the floor during Namaz. Neurological examinations, ESR, CBC, C-reactive proteins, blood glucose, liver function tests, BUN, UA, and X-rays were performed on each patient. Nerve conduction studies of the deep peroneal nerve, superficial peroneal nerve, posterior tibial nerve, and the sural nerve were performed. Needle electromyography was performed on the tibialis anterior, peroneus longus, abductor hallucis longus, extensor hallucis longus, gastrocnemius, and EDB muscles bilaterally in all patients. A control group of 25 individuals was also utilized. Statistical analysis was performed using the Mann-Whitney U test.

Results—Study group versus control results showed nerve conduction of the deep peroneal nerve to be extremely significantly ($p < .0001$) and amplitude to be very significant ($p < .0035$). Denervation potentials were only observed in the EDB muscle. When patients improved their feet positioning during Namaz, their symptoms improved.

Conclusion—Improper foot positioning during Namaz may contribute to anterior TTS secondary to prolonged stretching of the deep peroneal nerve.—*D.D-Q. Tran, D.P.M.*

♦ Tarsal tunnel syndrome and anterior tarsal tunnel are peripheral neuropathies due to compression of the posterior tibial and deep peroneal nerves, respectively. Systemic factors (diabetes mellitus, rheumatoid arthritis, seronegative arthropathy, myxedema) and local factors (soft-tissue masses, aneurysms, varicosities, biomechanics, trauma) may be causative factors.

It has been documented that trauma, such as severe ankle supination, can place excessive traction on the deep peroneal nerve, causing symptoms. This article focuses on trauma from prolonged stretching of the nerve secondary to foot position during Namaz. We may not commonly see the practice of Namaz in our own offices, but the concept of the article is well taken.—*S.A. Paukovitz, D.P.M.*

Painful Heel: MR Imaging Findings

Narváez JA, Narváez J, Ortega R, Aguilera C, Sánchez A, Andia E (Hospital Duran Reymals, Ciutat Sanitària y Universitaria de Bellvitge, Barcelona, Spain) *RadioGraphics* 20(2):333–352, 2000

Introduction—Heel pain is a common symptom presented by patients that is manifested by several anatomic structures. Unfortunately, it is often difficult to diagnose the precise cause. Magnetic resonance imaging (MRI) is a direct, noninvasive tool that can aid in the diagnosis as well as showing the extent and severity of the heel condition. In this article, there is a review of the anatomical structures and conditions that can lead to the symptom of a painful heel as well as the pertinent MRIs that are associated with these conditions.

Plantar Fascial Lesions—MRI can be used to evaluate the plantar fascia for inflammation, ruptures, and lesions that are seen in plantar fasciitis, plantar fascia ruptures, plantar fibromatosis, and plantar fascia xanthoma. The MRI shows such characteristics as size, shape, and interruptions in the intensity of the signal of the soft-tissue structures. These characteristics represent such things as edema, hematoma, inflammation, and rupture that are seen in conjunction with these conditions of the plantar fascia.

Tendinous Lesions—MRI is useful in assessing the tendons that can potentially cause heel pain. These tendons include the Achilles, the flexor digitorum longus (FDL), and the flexor hallucis longus (FHL). These tendons can lead to such conditions as insertional Achilles tendonitis and tendonitis and tenosynovitis of the FDL and FHL tendons. Through MRI these tendons can be assessed for size, shape, and changes in the signal intensity. These characteristics represent changes in the tendon consistent with inflammation, edema, increased amounts of synovial fluid in the tendon sheaths, and scar formation.

Osseous Lesions—Conditions leading to heel pain such as fractures, bone bruises, osteomyelitis, and calcaneal tumors can be diagnosed through the use of MRI. These conditions are seen on MRI as changes in the intensity of the signal in the medullary space. Each of the conditions has varying characteristics that can be seen on MRI that help distinguish them from other conditions.

Bursal Lesions—Lesions such as retrocalcaneal and retroachilleal bursitis, tarsal tunnel syndrome, and heel fat pad abnormalities can result from several factors including athletic activities and arthropathies. MRI can be helpful in diagnosing these conditions by showing characteristic changes in the amount of bursal fluid, the contents and boundaries of the tarsal tunnel, and variations in the heel fat pad.

Conclusion—Although MRI is usually not warranted for the symptom of heel pain, it can be very helpful in the diagnosis. After assessing a patient's history, physical findings, and MRI, it can be used in planning the treatment regimen for the diagnosis. If surgery is required to correct the condition, MRI can help plan out the procedure to be performed by mapping out the exact location of the lesion.—*L. Rowe*

♦ This article was a good comprehensive review of the various causes of heel pain and features seen on MR imaging. In atypical or recalcitrant heel pain, MR imaging is useful in identifying soft-tissue and osseous disorders. It is beneficial for surgical planning, and for identifying the exact location and extent of the pathology.

In most cases a thorough history and physical exam with standard radiographs are sufficient. Most times heel pain can be successfully treated conservatively, but when surgery is indicated, MR imaging can also aid in preoperative planning.—*S.A. Paukovitz, D.P.M.*

13   Tumor Pathology

Michael Rupp, D.P.M., M.D.

An Ulcerating Verrucous Plaque on the Foot

Ho J, Diven DG, Butler PJ, Tyring SK (Duke University Medical Center, Durham, NC; University of Texas Medical Branch, Galveston, TX; Milwaukee Medical Clinic, Milwaukee, WI)
Arch Dermatol 136(4):547, 550, 2000

Introduction—The term *verrucous carcinoma* refers to a well differentiated, slow-growing neoplasm with a tendency for local recurrence and no tendency to metastasize. It usually occurs in three major locations: the oral cavity, the anogenital region, and the plantar surface of the foot. The disease is characterized by a fungating, exophytic mass with numerous keratin-filled sinuses, often on the anterior weightbearing area of the sole of the foot.

Case Report—A 29-year-old African American man with long-standing type 1 diabetes presented with a 4-year history of a verrucous lesion on his foot. Hypertension, retinopathy, and nephropathy were present in addition to peripheral vascular disease that had resulted in leg amputation above the knee. The lesion on his foot had been stable in size for 3 years, but had intermittently ulcerated and healed; consequently, it had been diagnosed as a diabetic ulcer with a surrounding callus. Upon examination, a hyperkeratotic, partially ulcerated verrucous plaque on the plantar surface of his forefoot was discovered and no other verrucous lesions were noted. The lesion was excised down to subcutaneous tissue with negative intraoperative margins by frozen as well as permanent sections. To cover the wound, a split-thickness graft was applied. At 4 years, there has been no recurrence.

Discussion—Verrucous carcinoma (epithelioma cuniculatum) often presents as a nonhealing wart on the soles, palms, or other location that fails treatment. It rarely metastasizes and has a low mortality rate compared with other subtypes of verrucous carcinoma. Histologic diagnosis can be difficult—for which, a deep biopsy specimen of the lesion is needed. Moreover, multiple biopsy specimens are often necessary to establish the diagnosis. Treatment consists of wide local excision, but more serious cases may require amputation of a toe or even a foot. For minor cases, surgical curettage is sufficient.—*A. Duckworth*

♦ This paper demonstrates a fairly common but potentially treacherous clinical dilemma: a malignant tumor masquerading as a benign lesion. In this case the ulcerating but slowly progressing lesion was diagnosed by a number of clinicians as a complication of the patient's diabetes. Verrucous carcinoma can hide its malignant nature both at the time of physical examination and under the microscope. It lacks the typical microscopic features of squamous carcinoma, and a deep biopsy is needed to demonstrate the invasive nature of the lesion. Superficial biopsies may be nondiagnostic and misleading. The tumor can metastasize, but it usually does not. In advanced cases amputation may be necessary to completely remove the tumor.—*M. Rupp, D.P.M., M.D.*

Sentinel Node Biopsy for Staging of Aggressive Digital Papillary Adenocarcinoma
Malafa MP, McKesey P, Stone S, Dudley-Walker S, Cockerell CJ (Southern Illinois University School of Medicine, Springfield, IL; University of Texas Southwestern Medical Center, Dallas, TX)
Dermatol Surg 26:580-583, 2000

Introduction—Aggressive papillary adenocarcinoma is commonly found on the fingers and toes. This rare malignancy often has recurrence and metastases via lymphatic channels. The authors compare aggressive papillary adenocarcinoma to melanoma with regards to evidence of lymph node metastases affecting the prognosis. Routine lymph node dissection is limited to patients exhibiting lymphadenopathy due to the morbidity associated with the surgery. Therefore, the authors propose sentinel lymph node mapping and biopsy to stage the tumor and decrease lymph node dissection morbidity.

Methods—Sentinel lymph node mapping and biopsy were performed on a 44-year-old white male patient after excision of an aggressive digital papillary carcinoma of the second toe on his left foot. Radiocolloid was injected at the margins of the tumor site and mapped for lymphatic drainage. Hematoxylin and eosin staining and immunocytochemistry analysis were used to assess evidence of metastatic tumor cells in regional node biopsy.

Results—Lymphoscintography identified two sentinel nodes receiving drainage from the tumor site in the groin area. The sentinel nodes were negative for metastases and indicated no need for adjuvant therapy.

Conclusion—Aggressive papillary adenocarcinoma often has metastases via the lymphatic system. However, elective lymph node dissection for skin tumors is not routine because of the associated morbidity. Sentinel lymph node mapping is currently being used to stage melanoma which displays similar regional lymph node metastases as aggressive papillary adenocarcinoma. This method of lymph node mapping and biopsy has demonstrated almost no associated morbidity and proven accurate in staging regional nodes in patients with melanoma. Therefore, the authors propose this method for determining the stage of aggressive papillary adenocarcinoma with minimal associated morbidity.—*M. Garrison*

◆ This paper is interesting in several ways. The tumor presented as a chronic ulcer that occurred after trauma to the foot: a malignant tumor hiding behind a benign history. It also demonstrates that melanoma is not the only aggressive metastasizing skin tumor of the lower extremity. These fortunately uncommon tumors occur on the palms, soles, fingers, and toes and recur or metastasize in about one third of cases. The use of sentinel node biopsy in this case raises some of the problematic aspects of how to appropriately use new and not fully proven methods in clinical practice. Sentinel node biopsy has been used most widely in melanoma and breast carcinoma. Even in these settings, its ultimate role is unclear. The meaning of some of the tiny metastatic deposits found in sentinel nodes is not fully known. They may not be capable of growing into clinically significant lesions. More troubling is determining the benefit of the procedure to the patient. Proponents claim that the status of the sentinel node in melanoma is of prognostic importance, and that patients with a positive sentinel node are candidates for a full regional node dissection. Opponents note that there is significant morbidity associated with lymphedema after node dissection, but no proven therapeutic benefit associated with node dissection. There is no proven survival benefit with chemotherapy or interferon which might be used based on finding a positive sentinel node, so the benefit to the patient is difficult to define.—*M. Rupp, D.P.M., M.D.*

Venous Gangrene in a Patient with Adenocarcinoma of the Lung

Yang M-H, Fan FS, Chen P-M, Liu J-H, Chiou T-J, Wang W-S, Yen C-C
(Taipei Veterans General Hospital and National Yang-Ming University, Taipei, Taiwan)
Jpn J Clin Oncol 30(6):276–278, 2000

Introduction—It is not uncommon to see thromboemboli in cancer patients with mucin-producing malignant tumors. It is speculated that the serum anticardiolipin antibodies play an important role in the coagulopathy noted in cancer patients. Venous gangrene rarely plays a factor in the management of the cancer patient. This paper is a case presentation of a patient with adenocarcinoma of the lung complicated by venous gangrene of the foot.

Case Report—A 51-year-old female reported to the emergency unit in December 1998 with shortness of breath, dry cough, and an enlarging mass on the left chest wall. CT revealed bilateral effusion and a left pulmonary mass obliterating the bronchial tree with several nodular lesions bilaterally. The mass was subsequently excised and determined to be an adenocarcinoma with multiple metastatic lesions to the liver, right adrenal gland, and osseous structures. The patient was treated with two cycles of gemcitabine plus carboplatin and refused further treatment. In March 1999, the patient noted purplish discoloration of digits two through five on the left foot. Angiographic examination of the entire left extremity provided no evidence of arterial occlusion and a diagnosis of dry gangrene was made. A hemostatic screen revealed the patient was hypercoagulable with a prothrombin time of 15.3 s (control 12.5 s) and a partial thromboplastin time of 41.4 s (control 34.1). As evidenced by Doppler, thrombosis over the left femoral and popliteal veins provided the etiology of venous gangrene. Elevated serum titers for both IgM and IgG anticardolipin antibodies were detected by ELISA. The patient subsequently died 2 weeks later of sepsis despite broad-spectrum antibiosis.

Discussion—Mucin-producing malignancies of pulmonary origin commonly produce hypercoagulable states. Preponderance for cancer patients to be hyper-coagulable is expected with reports of protein C/protein S deficiency as well as decreased levels of antithrombin III commonly seen. Cancer cells have tissue factors that stimulate factor VII, thus initiating the extrinsic coagula-tion cascade. Furthermore, antiphospholipid antibodies are thought to interact with platelet phospholipids and the vascular endothelium, thereby inhibiting protein C activation and prostacyclin formation. Commonly elevated in cancer patients and therefore termed antiphospholipid syndrome, these antibodies predispose the patient to thrombosis. The authors therefore suggest that a serum screening for antiphospholipid elevation be considered in patients with malignancy to decrease the event of thrombosis. Studies have shown that morbidity in lung cancer patients increases dramatically with a thromboem-bolic event; however, in treating cancer associated thromboembolism it is suggested that low-molecular-weight heparin be considered instead of standard heparin.—*K.E. Van Voris*

♦ This paper demonstrates an unusual complication of paraneoplastic thrombosis. The development of thrombi by itself is not unusual in malignancy. Often the process is migratory. It appears in one part of the body only to resolve then reform in another location. This phenomenon is called Trousseau's sign after the physician who first noted the relation of migratory thrombophlebitis with visceral tumors. What is unusual is the progression to gangrene. In this case, antiphospholipid antibodies were detected. These promote thrombosis by inhibiting protein C, a natural anticoagulant. Resistance to activated protein C is common in malignancy. Recently there has been an interest in the tendency to thrombosis that accompanies inherited variations in factor V, so called Factor V Leiden, and other coagulation factors. At this point, there does not seem to be a significant increase in the incidence of these factors in cancer patients who develop thrombosis.—*M. Rupp, D.P.M., M.D.*

Infiltrating Basal Cell Carcinoma in the Setting of a Venous Ulcer

Lutz ME, Davis MDP, Otley CC (Mayo Clinic and Mago Foundation, Rochester, MN)
Int J Dermatol 39:519–520, 2000

Case Report—A 77-year-old man was referred with a 5-year history of a nonhealing right medial ankle ulcer that had not responded to multiple treatment modalities. His past medical history was positive for deep venous thrombosis in the right leg 30 years earlier and greater saphenous vein harvesting for coronary bypass grafting 28 years previously. Since that time, the patient has suffered from increasing right leg edema and stasis changes. The skin examination revealed a 3.0 × 3.5 cm ulcer adjacent to the medial malleolus with raised and rolled edges. There appeared to be healthy granulation tissue centrally with surrounding dermatitic changes. Noninvasive studies showed severe venous incompetence of the right popliteal and superficial veins. Arterial studies and transcutaneous oximetry were normal. CT scan showed no pelvic adenopathy and radiographs showed no underlying osteomyelitis. The biopsy of the ulcer edge and base showed infiltrating basal cell carcinoma. Mohs' micrographic surgery required three layers; the final extent of the ulcer was 7.8 × 6.9 cm. A split-thickness skin graft was placed.

Discussion—Basal cell carcinoma is the most common malignancy. It has the ability to disguise itself and appear in unsuspecting places. This case report demonstrates the difficulty in diagnosing a basal cell carcinoma in the setting of chronic venous insufficiency and ulceration. A biopsy should be performed if the ulcer is not responding to traditional treatment modalities or if it has an atypical appearance. It is not known whether the malignancy arises de novo or if it is a result of the ulcer itself. A study shows that up to 4% of ulcers have a malignant lesion. Squamous cell and basal cell carcinoma can both arise and ulcerate in the setting of stasis changes that may emulate or complicate a venous ulcer. This case shows the importance of considering a skin biopsy in nonhealing chronic venous ulcers.—*L.T. Rowe, B.S.*

♦ Malignant tumors can be hidden in what appears to be a benign lesion. Ulcers can have a variety of causes, and if an ulcer is not responding to treatment, biopsy is in order. Squamous carcinoma, basal cell carcinoma, melanoma, and other malignancies have all fooled experienced clinicians by presenting as ulcers of the lower extremity. Unusual infections can also present at times as an ulcer. Biopsy may be the only way to get to the right diagnosis.—*M. Rupp, D.P.M., M.D.*

γδ T-Cell Lymphoma of the Skin: A Clinical, Microscopic, and Molecular Study

Toro JR, Beaty M, Sorbara L, Turner ML, White J, Kingma DW, Raffeld M, Jaffe ES (National Cancer Institute, National Institutes of Health, Bethesda, MD)
Arch Dermatol 136:1024–1032, 2000

Introduction—T-Cell receptors (TCR) on the surface of mature T-cells consist of either a γδ or an αβ heterodimer expressed in association with the CD3 complex of proteins. Most mature T-cells express the αβ TCR and only about 5% express the γδ TCR. Among all of the cases of cutaneous T-cell lymphomas (CTCL), very few are of the γδ genotype and phenotype. The purpose of this study was to investigate three cases of γδ CTCL.

Methods—The subjects consisted of three males diagnosed with γδ CTCL who ranged in age from 46 to 74 years. Two of the subjects were Caucasian and one was African American. The subjects were evaluated by clinical examination, as well as microscopy and immunohistochemistry of biopsy specimens. In addition, polymerase chain reaction amplification for T-cell receptor gamma gene rearrangements and in situ hybridization for Epstein-Barr Virus (EBV) were performed on three biopsy sections to evaluate the role of EBV in the pathogenesis of γδ CTCL.

Results—The dermatological lesions were varied, and in some patients, more than one type of lesion was seen. All patients had a few scaly plaques. Two patients had multiple dermal pink to plum-colored tumors, some of which ulcerated and covered with hemorrhagic crusts. Two patients had painful indurated nodules and tumors, some of which healed with an atrophic scar and postinflammatory hyperpigmentation. All patients had lesions on their upper and lower extremities. All three exhibited an aggressive clinical course with resistance to multiagent chemotherapy and radiation.

On microscopic examination, one case presented with only epidermotropism, another case had only dermal involvement, and another case exhibited epidermal, dermal, and subcutaneous involvement. In this study, in situ hybridization for EBV RNA was performed in three biopsy specimens, but no evidence of EBV was found, suggesting that EBV does not play a major role in the development of primary γδ CTCL.

On immunohistochemical examination, all three cases were positive for CD3. Two cases were CD4/CD8 double negative and one case expressed CD8.

Molecular studies using PCR detected clonal T-cell receptor γ-chain gene rearrangement in all three cases. In addition, the tumor cells were negative for EBV RNA transcripts in all three patients by in situ hybridization.

Conclusion—γδ CTCL can exhibit diverse histological patterns, often in the same patient, including epidermotropism and dermal and subcutaneous involvement. The data suggest that γδ CTCL are EBV-negative clonal lymphomas that express a mature cytotoxic phenotype with frequent necrosis and/or apoptosis. γδ CTCL has preferential involvement of the extremities with necrotic tumors and subcutaneous nodules, and an aggressive clinical course. Because of poor clinical outcome, early diagnosis and aggressive therapy are indicated in these patients.—*B. Hoffman*

♦ Cutaneous T-cell lymphoma, which includes the older terms mycosis fungoides and Sezary syndrome, may be more common than is generally appreciated. There is evidence that it may be as common as the better known Hodgkin's disease. As in this case, multiple skin lesions are typical of the disease. Early lesions can easily be confused with dermatitis, but they do not respond to topical therapy. With time, lesions become more pronounced and systemic spread occurs. Some cases are associated with human immunodeficiency virus infection.—*M. Rupp, D.P.M., M.D.*

Primary Cutaneous B-Cell Lymphoma of the Leg in a Chronic Lymphedematous Extremity

Torres-Paoli D, Sánchez JL (University of Puerto Rico, School of Medicine, San Juan, Puerto Rico)
Am J Dermatopathol 22(3):257–260, 2000

Introduction—Several neoplasms have been described in the setting of lymphedema of an extremity. This report describes a case of cutaneous large B-cell lymphoma of the leg with chronic lymphedema.

Case Report—An 87-year-old white female with a history of lymphedema of the left leg secondary to filariasis presented with severely painful nodules on the affected leg and denied the presence of any constitutional symptoms. On physical exam, the leg showed severe edema with multiple erythematous brownish nodules of variable size from the knee to the dorsum of the foot. Few were ulcerated. Laboratory and radiographic studies were performed. A biopsy was also done on one of the nodules along with immunohistochemistry studies. Based on the results of the tests performed, a diagnosis of large cell B-cell lymphoma of the leg was made. The patient was treated with systemic chemotherapy and focal radiotherapy. The patient had an excellent response to the treatment and had no recurrence 6 months later.

Discussion—In 1984, Waxman et al. reported the first case of malignant lymphoma of the skin associated with chronic lymphedema (Waxman M, et al. *Arch Pathol Lab Med* 108:206–208, 1984). Since then several other reports have been made, often in association with breast and prostate cancer. They were all treated singly or with combinations of chemotherapy, radiotherapy, or amputation. All of these cases were shown to be of B-cell lineage. Large B-cell lymphoma is considered a primary B-cell lymphoma of the skin and expresses itself clinically as solitary or grouped plaques and tumors. They are located more frequently in the lower extremity of older women. Some of the characteristics of the neoplasm are CD19 and CD20 positive. Histopathologically, they present with dense, diffuse infiltrate of large cells in the entire dermis and subcutis, frequently with mitotic figures. The neoplastic cells resemble centroblasts or immunoblasts. Large B-cell lymphoma must be differentiated from anaplastic large cell lymphoma and nonlymphoid tumors. The association of these tumors with chronic lymphedema suggests some type of relationship that has spawned the development of several theories. In conclusion, the authors feel that there needs to be an awareness of the existence of lymphedema-related malignant lymphoma to prevent unnecessary surgery. Also, in contrast to primary large B-cell lymphoma of the leg, the prognosis of patients with lymphedema-associated lymphoma is relatively favorable.—*L.T. Rowe, B.S.*

♦ Podiatrists are well acquainted with the problems associated with edematous legs. This paper documents a rather unusual complication of chronic lymphedema. Neoplasms occurring in the setting of tissue damage are well known. Most common skin cancers tend to occur in sun-damaged skin. The nature of the clinical setting seems to be important in determining prognosis. Squamous carcinoma in sun-damaged skin rarely metastasizes. Squamous cancers occurring in sinus tracts associated with chronic osteomyelitis or in burn scars metastasize up to 30% of the time and can be fatal. In the case of the tumor presented in this paper, B-cell lymphoma, there appears to be a similar phenomenon in play. In the setting of lymphedema, cutaneous B-cell lymphoma has a better prognosis than in typical cases of B-cell lymphoma occurring in the leg. A better known malignancy occurring with lymphedema is angiosarcoma following removal of axillary nodes for breast cancer.—*M. Rupp, D.P.M., M.D.*

Aggressive Angiomyxoma: Irradiation for Recurrent Disease

Rhomberg W, Jasarevic Z, Alton R, Kompatscher P, Beer G, Breitfellner G
(Landes Krankenhaus Feld Kirch, Austria)
Strahlenther Onkol 176(7):324–326, 2000

Introduction—Aggressive angiomyxoma (AAM) is a fibromyxoid tumor found in the pelvic and genital soft tissues with a higher prevalence in females. The tumor tends to recur in a non-infiltrative manner in adjacent organs, despite clear borders on resection. The tumor does display dependency on different forms of hormones. Chromosomal translocation on 12q 14–15 is seen with AAM, an aberration common to a variety of mesenchymal tumors. This is a case report of a 27-year-old male, who received full radiation therapy due to frequent recurrences.

Case Report—Patient has a history significant for three radical resections of a tumor from the left lower leg. Tumor was presumed to be lipomyxoma. Due to the reoccurrences, the histology was reviewed and the diagnosis changed to AAM.

The tumor was located in the subcutaneous tissues of the left lower leg, just proximal to the medial malleolus. Due to the nonmalignant nature of AAM and additionally for cosmetic reasons, the tumor was resected without clear margins. Grossly the resected tissue had a nodular, gelatinous consistency with yellowish-gray coloring. Microscopic analyses using HE and Alzianblue staining revealed few collagen fibers, with an abnormally increased number of blood vessels. Vessels resembled venoles and to a lesser degree capillaries. No mitoses or karyotypic irregularities were visualized. The patient was subsequently referred to radiology for adjuvant radiation treatment.

Radiotherapy was administered five times a week for a total dose of 56 Gy within 6 weeks. Razoxane, 125 mg PO BID, was administered 5 days prior to initiating therapy and throughout the treatment. Skin necrosis developed within the radiation field, which was subsequently treated by plastic surgery. MRI 2 years post resection revealed no abnormalities, and no metastases.

Discussion—Mesenchymal tumors, as compared to carcinoma, are more difficult to identify in relation to dignity, grading, and infiltrating borders. To arrive at the correct diagnosis, other myxoid tumors such as myxoid neurofi-broma, angio-myo-fibroma, and lipofibroma must be kept as a differential.

The extrapelvic location of the AAM tumor as well as the occurrence in a male is rare. Radiotherapy is generally reserved for metastatic tumors, but due to the repeated recurrences in this case, radiotherapy was considered to control further growth. The follow-up time in this case is short, but longer than the previous time to reoccurrence.—*G. Grant*

♦ This lesion is more common in the genital tract and pelvis. Although it is classified as benign, it is locally aggressive and tends to recur. The microscopic appearance of the lesion is very benign, and it is easy to underdiagnose it as a less aggressive entity. This case makes an important point. When benign lesions recur unexpectedly, a reconsideration of the initial diagnosis may be in order. This should be applied to cutaneous spindle cell tumors. Dermatofibrosarcoma protuberans is easily misdiagnosed as dermatofibroma. Spindle cell melanoma can be difficult to accurately diagnose, particularly with a superficial biopsy. Correlation of biopsy results with the clinical course is always important.—*M. Rupp, D.P.M., M.D.*

Eccrine Sweat Gland Carcinoma: A Case Report and Review of Diagnosis and Treatment

Voutsadakis IA, Bruckner HW (Mount Sinai Hospital and Mount Sinai School of Medicine, New York, NY)
Conn Med 64(5):263–266, 2000

Introduction—Sweat gland carcinomas are rare and slow growing, but have the potential to reoccur and metastasize. Five-year survival rate is above 60% and many succumb to metastatic disease.

Case Report—A 48-year-old man presented with multiple left leg nodular skin lesions, left inguinal lymphadenopathy and a small 4-year-old lesion on his left foot. The lesion had begun to increase in size in the past year. The patient also had a history of skin lesions up to the knee and lower third of the left thigh as well as inguinal lymphadenopathy. Biopsy revealed poorly differentiated sweat gland carcinoma, which was treated with several chemotherapies resulting in short-lived effects. One year after diagnosis, radiation therapy of the left leg was begun. Two years after diagnosis, he developed thoracic spine metastases and a left pleural effusion as well as pulmonary masses. After many different combinations of chemotherapy, the disease overwhelmed the patient 5 years after diagnosis, leading to death as a result of progressive pulmonary disease.

Discussion—Eccrine sweat glands are present throughout the body except for the lips and parts of the external genitalia. Eccrine and apocrine carcinomas are malignancies that have a different biological behavior than squamous and basal cell carcinoma. Apocrine tumors have more decapitation secretion and have PAS-positive diastase-resistant material in the cells or lumina. Eccrine carcinoma usually shows areas of duct formation infiltrating through the dermis or islands of malignant cells. Both stain positive for carcinoembryonic antigen. There are four different histological types of eccrine carcinoma but with minimal biological differences. Differentiation, even between apocrine and eccrine carcinomas, is of little prognostic difference because both have similar natural histories. Mutations of p53 and of nucleotides (G:C to A:T) have been implicated. The primary treatment of sweat gland carcinoma is adequate excision with wide margins. In case of recurrence, re-excision or amputation is warranted. Radiation treatment may be effective in only local treatment. The role of chemotherapy is still questionable. After reviewing the literature, it seems that there is not an established effective treatment besides a wide surgical excision.—*F. Nejad*

◆ When the topic of aggressive skin lesions of the lower extremity comes up, melanoma is often where the discussion begins and ends. As shown in this case, there are other aggressive skin lesions of the foot and leg. In this case, the tumor was originally diagnosed as basal cell carcinoma of the foot. Basal carcinoma can occur on the foot, but it is relatively uncommon in that location. The tumor was apparently present for 4 years before it began to enlarge and develop satellite lesion, at which point the patient sought additional care. Earlier re-excision might have resulted in a better outcome without systemic metastasis.—*M. Rupp, D.P.M., M.D.*

Bizarre Parosteal Osteochondromatous Proliferation of Bone (BPOP): An Unusual Foot Mass in a Child

Gilmore A, Khoury J, Abdul Karim FW, Ballock RT (Case Western Reserve University; University Hospitals of Cleveland, Cleveland, OH)
Foot Ankle Int 21(5):404–407, 2000

Introduction—Bizarre parosteal osteochondromatous proliferation (BPOP) is a rare benign tumor with distinctive radiologic and histologic features. These lesions are found most commonly in the hands and feet. The lesion was first described by Nora et al. in 1983 (Nora FE, et al. *Am J Surg Pathol* 7:245–250, 1983) and then again in 1993 by Meneses et al. (Meneses MF, et al. *Am J Surg Pathol* 17:691–697, 1993). This case report presents an 8 year-old boy with a BPOP of his foot.

Case Report—A healthy 8-year-old boy presented with a 2-week history of a painful mass on the medial aspect of his right foot inferior to the talonavicular joint. The patient's first noticeable symptoms were an erythematous painful area over the medial aspect of the foot and a low-grade fever, all of which had resolved at the time of the first examination except the pain. The patient denied any history of trauma. Upon palpation of the area, no significant mass was appreciated.

Radiographs were taken which showed a mineralized mass at the inferior aspect of the talonavicular joint, which was well marginated, arising from the cortical surface of the bone without any alteration to the underlying bone. The CT scan that was taken suggested an osteochondroma.

An excisional biopsy was performed. A large, fragmented, calcified mass was discovered inferior to the talonavicular joint with a bony stalk coming from the subchondral bone of the talus. It appeared to have a thin cartilage cap with a firm nodular surface. Histopathologically, the mass exhibited the distinctive characteristics of BPOP. Based on the radiographic and histologic specimen, a diagnosis of BPOP was made.

Discussion—A BPOP is a benign lesion that tends to recur with an atypical histologic appearance. The lesion tends to occur equally in men and women from 8 to 73 years of age but is predominantly seen in the 3rd and 4th decade. Clinical symptoms include a painless mass with an occasional associated erythema that can last from a few weeks to years. The BPOP arises from the cortex by a pedicle without disrupting the underlying bone or architecture of the surrounding cortex. Radiographically, the well defined mass can be up to 3 cm in diameter. Grossly, the mass can resemble an osteochondroma in its size and cartilage-covered bony matrix, but histologically, it can be differentiated. The differential diagnosis of BPOP is osteochondroma, dysplasia epiphysealia hemimelia, parosteal osteosarcoma, myositis ossificans, florid reactive periostitis, and subungual exostosis. The recommended treatment of BPOP is simple excision, although there is a high rate of recurrence, but there have been no reports of metastases.—*L.T. Rowe, B.S.*

♦ This case demonstrates a very important point. The accurate classification of bone tumors relies on a combination of clinical, radiographic, and pathologic features. Benign enchondromas of the hands and feet often have a microscopic appearance suggesting a low-grade chondrosarcoma. Radiographic findings are very useful in making the distinction. Florid reactive periostitis of the bones of the toes can cause a painful mass that on biopsy shows a haphazard fibrous proliferation with mitotic activity which may resemble a sarcoma, but the radiographic features are benign. Another important point in this case is that not all lesions reported as benign are totally cured by excision. BPOP may recur one or more times in up to half of cases.—*M. Rupp, D.P.M., M.D.*

Popliteal Lymph Node Metastasis from Primary Cutaneous Melanoma

Thompson JF, Hunt JA, Culjak G, Uren RF, Howman-Giles R, Harman CR
(Royal Prince Alfred Hospital; University of Sydney, Sydney, NSW, Australia)
Eur J Surg Oncol 26:172–176, 2000

Introduction—The popliteal lymph nodes primarily drain the deep tissues of the lower leg and foot. In some individuals, there is direct drainage from the skin to the popliteal lymph nodes. Because of this, some metastases from cutaneous melanomas will metastasize directly to these nodes.

Methods—The study was a retrospective chart analysis involving 14,866 patients over 30 years in Sydney, Australia. Of these, 4260 had primary cutaneous melanomas distal to the knee. Those with metastasis to the popliteal lymph nodes were identified and further analyzed.

Results—Thirteen patients were recorded as having metastases to the popliteal lymph nodes. Eight of the 13 patients developed distant metastases. Seven of 13 died and six were clinically disease free at the last follow-up. Nuclear medicine lymphatic mapping data (lymphoscintigraphy) were analyzed for 236 patients with melanoma distal to the knee. Seventeen of these patients had direct drainage to the popliteal nodes. Six of 17 patients had popliteal biopsy performed, with one having metastatic disease in the node.

Discussion—Lymphoscintigraphy is performed by injecting radioactive tracer into areas around the primary biopsy site and mapping the channels to see their drainage patterns. It has shown that there is great variability in pathways taken by lymph channels. It has been shown that lymph draining to the popliteal nodes can originate from anywhere on the foot. Popliteal nodes are rare sites of metastasis. Preoperative lymphoscintigraphy will help identify patients with potential to metastasize to these nodes.—*D. Clement*

♦ One might well assume that the popliteal nodes are the logical place for melanomas on the foot to metastasize to initially. As this paper shows, that assumption is false and popliteal nodes are only rarely involved. It turns out that the popliteal nodes primarily drain the deep tissues rather than skin. Melanoma of the foot is more likely to metastasize to groin nodes. This suggests that sampling of the politeal nodes in melanoma patients should be based on strong clinical evidence, or at least lymphoscintigraphy demonstrating drainage to the popliteal nodes. The danger of lymph node dissection in the leg is the significant morbidity that accompanies the resultant lymphedema. With the advent of more limited sentinel node biopsies, the removal of lymph nodes in melanoma has increased. Some clinicians propose that sentinel node biopsy should be the standard of care in melanoma, but the issue is still controversial.—*M. Rupp, D.P.M., M.D.*

Lymphatic Mapping and Sentinel Lymph Node Biopsy in Patients with Melanoma of the Lower Extremity

Hettiaratchy S, Dheansa B, Powell B (St. George's Hospital, London, UK)
Plast Reconstr Surg 106(3):734–735, 2000

Introduction—There have been claims that patients with positive sentinel nodes and primary less than 3 mm thick have disease confirmed to the sentinel nodes. With further investigation, such hypothesis may not be correct.

Methods—One hundred ninety patients with melanoma of various sites underwent sentinel node biopsy. This was then sent for staging and pathological analysis.

Results—Twenty-six patients came up with positive sentinel nodes (13.7%), and went on to regional clearance lymphectomy. Two patients had disease involving nonsentinel lymph nodes. One of the patients had a primary tumor of 4.4 mm and the other had a primary tumor of 2.1 mm on his back with two out of 18 other nodes in the axilla area testing positive for melanomas.

Conclusion—Depth of primary tumor may not be a reliable indicator of the status of the rest of the lymph node basin.

Discussion—By separating positive sentinel nodes into various stages of tumor invasion, it was found that the likelihood of nonsentinel node involvement could be predicted by the degree of micrometastatic invasion of the sentinel node itself. This may be the most accurate way of determining the status of the whole lymph node basin.—*S.B. Heninger*

◆ The idea of sentinel node biopsy in melanoma is elegant. Inject a radioactive tracer in the area of the tumor, then use a detector to pinpoint the location of the lymph node to which the radioactive tracer drains. This enables the surgeon to precisely remove the node most likely to be involved with tumor. A complete lymph node dissection with the increased risk of lymphedema can be avoided if the sentinel node is free of tumor. There are, however, problems. The tracer may go around a node completely blocked by tumor and a false-negative biopsy may result. Occasionally, a melanoma may drain to an aberrant node outside of the expected drainage area, or to an interval node between the melanoma and the expected location of the draining nodes. On the whole, lymphatic mapping can accurately identify the sentinel node in a great majority of cases. Sentinel node biopsy is reserved for melanomas over 1 mm in thickness. Melanomas of this size are expected to have spread to the sentinel node in about 20% of cases. For thinner lesions, the incidence of metastasis is much lower.—*M. Rupp, D.P.M., M.D.*

Malignant Melanoma of the foot and Ankle

John KJ, Hayes DW Jr, Green DR, Dickerson J (Broadlawns Medical Center, Des Moines, IA; Scripps Mercy Medical Center, San Diego, CA)
Clin Podiatr Med Surg 17(2):347–360, 2000

Background—Malignant melanoma is a neoplasm of pigmented-producing melanocytes or their precursor cells. In adults, melanocytes normally reside in the basal layer; however, if malignancy develops, they can spread to other layers of the skin or mucosal lining.

In the United States, 90% of the malignant melanomas present in Caucasians. Patients of African, Asian, and Hispanic decent are least susceptible. The most common site for women is the lower extremity, whereas men have lesions on the trunk, head, and neck. Most cases occur in the 4th, 5th, and 6th decades of life. About 30% of all melanomas occur on the lower extremities, with 5% occurring on the foot. Forty-nine percent of the lesions occur on the dorsum of the foot, 40% on the plantar surface, and 11% subungually. Subungual presentation is more prevalent in dark-skinned individuals.

Ultraviolet light is the main cause of malignant melanoma. Areas of skin exposed to direct sunlight have a high correlation with melanoma. Other factors include genetic factors and female hormones.

Clinical Features—Malignant melanomas are asymmetrical with jagged and irregular borders. Their color fades off into the surrounding skin. In addition, melanomas range from blue to black with shades of red and pink. The diameter of melanomas is greater than 6 mm, whereas benign pigmented lesions have diameters less than 6 mm. Finally the appearance of elevation increases the suspicion of malignancy.

A way to remember the clinical features of malignant melanoma is the pneumonic "ABCDEs of Melanoma." A stands for asymmetry, B for border irregularity, C for color variation, D for diameter greater than 6 mm, and E for elevation above the level of the surrounding skin. One common factor in melanomas is their changing nature. Any pigmented lesion that undergoes a change in size, configuration, or color should be considered a melanoma and a biopsy should be taken.

Classification—There are four basic growth patterns of melanoma. Differentiating these patterns is important in understanding their course, preferred treatment plan, and prognosis.

1. *Superficial spreading melanoma* is the most common pattern representing 70% of all lesions. They develop rapidly from preexisting nevus in a radial direction, which attributes to their flat appearance.

2. *Nodular melanoma* is the second most common growth pattern and occurs in 15–30% of patients with melanoma. It is characterized by rapid vertical growth that invades the dermis. This malignancy is the most aggressive and has a significantly worse prognosis. They start de novo rather than from a pre-existing nevus and are more common in men. Lesions have an elevated appearance.

3. *Lentigo maligna melanomas* have prolonged horizontal growth pattern and are slow to metastasize. They appear on sun-exposed skin and are uncommon before 50 years. They develop on pre-existing benign lesions called Hutchinson's freckles and appear as large, flat lesions with notched borders and tan to brown coloration. As the disease progresses, the lesion may develop a vertical growth phase and eventual metastasize.

4. *Acral lentiginous melanoma* characteristically occurs on the palms or soles, or beneath the nail beds; however, not all plantar lesions are acral lentiginous melanomas. Dark-skinned individuals are more susceptible to these lesions. Twice as many women are diagnosed with this type of melanoma then men. The pattern resembles lentigo maligna but the lesion moves more quickly into vertical growth phase and can ulcerate.

Subungual melanomas can present in any of the four growth patterns. Seventy-five percent involve the great toe or thumb and are seen in dark-skinned individuals. They can be differentiated from benign lesions by a brownish discoloration of the nail bed and surrounding tissue.

Amelanotic melanomas are composed of melanoblasts, the precursor cells of melanocytes. Between 2% and 8% of all diagnosed malignant melanomas are amelanotic in nature. Their aggressive nature is due to their undifferentiated nature. Also, these lesions are misdiagnosed or often diagnosed at advanced stages, leading to a poor prognosis.

Pathologic Staging—The prognosis of malignant melanoma is inversely proportional to the depth or vertical invasion of the primary tumor. Clark developed a microstaging system based on the anatomic level of invasion of the tumor. In level I, the tumor cells are above the basement membrane and within the epidermis. In level II, the cells have broken through the basement membrane and have extended into the papillary dermis. In level III, the cells fill the papillary dermis and reach the papillary/reticular dermis. At level IV, the cells are mixed between bundles of collagen in the reticular dermis. Finally, at level V, the tumor cells have invaded the subcutaneous tissue and beyond.

Breslow correlated the depth of the tumor with the prognosis and severity of the disease. Stage I includes tumors less than 0.76 mm. These have the best prognosis and recurrence is rare. Tumors that are 0.76–1.5 mm thick are stage II with intermediate prognosis. Lastly, stage III tumors are greater than 1.5 mm and frequently recur and metastasize. A fourth stage has been added to designate tumors greater than 4.0 mm.

The TNM classification combines the Clark and Breslow classification to more accurately state tumors. T stands for primary tumor; N is for assessment of regional lymph nodes; M classifies the level to which a tumor has metastasized. This five-stage TNM system is internationally recognized system for staging malignant melanoma and is currently the most recognized system among pathologists.

Treatment—Excision of the primary lesion is the treatment of choice for cutaneous malignant melanoma. Some advocate excising a radius of 5 cm surrounding the lesion. Others believe the margin depends on the depth of the lesion. Any lesion less than 0.76 mm should be excised with 1-cm margins. Lesions greater than 0.76 mm should be excised with a margin of 3–5 cm. Full excisions should be taken in order to avoid missing a portion of the deep malignancy. Biopsy should be taken to the level of the fascia, up to, but not including, the periosteum. The specimens should be sutured at a designated margin in order to orient the specimen should further excision be required. The specimen is sent to a pathologist in formalin.

Melanomas located on the toe require amputation at the metatarsophalangeal joint. Subungual melanomas are associated with local recurrence, in-transit metastases, and nodal metastases regardless of the tumor depth. Elective lymph node dissection or sentinel node mapping should be considered with all subungual melanomas. After the regional lymph nodes, the most common sites for metastases are liver, lung, brain, bone, and visceral organs.

Conclusion—Malignant melanomas are deadly skin disorders if not detected early and treated aggressively. Podiatrists who are aware of the manifestations of this malignancy, the prognoses of the different stages, and the treatment available, will have the most success in controlling cutaneous malignant melanoma of the foot and ankle.—*O.T. Wang, D.P.M.*

◆ This review highlights many important aspects of melanoma. Early excision, while the melanoma is still thin, is the treatment of choice. This requires skill in the recognition of atypical pigmented lesions and a liberal approach to the timely removal of such lesions. There is no proven therapy beyond early excision. Lymph node dissection, interferon, and chemotherapy are all options, but none of these options appears to have a proven survival benefit.—*M. Rupp, D.P.M., M.D.*

14 Pediatric Manifestations of the Foot

RICHARD M. JAY, D.P.M.

Things You May Not Know About Pediatrics

Perkin RM, Van Stralen D (Loma Linda University Children's Hospital, Loma Linda, CA)

JEMS 25(3):38–49, 2000

This article discusses 20 differences between children and adults which may be beneficial in the management and evaluation of pediatric patients.

1. Children are psychologically immature and may respond inappropriately to illness or injury as a result of their anxiety. In a child who is suffering from psychological stress, it may be difficult to differentiate between physical signs produced by fear and those produced by injury or sickness. A stressful situation can cause such physiologic reactions as tachycardia, tachypnea, hypertension, prolonged crying, shaking, breath-holding spells, poor peripheral perfusion, and prolonged capillary refill time. It is important to try to gain the confidence of the child to reduce anxiety and obtain a more accurate assessment.

2. When evaluating an infant's level of consciousness (LOC), one must keep in mind that infants are near-sighted and tend to focus on objects that are 1–2 feet from their face. As a result, poor eye contact and poor visual tracking are good ways to assess LOC in infants. In children, one must make sure to question the child using a vocabulary that the child can understand.

3. Child abuse is a leading cause of childhood death especially in the 1 year of life. Inflicted head injury from "shaken-baby syndrome" is the most frequent cause of traumatic deaths for infants and its presentation can be

confusing because external evidence may not be present. Any infant who has seizures, lethargy, or an altered LOC should be examined for signs of inflicted brain injury.

4. Spinal cord injury in pediatric patients may not be visible on radiograph, particularly because a child's cervical spine does not reach maturity until about age 8. Pediatric patients are predisposed to spinal cord injury because they have hypermobility and ligamentous laxity.

5. Vital signs in children have different "normal" values than in adults. For instance, tachycardia and tachypnea are more normal for injured or sick children than for adults. However, tachycardia is also frequently the first sign of shock; therefore, any heart rate over 160 must be explained.

6. Children depend on normal heart rate to maintain cardiac output. Bradycardia (<60 bpm) is associated with inadequate cardiac output. One must aggressively treat bradycardia in pediatrics even if blood pressure is normal. Ventilate with 100% oxygen, do chest compressions, and give epinephrine if necessary.

7. Bradycardia may be the first sign of hypoxemia in an infant. Central cyanosis (blueness of lips and mucus membranes) is not a reliable or early indicator of hypoxemia.

8. Newborn infants have difficulty breathing through their mouths when nasal passages are occluded; thus, maintaining an open nasal airway is extremely important for an infant. Breathing can be compromised with nasal congestion, increased secretions or the presence of a nasogastric tube.

9. The pediatric airway differs from that of an adult. There is a proper technique to opening, maintenance, and intubation of the pediatric airway.

10. Grunting on exhalation in an infant usually indicates a medical emergency. Diseases with reduced lung compliance exhibit grunting as do nonrespiratory disorders such as peritonitis, hemmorhage, and appendicitis.

11. During infancy, inhibitory responses predominate so that upper airway obstruction may trigger reflexes that produce apnea rather than respiratory stimulation.

12. Special care must be taken when restraining children to spinal boards because they have very compliant chest walls which may impair chest wall movement.

13. A child's liver and spleen are vulnerable organs which can be easily damaged by blows to the abdomen. Palpate the abdomen to detect pain and/or rigidity in the injured child.

14. The horizontal insertion of the diaphragm in infants (in adults, it is oblique) tends to draw the ribs inward during spontaneous respiration

which wastes work. One must monitor a child's respiration very carefully when he or she is on a spinal board.

15. The fact that children have a thin epidermal layer and a high body-surface-to-mass ratio has several implications. One, they are vulnerable to rapid loss of body heat and have a higher risk of hypothermia than do adults. Two, children require a different burn diagram than adults. Three, efforts to help a child preserve body heat should focus on large surface exposures such as the head. And four, thermoneutral temperature for infants (the temperature at which they do not expend energy warming or cooling the body) is at 80° while for the adult it is 70°. Thus, an exposed infant can develop hypothermia in an air-conditioned room.

16. A persistent cough (3–4 weeks) is abnormal and requires further evaluation.

17. Apnea may be the only clinical manifestation of seizure in neonates, infants, and young children.

18. Fewer than half of full-term infants cough when stimulated. Irritant receptors in the large airways stimulate cough due to mechanical irritation and respiratory infection and they also prevent aspiration of foreign materials into the airways. The absence of cough may result in aspiration pneumonia.

19. There is no federally mandated curriculum to train prehospital care providers in emergency pediatrics.

20. Children with airway obstruction have a prolonged inspiratory duration, and you may hear strider. One should reduce airway swelling with cool air, humidified oxygen, or mist generated by a hot running shower. Very cold air can cause bronchospasm. Also, do not give bronchodilators because this may cause swelling of the blood vessels and worsen obstruction.—*B. Hoffman*

America's Tragedy: Pediatric Trauma

Roback MG (University of Colorado Health Sciences Center, The Children's Hospital, Denver, CO)
Emerg Med Serv 29(4):61–65, 2000

Introduction—Trauma is the leading cause of death and disability in children with motor vehicle collisions (MVC), causing 80% of these injuries. Trauma-related death can occur in three different time intervals: seconds after the event, minutes to hours after the event, and days to weeks following the event. Death within seconds after the accident is usually due to extensive injuries that do not allow time for the start of resuscitation. Minutes to hours after the trauma, called the "Golden Hour," permits time to begin aggressive resuscitation. Lastly, complications, sepsis, organ failure, and brain death are the usual causes of death days to weeks following the traumatic event.

Objectives—How aggressively a pediatric patient is worked up and treated depends on the mechanism of injury. High-risk mechanisms include greater magnitudes of force, falls greater than 20 feet, fires causing burns or asphyxia, and penetrating trauma. MCVs of high-risk include ejections from the car, rollovers, being improperly restrained, or not being restrained at all. Assessing a pediatric trauma also involves knowing the speed and extent of vehicle damage, medical status of other accident victims, and patient's position in the car.

Knowing where to send the pediatric patient is crucial. The Regional Pediatric Trauma Center (RPTC) is the best first choice followed by a level I trauma center with pediatric commitment (LI-P). If these first two facilities are not accessible, a level II trauma center with pediatric commitment (LII-P) is a third option. A child in traumatic arrest or whose airway cannot be secured should be sent to any nearby trauma center. Knowing the transport time and how much time can be tolerated to get the patient to the facility is equally important.

There are many differences between the pediatric and adult trauma patient. Children can have more internal organ injuries without having associated bony fractures since their skeleton is not yet fully developed. Pediatric patients also have a higher risk of hypothermia and cervical injuries. They may show minimally altered vital signs despite their trauma emergency. Therefore, knowing how to assess the extent of the trauma is crucial. Approaching these patients requires doing a primary survey and addressing any life-threatening conditions (resuscitation phase) they might have. After the patient is stabilized, a secondary survey, or head-to-toe examination, should be performed. Finally, the definitive care phase requires the pediatric patient be managed by a surgeon and the child be transferred to the appropriate pediatric trauma center.

There are many common errors that occur in pediatric trauma care settings. Sometimes physicians fail to open and maintain the airway or to immobilize the cervical spine. Failing to recognize and treat internal hemorrhaging and giving inadequate fluid resuscitation are other common errors.

Conclusion—When caring for a pediatric trauma victim, transporting the child to an appropriate medical facility is vitally important. The patient should then be immediately assessed for the ABCs of resuscitation. Being aware of the anatomical differences between pediatric and adult patients, having pediatric sized equipment, and avoiding the common errors will help increase the potential for treatment success.—*G.H. Jhala*

Surgical Treatment of the Cleft Foot

Tani Y, Ikuta Y, Ishida O (Hiroshima University School of Medicine, Hiroshima, Japan)
Plast Reconstr Surg 105(6):1997–2002, 2000

Introduction—About 0.009% of children are born with cleft foot. Clinically, they may have cleft skin or ray deficiencies. The goal of surgically reconstructing a cleft foot include closing the cleft, keeping the feet symmetrical, and preventing collapse and valgus formation of the toes. The three most common surgical procedures for treating cleft foot are primary simple closure of the cleft, application of a double-pedicled flap, and insertion of a silicone block. This study evaluated the results of these procedures on 32 cleft feet.

Patient Profile—Twenty-one patients, ages ranging between 7 months and 6 years, were treated surgically for cleft feet. They were classified based on the number of central ray deficiencies they had: zero, one, two, or three deficiencies. Patients with zero to one central ray deficiency were treated with primary simple closure of the cleft. In patients with three to four deficiencies, eight were given primary closure, seven were given a double-pedicle flap, four were given silicone blocks, one was given a toe transfer, and five had concomitant syndactyly surgery. Only 14 patients had follow-up.

Surgical Procedure—The simple closure of the cleft was involved a dorsal zigzag incision and a plantar straight incision. A triangular flap was sutured across the interdigital space. For the double-pedicle flap procedures, a flap created from the cleft area was turned into a third toe and the dorsal skin defect was filled with a skin graft. The silicone block insertion involved expansion of the dorsal skin for several weeks and insertion of the block into the space. No skin graft is necessary.

Results—A procedure was considered successful if there was postoperative widening of the cleft, hypertrophic scarring, pigmentation of the skin graft, and overlapping of the toes. Gait and ulceration risk were also evaluated. The valgus deformity of the first toe and the distance between the first and fifth metatarsals were assessed by X-rays. A 10-point system was used to evaluate these patients. All nine patients with zero to one deficiency were grade as excellent. Of the patients with two to three ray deficiencies treated with double-pedicle flaps, four were rated as good, three were rated as fair, and one was rated as poor. Three patients given the silicone block insertions were graded as excellent and one was graded as good. No silicone synovitis or fragmentation occurred.

Discussion—Primary simple closure works well for patients with zero to one central ray deficiency because they have soft tissue in the central forefoot. On the other hand, this procedure cannot maintain the width of the forefoot in patients with two to three central ray deficiencies. For patients with more severely deformed cleft feet, the silicone block technique allows the foot to maintain the width and correct the deformity. The main postoperative complications are silicone rejection and synovitis. Also, as a child ages and his or her foot grows, a larger silicone block may need to be implanted. Therefore, silicone block implantation into the foot appears to be a safe and effective treatment option for cleft foot.—*G.H. Jhala*

◆ The authors present an interesting finding using a silicone block to maintain the distance across the width of the forefoot. One of the major complications with surgical procedures to correct cleftfoot is the narrowing of the forefoot that creates difficulty with shoe gear. Eventually, if left untreated, the medial and lateral columns start to roll into a varus on the fifth and a valgus on the first great toe. Eventually, this leads to a severe valgus deformity of the great toe and an increased varus deformity of the fifth. With the use of a block and tissue expander to close over this silicone block, the width of the forefoot is maintained and proper shoe gear can be utilized. Care must be taken, however, with the use of any type of implanted device in children, especially if it is too large. Foreign-body reaction and silicone synovitis can occur with any implantation, especially if the implant is too large and subjected to excessive motion.—*R.M. Jay, D.P.M.*

Resistant Talipes Equinovarus Associated with Congenital Constriction Band Syndrome

Hennigan SP, Kuo KN (Rush-Presbyterian–St. Luke's Medical Center and Shriners Hospital for Children, Chicago, IL)
J Pediatr Orthop 20(2):240–245, 2000

Objective—To review 28 children who had clubfoot with ipsilateral constriction bands to determine whether the location and severity of the bands, as well as the presence of neurologic deficit, influenced the treatment and outcomes of those patients.

Methods—All 28 patients conformed within the Patterson's criteria, which include the appearance of a constriction ring seen alone or in combination with deformity of the distal part of the limb. The locations of the constrictor bands were divided into four zones. The severity of the bands were also considered and placed into four different grades. Zone 1 bands occurred between the greater trochanter and the knee and accounted for three of the 135 bands total (2%). Zone 2 bands occurred between the knee and the ankle accounting for 67 of the 135 total bands (50%). Zone 3 bands occurred between the ankle and the metatarsophalangeal joints accounting for 14 of the 135 bands total (10%). Zone 4 and were limited to the toes and accounted for 51 of the 135 total bands (38%).

The severity of the bands was also considered and consisted of four grades. Grade 1 bands were subcutaneous, not to the level of the fascia, and accounted for a total of four bands (3%). Grade 2 bands were to the level of the fascia but did not compromise circulation to the distal extremities and accounted for 25 bands (19%). Grade 3 bands were to the level of the fascia but compromised distal extremity circulation, necessitating surgical release of the bands, and accounted for 45 bands (33%). Grade 4 bands included all congenital amputations accounting for 61 bands (45%).

These patients were also divided into two groups. Group A included children without documented neurologic deficit, totaling 21 children with 26 clubfeet. Group B included those patients with documented neurologic deficit, accounting for 10 patients with 11 clubfoot deformities.

Results—The average follow-up of the 28 patients was 112.5 months. In group A, 21 patients with 26 clubfeet underwent a total of 37 surgeries, averaging 1.4 surgeries per clubfoot. Clinical results were good for 15 patients with 19 clubfeet. Five patients with five clubfeet had fair results. Two patients with two clubfeet had poor results. One child had a severe postoperative infection ultimately required an amputation.

Group B had 10 patients with 11 clubfeet that required 41 surgeries, averaging 3.7 surgeries per clubfoot deformity. Four patients had good results. Two patients had fair results. Five patients had poor results, with one of the patients ending up with an amputation. None of the patients in group B regained muscle function that was absent preoperatively.

Conclusion—The zoning of the constriction bands, as well as neurologic deficiency, apparently played a significant role in the final outcome of the foot deformity. Those patients in group B with the neurologic deficit ultimately needed more surgeries to help correct the deformity, with the outcome not being as good as group A without the neurologic deficiencies.—*Q. Solomon*

♦ Although constriction syndromes are rare, when they are present, they can lead to neurologic problems as well as muscular defects of the leg. The constriction band that is of most concern is that in zone 2. This lies between the ankle and the knee and, depending upon the grade of severity, will indicate whether or not there will be neurologic deficit. The constriction band creates a compression on the nerve, which can lead to a possible compartment syndrome or direct neuroptmesis. With any of these constriction bands, the earlier the treatment and the more of a complete soft-tissue release will yield a better long-term effect on the clubfoot syndrome.—*R.M. Jay, D.P.M.*

Function After Correction of a Clawed Great Toe by a Modified Robert Jones Transfer

Breusch SJ, Wenz W, Döderlein L (Orthopaedic University Clinic, Heidelberg, Germany)

J Bone Joint Surg 82-B(2):250–254, 2000

Introduction—This retrospective cross-sectional study reviewed 51 patients who underwent a modified Jones transfer as treatment for a clawed hallux in conjunction with a cavus foot type deformity. Preoperatively, all patients had dorsal corns and/or pressure symptoms under the first metatarsal head. Thirty-six of these patients were diagnosed with a cavus foot with progressive neuromuscular disorder. Ten were diagnosed with a cavus foot with a static neuromuscular disorder and five were of other causes.

Method—A modified Robert Jones extensor hallucis longus (EHL) tendon transfer was performed by passing the distal end of the tendon through a horizontal drill hole in the neck of the first metatarsal. The tendon was sutured to itself under physiologic tension by placing the ankle in full extension with passive dorsiflection of the first ray. In patients with a rigid plantarflexed first ray, an extension osteotomy of the first metatarsal was also performed and fixed with K-wires (in 58 feet). The interphalangeal joint (IP) was resected and fused via percutaneous crossed K-wires. A transfer of the peroneus longus (PL) to the peroneus brevis (PB) was performed in 24 feet. A tibialis anterior tendon transfer was performed in 36 feet and a split-transfer was performed in 11 feet. The mean follow-up time postoperatively was 42 months.

A multivariant regression analysis of the data was performed and significance was performed via the Fisher's exact test. Postoperatively, subjects were evaluated clinically and radiographically for range of motion, pain, union, gait disturbances, elevation of the first ray, and satisfaction.

Results—Overall patient satisfaction was 86%. Common complications included catching of the big toe, asymptomatic nonunion, metatarsalgia, and hallux limitus. PL transfer associated with elevation of the first ray was noted to be significant ($p < .0001$). There was no correlation between nonunion of the IP joint and hallux limitus/flexus.

Discussion—The Jones tendon transfer was effective for the correction of hallux claw toe with high patient satisfaction. PL transfer should be used with caution as overcorrection can result and cause transfer symptoms.—*D.D.-Q. Tran, D.P.M.*

♦ The authors address the reduction of the pulling of the great toe by modified Robert Jones tendon transfer. They transfer the extensor hallucis longus to the neck of the first metatarsal along with a release of the plantar fascia. This also includes a fusion of the IP joint of the hallux. Certainly, the procedure is not a new technique and has been described by many authors previously, but again, this article does not address certain very important concerns. One of the greatest concerns is that too much elevation of the first ray will further induce a hallux limitus. The radiographs in this report certainly demonstrate this and they discuss it to the point where they talk about a "roll- out." This is apparently a supination of the foot to avoid the jamming of the great toe on the first metatarsal. I do think that this is a result of the procedure, but certainly the supination that the authors call "roll- out" can be limited by the use of an insert. The pull of the peroneus longus still needs to be maintained to allow the first ray to purchase the ground. Either casting with an insert and posting the valgus deformity present preoperatively will reduce the flexion deformity of the IP joint. If clawing is that significant, I do not agree with the authors to maximally dorsiflex the first ray, but rather believe it should be supported with the transfer to create a slight elevation and fuse the IP joint, rather than forcibly elevating the first ray and thereby inducing the hallux limitus. — *R.M. Jay, D.P.M.*

Haglund's Syndrome: Disappointing Results Following Surgery—A Clinical and Radiographic Analysis

Schneider W, Niehus W, Knahr K (Orthopaedic Hospital Vienna-Speising, Vienna, Austria)
Foot Ankle Int 21(1):26–30, 2000

Introduction—Haglund's deformity, also known as pump bump, is an osseous deformity of the posterior superior aspect of the calcaneus that typically occurs secondary to friction between the calcaneus and the shoe counter. The purpose of this study was to determine whether clinical findings and radiographic angles were useful in determining the risk factors and predictors for surgical outcome and rehabilitation time.

Methods—A retrospective study was conducted on 49 surgical cases of Haglund's deformity. Clinical analysis was based on the ankle hindfoot system which evaluates many variables such as pain, gait, ankle range of motion, foot type, preoperative conservative treatment, postoperative complaints, and overall satisfaction. Radiographic analysis was based on multiple angles and measurements which help determine the severity of the deformity as well as the area of resection required. The surgical technique consisted of removal of a triangular shaped wedge from the posterior superior aspect of the calcaneus.

Results—Thirty-four patients reported relief of pain and seven patients noted some improvement. One patient described no change while seven patients felt their symptoms had worsened. Forty-three patients would undergo the operation again while seven would not. The majority of the foot types were

normal with only one cavus foot and no flatfeet. The average time of rehabilitation was 2 months until patients could wear normal shoes, 5 months to
resume full sporting activity, and 6 months until there was complete pain relief.

Discussion—Seventy-three percent of the patients were satisfied with the
surgery which is an unacceptable outcome for a procedure that is considered
by most as minor; 14.3% of the patients would not undergo the surgery
again. The most frequent reason for dissatisfaction was the extended length
of rehabilitation followed by persistent postoperative pain. No specific foot
type including the cavus foot (the most common type seen with Haglund's
deformity according to past studies) could be confirmed as a risk factor
for the deformity or a predictor for surgical outcome. Also, the popular
hypothesis that compensated rearfoot varus, compensated forefoot valgus,
and rigid plantarflexed first ray are precursors to Haglund's could not be
confirmed. Lastly, the data show that neither clinical findings nor radiographic
measurements are reliable predictors of surgical outcome.

Conclusion—The surgical treatment of Haglund's deformity often yields
less than satisfactory results. The patient should be made aware of the
potential for a lengthy rehabilitation time. All conservative treatment should
be exhausted before attempting surgery.—*D. Carmack*

♦ The authors speak of a disappointing result following surgical procedure to reduce
a Haglund's deformity. Fewer than 75% of the patients were satisfied. I do concur
with the author that often, not only with Haglund's deformity, but with other minor
surgical procedures of the foot, surgery is entered into lightly by the patient. In
addition, the physician, all too often, does not give the full long-term course of
rehabilitation. It is not uncommon for discomfort with these posterior ostectomies
to last 3–6 months. If patients know of the long-term recovery potential, they may
not be as anxious to proceed with the sugery. For this reason, I strongly recommend
conservative approaches until failure and then the patient would realize the severity of
the condition and not take the surgical recommendations lightly.—*R.M. Jay, D.P.M.*

Surgical Treatment of Severe Hindfoot Valgus by Medial Displacement Osteotomy of the Os Calcis in Children with Myelomeningocele

Torosian CM, Dias LS (Fox Valley Orthopaedic Institute, Geneva; Northwestern
University Medical School, Children's Memorial Hospital, Chicago, IL)
J Pediatr Orthop 20(2):226–229, 2000

Introduction—Pedal deformities are the most common abnormalities in
children with myelomeningocele. Valgus deformities of the hindfoot and ankle

become prevalent as the child matures, begins to ambulate, and gains weight. Hindfoot valgus is most likely caused by muscle imbalances, weightbearing, and the effects of gravity on the partially sensate or insensate foot. Bracing and shoe wear become more difficult as the deformities progress. Surgery is indicated when the deformity is severe, rigid, and associated with pain, difficulty with brace wear, and ulceration.

Several authors attempted correction of these deformities with extra-articular subtalar arthrodesis or triple arthrodesis; success was variable. If the valgus deformity is in the subtalar joint and calcaneus, a medial displacement calcaneal osteotomy may be indicated to correct hindfoot valgus, while preserving subtalar motion. A retrospective review of the medial displacement osteotomy of the os calcis was performed to determine the effects of the procedure on pain relief, bracing, and degree of hindfoot correction, and to assess overall patient satisfaction.

Methods—Thirty-eight procedures were performed on 27 patients with myelomeningocele and concurrent hindfoot valgus associated with pain, difficulty with bracing, and ulceration. The authors performed a medial calcaneal displacement osteotomy and followed patients both clinically and radiographically for at least 24 months.

Results—Outcomes were analyzed clinically by the degree of hindfoot valgus and by the presence of pain, pressure sores, and problems with brace and shoe wear. A good result, defined by less than 5° valgus with no pressure sores or difficulty with brace wear, was obtained in 82% of patients. Five patients (13%) were rated as poor, due to inadequate displacement, recurrent ulceration, or residual supramalleolar valgus.

Discussion—The medial sliding calcaneal osteotomy is a simple and effective treatment for hindfoot valgus in pediatric patients. It provides excellent correction, while preserving subtalar joint motion.—*T.C. Melillo, D.P.M.*

♦ This article addresses a reduction of a hindfoot valgus by a medial displacement osteotomy of the calcaneus. This is similar to the Koutsogiannis procedure. I do feel that this sliding type of osteotomy is certainly indicated for flatfoot procedures, but should not be considered a procedure of primary choice. The intent of the procedure is to reduce the heel valgus and allow the forefoot to supinate upon the rearfoot. The end result will be an increase in the calcaneal inclination and the first ray will be able to set upon and purchase the medial surface. In order for this to occur, adequate dorsiflexion must occur at the ankle joint, so as not to occur at the midtarsal or subtalar joints. Consideration of tendo Achillis lengthening should be a prerequisite. Along with this, either the sliding osteotomy or Dwyer procedure is a good choice. The other consideration with all of this in mind is to plantarflex the first ray on the rearfoot, thus supinating the forefoot on the rearfoot. This is accomplished by the use of the peroneus longus to bring the first ray down. The only way this will occur is through a stable lateral cuboid, and stability of the cuboid is determined by the inversion component of the subtalar joint and the alignment of the heel into a slight varus position. Reduction of the valgus would increase the pull of the peroneus longus, but all of this must be considered after the tendo Achillis is lengthened to gain dorsiflexion. — *R.M. Jay, D.P.M.*

Return to Athletic Activity After Foot and Ankle Surgery: A Preliminary Report on Select Procedures

Saxena A (Palo Alto Medical Foundation, Palo Alto, CA)
J Foot Ankle Surg 39(2):114–119, 2000

Objective—This study establishes parameters to differentiate competitive athletes and sports enthusiasts from recreational athletes, examines the results of foot and ankle surgery in athletes, and reports time frames for return to activity (RTA) based on selected procedures.

Methods—Athletes were defined as professional, varsity college and high school, runners amassing 25 miles per week, or competitive sports enthusiasts who exercise 6 hours per week; excluded were individuals who exercise irregularly. Retrospective chart review was conducted on 138 surgical patients from 1990 to 1997, available for follow-up examination 1 year postoperatively. Noted were the procedure, follow-up duration, complications, and the athlete's ability to return to practice sessions. Athletes were asked if they experienced limitations from the surgery and if they considered it a success.

Results—Beyond sports enthusiasts, the population included 11 professional (avg RTA 6.6 weeks), six college (avg RTA 9.7 weeks), and 18 high school athletes (avg RTA 8.4 weeks) representing various sports (running, soccer, triathlon, other). The average patient age was 32.8 years (68 male, 70 female). Twenty-eight Achilles procedures included peritenolyses (eight runners, avg RTA 4 weeks) plus debridement (four athletes, avg RTA 9.75 weeks), and tendocalcinosis or retrocalcaneal exostosis/bursitis (17 athletes, avg RTA 13.8 weeks). Forty-four bunionectomy procedures included 31 first metatarsal osteotomies: 10 Austin, 13 Hohmann, eight Ludloff, with five concomitant Akin procedures (avg RTA 8.9 weeks). There were two cheilectomies and two isolated Akins, plus soft-tissue procedures. Screw fixation was used in 42 of these patients. Seven athletes had Valenti procedures for hallux rigidus (avg RTA 5.5 weeks). Six athletes had hallucial sesamoidectomies (avg RTA 7.4 weeks). Seven athletes had Morton's neurectomies via dorsal approach (avg RTA 4 weeks). Of 48 rearfoot procedures, the average RTA for ossicle excision was 9.1 weeks. Seven athletes had Brostrom-type lateral ankle stabilization procedures (avg RTA 10 weeks), and seven had open reduction and internal fixation for Jones or navicular fractures (avg RTA

11.3 weeks). Overall, there were no cases of infection or reflex sympathetic dystrophy. One hundred thirteen patients believed their surgery a success, 23 athletes increased their activity level, two had a decrease in desired activity level, two had revision surgery, and eight had symptomatic screws removed.

Discussion—This paper encourages others to employ its guidelines to help select procedures that will return athletes to their desired level of activity. Athletes are typically more motivated to follow postoperative management than the average patient, making a faster return to desired activity, though this comparison remains to be studied. The literature shows that athletes' return to competition is highly variable, depending on seasonal injury and other factors. The minimal complications demonstrated by this study imply that athletes are healthy and compliant with postoperative care. Most athletes are managed with removable/functional cast bracing. The results of this study indicate that athletes may undergo foot and ankle surgery without inhibiting their career, and in some cases may increase their level of activity.—*D. Collman*

Talo-navicular Arthrodesis for Residual Midfoot Deformities of a Previously Corrected Clubfoot

Wei SY, Sullivan RJ, Davidson RS (Children's Hospital of Philadelphia, University of Pennsylvania School of Medicine, Philadelphia, PA)
Foot Ankle Int 21(6):482–485, 2000

Introduction—Following surgical or nonsurgical correction of clubfeet, many residual deformities may ensue. These often include avascular necrosis, triangulation of the navicular, and subluxation of the talonavicular (TN) joint. This article investigates the use of TN joint arthrodesis to correct one or more of the residual deformities associated with clubfoot correction.

Methods—A retrospective study of 19 consecutive TN fusions from 1991 to 1996 were reviewed. The 16 patients who underwent the TN fusion had a history of a painful TN joint secondary to one of the aforementioned residual deformities after a previous clubfoot correction. The average age of the patients was 11 years and the average time period since the initial correction was 10 years. A TN fusion was done only on cases in which the hindfoot was adequately aligned during the previous clubfoot correction. The incision from the previous clubfoot correction was used and a medial release was performed as necessary. The articular cartilage was removed, avoiding shortening of the medial column, and was fixed with either Kirschner wires, screws, or staples. Lateral column shortening and/or bone graft at the fusion site was performed as needed. Each of the patients answered a standardized questionnaire based on Atar's objective rating system for clubfoot surgery to assess their satisfaction. A physical and radiographic examination was also performed.

Results—All 15 patients reported being satisfied with the surgical outcome, with 14 of them being completely satisfied. An average score of 76 out of 100 was attained on the Atar's objective rating system. An approximately equal number of feet were divided between losing their subtalar motion, maintaining 15° of motion, and achieving at least 15° of motion. All patients were able to dorsiflex their ankle joint to neutral. Radiographically, the talus–first metatarsal angle on the AP went from an average of 18.6° to 3.7° while on the lateral view it went from 31.0° to 16.1°. The talus–calcaneus angle did not change. There were two postoperative complications that resulted in further surgery.

Conclusion—The talonavicular arthrodesis for residual clubfoot deformities provided satisfactory pain relief and improvement of the talus–first metatarsal angles, especially when combined with a calcaneal osteotomy. This study contrasts previous studies of TN arthrodesis performed in adult patients. These previous studies showed loss of subtalar range of motion and thus trouble with ambulation. This study showed that when this procedure is performed on children, some subtalar joint range of motion is maintained. This may minimize future osteoarthritic changes in adjacent joints.—*L. Rowe*

♦ This article is quite good with regard to the recurrent residual midfoot deformity seen in talipes equinovarus. What is noted is one of the following: either a talonavicular joint that leaves the foot into a cavus position or severe talonavicular arthritis as well as a possible subluxation of the talonavicular joint. Postoperative and long-term findings leave the child in a residual cavus deformity. Usually what is noted is a flat-topped talus and arthritic changes. This is due to the lack of dorsiflexion at the ankle joint; the change will end up in the talonavicular joint. We consider either osteotomies, midfoot fusions, or the talonavicular fusion, as described, as the recommended treatment of choice for these residual deformities.—*R.M. Jay, D.P.M.*

The Viladot Implant in Flatfooted Children

Black PRM, Betts RP, Duckworth T, Smith TWD (University of Connecticut; Hartford Hospital, Hartford, CT)
Foot Ankle Int 21(6):478–481, 2000

Introduction—It is believed that adult anterior knee pain, hip pain, and back pain can all be correlated with a pediatric flatfoot. In 1991, Viladot described a surgical procedure utilizing a silastic implant to control talar position by preventing subluxation of the head of the talus off of the calcaneus. Viladot reported successful results in 234 cases with insertion of the implant into the sinus tarsi accompanied by tibialis posterior tendon advancement and soft-tissue correction. A bi-incisional approach was used to access the sinus tarsi. In an attempt to reproduce Viladot's results, 22 implants over a 3-year period were inserted using the technique described by Viladot.

Methods—In maintaining Viladot's criteria, 15 children ranging from 5 to 14 years old with painless flatfeet underwent surgical correction. A total of 22 implants were inserted via a bi-incisional approach. Through the medial incision, using a wide periosteal flap, the tibialis posterior tendon was advanced to the navicular. The rearfoot valgus was corrected by lever through the sinus tarsi and soft-tissue adjustment. The lateral approach allowed the Viladot implant to be passed through the sinus tarsi from lateral to medial with forceps. The Viladot implant resembles a wineglass and in the sinus tarsi the footplate lies medially and the barrel laterally. Postoperative care consisted of a below-knee cast for 1 month with subsequent rehabilitation.

Results—Optical center of pressure plot, radiograph, and clinical results were all considered in 22 feet of 15 children. Clinical improvement was achieved in seven patients who regressed in 6 months. Seventy-three percent of patients reported significant pain, while 9% described little discomfort. Per patient report, the only improvement from the surgery was decreased shoe expense.—*K. Van Voris*

◆ This is a very interesting viewpoint on this procedure. The authors reviewed 22 cases of flatfoot correction utilizing the sinus tarsi implant. They compared it to Viladot's 234 patients. The authors describe doing a tibialis posterior advancement and immobilizing the patient for 1 month and then starting rehabilitation. The implantable silicon plug is put in at this time. Their results were quite poor and they have a 32% clinical improvement as compared to Viladot's 100% improvement. Furthermore, 36% of the implants had to be removed, whereas in Viladot's study only 0.5% of the implants had to be removed.

I found this article quite alarming. The authors, right at the onset of the article, write on the children with painless flatfoot deformities. Certainly when entertaining any procedure, especially for flatfoot, one would wait until some symptoms of pain were present. Personally, I have had over 20 years of experience utilizing sinus tarsi implants, and all of them have been quite successful with a minimal removal rate and close to 100% improvement. The parents and children have both been pleased and the results have been excellent. Along with the procedures, the majority of them did have an equinus with the flatfoot and a tendo Achillis or Gastroc lengthening was done simultaneously. I do think that one of the problems with this paper, besides suggesting surgery for children who are asymptomatic, is that the posterior complex was not addressed in reference to the amount of dorsiflexion that was available at the ankle. Certainly, tightening of the posterior tibial tendon was the answer to reduce flatfoot deformities as originally described by Kidner in the early 1900s.—*R.M. Jay, D.P.M.*

Relapse in Staged Surgery for Congenital Talipes Equinovarus

Uglow MG, Clarke NM (Southampton General Hospital, Southampton, Hampshire, UK)

J Bone Joint Surg 82-B(5):739–743, 2000

Introduction—Surgical treatment of talipes equinovarus (TE) with single-stage primary correction has been cited to be associated with complications such as dehiscence, necrosis, infection, and wound slough. This prospective study utilizes a two-stage procedure for TE correction and evaluates relapse and associated wound complications compared to single-stage procedures.

Methods—Ninety-one recalcitrant TE feet in 86 patients were studied. Preoperatively, all subjects were graded for deformity severity using the classification system developed by Dimeglio et al. Each subject underwent a two-stage surgical correction procedure. The first stage is the plantar medial release with the incision starting proximally at the level of the mid-os calcis and extending dorsal distally at the level of the base of the first metatarsal. Underlying structures were released/divided as in the single-stage procedure. Two weeks after the first stage, the second stage is performed pending good healing. This posterolateral release is similar to the single-stage procedure with the incision being oblique and starting proximally at the mid-calf level and terminating distally between the tendo Achillis and the lateral malleolus. All subjects are managed postoperatively with long-leg casts and night splints. Postoperative reassessment with the Dimeglio grading is also performed.

A relapse of the deformity is considered if additional surgery is required for correction. Relapse trend was assessed using the Cochrane-Armitage test.

Results—Relapse trend with increasing deformity severity was statistically significant. The overall rate of re-operation was 30.8%. No feet were noted to be worse than preoperatively. Improvement in deformity grading was appreciated postsurgery. The rate of infection was 1.1% of cases and 0.5% of wounds. No slough or necroses were encountered.

Discussion—Exact incidence of wound complications following primary TE correction is not known, although it has been suggested to be less that 4%. A two-stage surgery appears to be effective in reducing wound complications or at worse does not present with less favorable results than other forms of surgery. Pre- and postoperative grading suggests that correction is less and the need for further surgery is greater in higher grade levels of deformity.—*D.D.-Q. Tran, D.P.M.*

♦ The authors present their findings using a two-incisional approach regarding the clubfoot deformity. They found that with severe deformities in plantarflexion of the foot and severe clubfoot deformity, surgical reduction will yield an increase in wound complications in the child's foot. By staging the procedures, as other authors have prescribed, wound formation is minimized. It would seem with gradual reduction of the deformity, timed over a 3- to 4-month period, the risks of wound problems would decrease; however, the authors did not find an appreciable difference between the posterolateral and medial approach. Those children with severe deformities do wind up with a delayed healing at the operative site.—*R.M. Jay, D.P.M.*

Injuries in Youth Soccer: A Subject Review

Anderson S, Griesemer B, Johnson M, Martin T, McLain L, Rowland T, Small E (Committee on Sports Medicine and Fitness)
Pediatrics 105(3):659–661, 2000

Background—Soccer, known as football internationally, is one of the most popular team sports played in the world. In the United States, it is a growing sport, but along with its increased participation comes a higher incidence of injury. By reviewing the spectrum of soccer-related injuries, it is suggested that selective rule changes be made with the desire of reducing the risk of injury.

Methods—Of the 18 million or so American participants, roughly 3 million are youth soccer players. Nonfatal soccer injuries affect up to 5.2% of these young players; up to 80.9% of whom damage their lower extremity. The following is a breakdown of percentages of all injuries: 2–7.1% occur at the groin, 1.8–21% at the hip and thigh, 10–26% at the knee, 13–23.1% at the ankle, and 0.3–28% of all soccer-related injuries affect the foot.

Indoor soccer players are 6.1 times more likely to sustain an injury, possibly because of the hard playing surface, artificial turf, and the presence of walls bordering the sidelines. With indoor play, player-to-player contact accounts for 31–70.3% of harm done, whereas similar outdoor contact accounts for 43–60.9% of injuries. Nearly half of these are a result of tackling, and one study shows that the goalie position shares a disproportionate amount of these contact-related injuries.

Older players, with both boys and girls, show higher rates of injury, as do players with relatively poor muscle strength. The typical soccer-related injury is a soft-tissue contusion. Fractures account for only 3.5–9% of injuries, and sprains, strains, dislocations, tendinitis, overuse, and heat-related injuries are not uncommon. With the skeletally immature athletes, calcaneal apophysitis is common and attributed to running with cleated shoes without necessary heel padding. Modified activity, improving calf flexibility, and using heel pads address this problem.

Heading the ball has been looked at closely by researchers. A controlled study in Norway showed mild to severe deficits in attention, concentration, and memory in 81% of adult players who have played since their youth. Others have voiced concern of cognitive impairments in youth with much shorter exposure to heading. Lastly, soccer proves to be the second leading cause of orofacial and dental sports injuries.

Conclusion—This review shows that the rate of soccer-related injuries is comparable to that of other contact sports and that most injuries result from player collision. Most injuries are soft tissue in nature and occur in the lower extremity. The authors recommend the following: protective mouth guards and eye-wear be used, the impact of heading the ball be explored, violent and aggressive behavior be discouraged, and rules be adjusted to minimize accidents and injuries. All things considered, soccer still remains an integral part of youth activity and fitness that pediatricians should encourage.—*C. Jacka*

♦ This article is an overview of the injuries sustained in soccer. The frequency type and causes of injury are included and, upon reviewing the article, it is interesting to note that up to 28% of all injuries of the lower extremity are related to the foot and 13–20% are related to the ankle. In addition, 10–20% of these injuries are related to the knee. The article discusses other injuries to the body and the attempt to change the rules of the sport to prevent some of these injuries, for example, the spearing rule in football, will reduce head and neck injuries. In our profession, we can limit the number of injuries with a simple modification of shoe gear. It has been documented that the soccer cleat is a poor stabilizing boot for any type of foot. With the child who is prone to hyperpronation, modifying this shoe with an over-the-counter insert or orthoses will minimize fatigue and stress overuse injuries.—*R.M. Jay, D.P.M.*

High School Cross Country Running Injuries: A Longitudinal Study

Rauh MJ, Margherita AJ, Rice SG, Koepsell TD, Rivara FP (University of Washington, Seattle, WA; Washington University, St. Louis, MO; Jersey Shore Medical Center, Neptune, NJ; Harborview Injury Prevention and Research Center, Seattle, WA)
Clin J Sport Med 10(2):110–116, 2000

Introduction—Participation in high school athletics is increasing. There have been many studies that have evaluated the risk of injury in the traditional sports of football, basketball, soccer, and wrestling. Cross country, which in the United States ranks as the seventh most popular sport, has had very little research to estimate the risk of injury.

Methods—This is a prospective-longitudinal study of 23 high schools in western Washington state between 1979 and 1994. Of these teams, there were 1,202 girls and 2,031 boys. The athletic coaches were required to take a class that informed them of the details of the study. They were then required to report every day the incidence of injury. In addition, each subsequent injury, severity, site of injury, and the setting in which the injury took place (practice or meet) for girls and boys was reported. Four time-loss classifications were used to determine the severity: 1) 1–4 days missed, 2) 5–14 days missed, 3) 15 or more days missed, and 4) out for season injuries.

Results—Overall there was an injury rate of 1,622. Girls had a higher injury rate than boys for both initial and subsequent injury. The most common initial injury sites for girls were hip, shin, and feet. The most common initial injury sites for boys were knee, shin, and ankle. The most common reinjured sites overall were shin, knee, and foot. Girls had a higher incidence of reinjury to the knee, calf, and foot. Girls had a tendency to become injured more in meets than boys; however, there was not much statistical difference between practices and meets among girls' setting of injury. The boys, on the other hand, had a 50% greater risk of injury during practices. The amount of time missed for girls was higher in class 1 (1–4 days missed), class 2 (5–14 days missed), class 3 (>15 days), and class 4 (out for the season) than boys. In fact, girls had two times greater risk for class 4 injuries.

Conclusion—Girls have a much higher propensity towards injury, both initial, and subsequent injury in high school cross country. The shin is the most common initial and subsequent site of injury in cross country runners.—*T. Marshall*

◆ This article concerning the incidence of injuries in young athletes was put together quite well. Most importantly, it was noted that the female athlete is prone to a greater risk of injury than her male counterpart. Injuries in cross country training and events were significantly higher and the risk ratio was greater in females than in males. The authors compared initial injuries and subsequent injuries and found that females are at greater risk than males in both categories.

What is most important to cull from this article is that no matter what the causes of the injury, in all areas of the lower extremity, females are at greater risk than males. The practitioner needs to address the entire musculoskeletal system prior to any child entering into any athletic endeavor. Certainly if there are some minor variances within the biomechanical examination, whether it be excessive subtalar range of motion or limited motion, or if the Q-angle is increased in the knee, the findings should be addressed even if the patient is asymptomatic. Preventive treatment from the standpoint of the podiatrist should include standard over-the-counter supports or custom-molded biomechanically constructed orthoses. This study is a great template for any practitioner who is planning on doing any further lower extremities studies with young athletes in various sports. — *R.M. Jay, D.P.M.*

15 Plastic Surgery and Reconstruction

GARY P. JOLLY, D.P.M.

Forefoot Reconstruction by Reversed Island Flaps in Diabetic Patients

Pallua N, DiBenedetto G, Berger A (University of Aachen School of Medicine, Aachen, Germany; University of Hannover Medical School, Hannover, Germany)
Plast Reconstr Surg 106(4):823–827, 2000

Background—Diabetic patients with unstable or complicated ulcers have been treated conservatively until the mid-1980s with poor results. These patients would eventually develop wound dehiscence, tissue necrosis, and infection that lead to amputation. Even though early surgical treatments have become favorable lately, there are still a lot of patients with large ulcers on both the dorsal and plantar aspects of their feet. Free-tissue transfer has been reported for treatment of diabetic ulcers; however, no study has looked at reversed island flaps of the foot for these patients. This article reviews the treatment of diabetic ulcers with reversed island flaps in diabetics.

Methods—Twelve diabetic patients with ulcers on the dorsum and plantar aspects of their feet underwent reconstructive surgery. They all had received previous conservative treatment or had undergone surgical treatment with skin graft that failed. All patients underwent foot angiogram and a Doppler evaluation of the dorsalis pedis artery, the plantar arteries, and their communicating branches. Wide debridement of the lesions was performed prior to application of flaps. A one-stage operation was done for ulcers and a two-stage operation was performed on patients with tumors. Dorsal ulcers were reconstructed with a reverse dorsalis pedis flap with retrograde arterial inflow from the proximal communicating branch and plantar ulcers were reconstructed using a reversed medial plantar flap, with retrograde arterial inflow from lateral plantar artery after division of the posterior tibial artery proximal to its distal bifurcation. Skin grafts were placed over the donor sites in all cases.

Results—In the dorsalis pedis group, the flaps survived entirely. A skin breakdown at the donor site area was evident in two patients 3 weeks after the surgical procedure. The patients began walking 3 weeks post-operatively.

In the medial plantar group, two patients had temporary donor site pain with walking 2 months postoperatively. This was probably due to absence of plantar fascia, which was harvested with the flap. There was one case of skin breakdown at the flap donor site 4 weeks postoperatively. Again at 3 weeks postoperatively, the patients began walking without special shoe gear.

Discussion—A thorough preoperative evaluation of the distal arteries is mandatory for all patients before raising the flaps. Debridement with skin grafting is still the most widely used technique because of the ease of treatment. However, when deep structures are exposed or damaged, local or distal flaps are the option of choice. Free flaps have also been used for coverage of large ulcers in diabetic patients with good results. The distally based island flaps used in this study provide a good result for medium-sized defects of the forefoot.—*O.T. Wang, D.P.M.*

♦ This study looked at the feasibility of using distally based (reverse-flow) tissue flaps to cover forefoot defects in diabetic patients. This paper is significant in that this was the first study of its kind. Although reverse-flow island flaps raised on the dorsalis pedis and the medial plantar artery have been well described in the literature, their use in diabetics, who frequently manifest vascular disease within the small vessels of the foot, has never been described.

Twelve patients were reported, seven with dorsal defects and five with plantar ulcers. These ulcers were unstable, having failed to remain closed despite previous treatment. Preoperatively, all patients underwent Doppler exam and angiography to confirm patent collateral flow between the dorsalis pedis, and the plantar vessels via the perforators in the first interspace. All flaps survived, and only several minor complications were reported.

This article is one of the most significant papers to be published on treating medium-sized defects of the forefoot in diabetics. Prior to this report, free flaps were the only method of closing these wounds. Although islands, based on the digital artery, are effective for small defects, sacrifice of the entire toe is necessary to close larger wounds. — *G.P. Jolly, D.P.M.*

The Medial Crossover Toe: A Cadaveric Dissection

Deland JT, Sung I-H (Cornell University Medical College, Hospital for Special Surgery, New York, NY; Hanyang University Hospital, Seoul, Korea)
Foot Ankle Int 21(5):375–378, 2000

Introduction—Medial deviation of the second toe is a fairly common clinical entity. Since no thorough dissection of a medial crossover second toe has been performed, the pathologic anatomy has remained unclear. A cadaveric dissection of a medial crossover toe was carried out in this report to better understand the anatomical abnormalities found in this disorder.

Methods—Anatomical dissection was performed on two cadaveric specimens from the same individual: one with crossover second toe and one with a normal alignment of the second toe.

Results—The dissection revealed several findings: medial deviation of the extensor tendons; rupture of the fibular collateral ligaments and contracture of the medial collateral ligaments; medial displacement of the flexor tendons; and medial displacement and lateral thinning of the flexor plate. No deformities of the second metatarsal head or base of the proximal phalanx were identified.

Discussion—These findings explain the difficulty encountered in achieving a successful long-term correction of a medial crossover toe with soft-tissue procedures alone. Deviation and attenuation of the plantar plate and collateral ligaments destabilize the metatarsophalangeal joint, and make correction of the deformity more difficult.—*T.C. Melillo, D.P.M.*

◆ This is a landmark paper, dealing with the unstable second metatarsophalangeal joint. A cadaveric dissection revealed lateral attenuation of the plantar plate and lateral suspensory ligaments, resulting in medial displacement of the plantar plate, and more importantly, the flexor tendons. The findings reported in this paper clearly show the folly of attempting to treat the crossover toe by digital arthroplasty, capsulotomy, and extensor tendon lengthening.

Because only one dissection was reported, the reader should be aware that variations in pathology are possible. This author has had occasion to see crossover toe without any damage to the plantar plate, and only attenuation of the lateral suspensory ligament. It should also be noted that in the hand the lateral suspensory analog is called the accessory suspensory ligament, and is in fact, smaller than the collateral ligament. However, in the metatarsophalangeal joint, the accessory ligament is actually much larger and stronger than the collateral ligament and should not be referred to as accessory. This difference is size is the result of the difference in joint function. In the hand, the metatarsophalangeal joint functions in flexion, whereas in the foot, the joint functions in hyperextension.—*G.P. Jolly, D.P.M.*

Medial Plantar Flap Based Distally on the Lateral Plantar Artery to Cover a Forefoot Skin Defect

Oberlin C, Accioli de Vasconcellos Z, Touam C (Hospital Bichat, Paris, France)
Plast Reconstr Surg 106(4):874–877, 2000

Objective—This is a case report on the use of a variant surgical technique based on a medial plantar skin flap based distally on the lateral plantar artery.

Methods—The following surgical technique was published by Martin et al. in 1991 (Martin D, et al. *Ann Chir Plast Esthet* 36:544, 1991). Martin et al. proposed several new flaps based on the concept of "reverse-flow Y-V pedicle extension of a flap. The idea was to raise a flap on a branch of a Y like a vascular bifurcation. The section of the trunk of the bifurcation turns the Y to a V vascular pattern, which allows for the distal mobilization of the flap on the remaining branch of the V" (Martin D, et al. *Ann Chir Plast Esthet* 39:403, 1994). This approach permitted adequate distal advancement of an island flap with a size up to the entire instep area.

Results—No results were given.

Conclusion—This technique proposes an instep island flap based on the lateral plantar artery. The inflow and outflow of blood is assured by the anastomosis between the dorsalis pedis and lateral plantar vessels. This approach allows for the transfer of similar tissue and provides adequate coverage of the weightbearing zone of the distal forefoot.—*Q. Solomon*

♦ The authors describe a retrograde flap based on the lateral plantar artery, which relies on the integrity of the collateral flow between the dorsalis pedis artery and the plantar perforators and the plantar arch. To increase the arc of rotation of the flap they sever the posterior tibial artery. This technique is described in one 25-year-old patient who suffered a soft-tissue loss to the forefoot. While this is a most interesting approach, its use in patients with vascular compromise would be contraindicated. The posterior tibial artery plays a major role in the perfusion of the foot, so other methods of soft-tissue replacement should be considered, such as free flaps, reverse flow sural artery islands, and toe fillet flaps, which can be converted to islands to increase their reach. Given the alternatives to posterior tibial artery sacrifice, the popularity of this flap is likely to be limited.—*G.P. Jolly, D.P.M.*

Tensor Fasciae Latae Perforator Flap for Reconstruction of Composite Achilles Tendon Defects with Skin and Vascularized Fascia

Deiler S, Pfadenhauer A, Widmann J, Stützle H, Kanz K-G, Stock W
(Ludwig-Maximilians-University of Munich, Munich, Germany)
Plast Reconstr Surg 106(2):342–349, 2000

Introduction—Large defects in the skin overlying the Achilles tendon and in the tendon proper must be reconstructed using a well vascularized graft. Several sites, including the forearm and the tensor fasciae latae muscle and fasciae latae, have been previously described with accompanying benefits and drawbacks.

A new flap graft is proposed for reconstruction of the tendon and overlying skin. This is a free vascular flap derived from the current tensor fasciae latae flap design. Several benefits of this new flap include:

- The tensor fasciae latae muscle is left intact, avoiding instability in the knee.
- Protecting the perforating arteries allows for a thin, well vascularized skin–subcutis–fasciae latae flap, which will reconstruct the defects in the tendon and skin.
- Protecting the lateral cutaneous nerve of the thigh enables the surgeon to preserve sensation in the graft site.
- As a general rule, the donor site is closed primarily avoiding conspicuous scarring.

Patients and Methods—Five patients underwent tensor fasciae latae perforator flap transplant to repair defects in the skin and underlying tendon. The defect was excised with large margins. The graft was lifted ipsilateral to the defect and placed so as to double the fascia latae and repair the tendinous defect. The lifted artery was anastomosed end-to-side to the posterior tibial artery; concomitant veins were joined to the posterior tibial vein either end-to-end or end-to-side.

Postoperative management included a nonweightbearing cast for 4 weeks, followed by a walking cast for 2 weeks, after which physical therapy was initiated. Patients were examined an average of 20 weeks post-transplant, when several criteria were reviewed.

Results—All patients were pleased with the aesthetic outcome at the donor site. The patients had no resulting knee instability or painful scarring. The recipient site was normal, allowing for full function of the ankle and activities of daily living. Plantarflexion strength of the foot was 50–71% normal, as verified with a heel raise test. All patients had noticeable excess tissue in the narrow region of the tendon; three patients subsequently requested debulking procedures, resulting in a more pleasing outcome.

Discussion—The disadvantages of other free flaps and lack of good functional results from conservative treatment or rotational flaps, in the repair of large defects, led to the search of a more appropriate flap for this area. Recipient site was noted to be nontender, with acceptable sensation to touch and pain. Reduced strength noted in the Achilles tendon was within the reported range of other studies. The authors believe the tensor fasciae latae perforator flap is a viable option in the treatment of large defects to the Achilles tendon and overlying skin.—*G. Grant*

♦ This paper describes a technique for composite replacement of the Achilles tendon and its overlying skin. This area, despite lying between the posterior tibial and peroneal arteries, is a rather difficult one to cover, particularly when there is an associated functional deficit. In this paper, a fasciocutaneous free flap is developed, based on perforators to the fascia latae, which come off the ascending branch of the lateral circumflex branch of the femoral artery. This flap produces a good cosmetic result both at the recipient and donor sites and does not produce a functional loss in the thigh. It was reported to function well when integrated into the Achilles tendon. However, in their series of five patients, the strength of the triceps was only 52% of the unaffected limb. This would hardly seem to be an acceptable functional outcome. Perhaps this flap in conjunction with a flexor hallucis transfer would produce the superior cosmetic outcome that the authors report with a more acceptable functional result. — *G.P. Jolly, D.P.M.*

Extensor Digitorum Brevis Free Flap: Anatomic Study and Further Clinical Applications

del Piñal F, Herrero F (Hospital Mutua Montañesa, Santander, Spain)
Plast Reconstr Surg 105(4):1347–1356, 2000

Introduction — The extensor digitorum brevis (EDB) is a muscle flap that has been used as a pedicle or free flap to restore vascularization, sensation, and structure to injured areas. This article further discusses the uses of the EDB to repair injuries in the hand and Achilles tendon.

Case Reports — There are several uses of the EDB. In case 1, this muscle was used as a flow-through free flap to provide complete revascularization and neural restoration of the hand following a severe crush injury. Immediately following the procedure, the hand regained warmth, sensation, and structure. In case 2, a combined EDB-deep peroneal nerve was used to repair an adhered palmar skin graft following a heating press injury. The patient achieved a normal Tinel's sign, sweating, and pain sensation. In case 3, the EDB was used to repair a closed ruptured Achilles tendon. This "T-interposed EDB" used 1.5 cm of the donor anterior tibial artery interposed into the posterior tibial artery. In case 4, a bilobed dorsalis pedis fasciosubcutaneous–EDB combined flap was used to restore structure and function following debridement for compartment syndrome of the hand.

Materials and Methods — Dissection was performed on both feet of 13 fresh cadavers to evaluate the anatomical relationship of the lateral tarsal artery to the EDB. First, the lateral tarsal artery was isolated and freed laterally. Superficial surface dissection was performed while preserving the superficial peroneal nerve and EDB peritenon. Next, deep surface dissection was done and the tendons were cut distally. The lateral tarsal artery was then ligated laterally and the EDB was elevated from its origin.

Results — In all specimens, the lateral tarsal artery and venae comitantes were shown to be the main blood supply to the EDB. When attempts were made to cover the Achilles tendon with the proximally pedicled EDB, several EDBs did not reach the calcaneus–Achilles junction. Two specimens did not have an anterior tibial artery, but this absence was taken over by the perforating peronal artery. This perforating peroneal artery formed a dorsalis pedis artery and lateral tarsal branch. However, these branches were shorter than normal, thereby limiting the uses of the T-interposed EDB.

Conclusions—The dorsalis pedis artery should only be used if the perforating peroneal artery has strong pulses and provides complete revascularization with dorsalis pedis occlusion. The anterior tibial artery is a good choice for interposition because it has a wider diameter so more blood flow can be achieved. In addition, the EDB is a perfect match for hand defects and resists shearing forces well. Because of this, the EDB is a first choice for palm and sole defects that have an associated gap and the authors feel it is an excellent choice for repairing small defects.—*G.H. Jhala*

◆ This paper describes the development of a free flap for small, defects, based on the lateral tarsal artery and the extensor digitorum brevis muscle belly. In the authors series, they report on the use of the muscle with varying pedicle lengths, for use in defects in the hand. For use in the foot, they describe a technique for harvesting the muscle, the lateral tarsal artery, and a small section of the dorsalis pedis artery, as a "T." The dorsalis pedis artery was then reapproximated end-to-end. It is here that this elegant little muscle flap would seem to have its greatest serviceability in the foot.

This flap could be used to cover defects of the posterior heel or the malleoli, by anastomosing the flap to either the posterior tibial artery or to the peroneal artery. Local muscle flaps, such as the abductor hallucis or abductor digiti minimi, have limited arcs of rotation, particularly the digiti minimi. This free flap would certainly seem to be a viable alternative to a latissimus dorsi or gracillis flap, which would offer too much bulk for small defects.

The greatest danger with this flap and its use in the foot is that in harvesting, the dorsalis pedis artery is exposed to injury, and in anastomosing it to either the posterior tibial or to the peroneal artery, the potential for compromise exists as well. Therefore, competence in microvascular surgery is still a prerequisite for anyone contemplating this procedure.—*G.P. Jolly, D.P.M.*

Filleted Toe Flap for Chronic Forefoot Ulcer Reconstruction

Lin C-H, Wei F-C, Chen H-C (Chang Gung Memorial Hospital, Taipei, Taiwan)
Ann Plast Surg 44(4):412–416, 2000

Introduction—The varying locations of forefoot defects require consideration of several reconstructive parameters. Dorsal forefoot defect reconstruction requires thin, resurfaced tissue, while plantar forefoot defects demand sensate, stable, and durable skin flaps. In the case of plantar forefoot lesions, a V-Y advancement flap or a rotation flap can allow small-defect resurfacing, while a free flap is usually required for large-defect resurfacing. Filleted toe flaps, previously reported for use in reconstruction of weightbearing areas of the foot, have been elevated as island flaps and proven reliable for forefoot defects. Justification for the filleting procedure can be obtained by observing that underlying structural abnormalities in forefoot lesions essentially render the toe useless distal to the lesion.

Methods—A total of nine patients (mean age, 55.7 years) with forefoot ulcers, treated with filleted toe flaps, were followed for 1–7 years. Wound etiologies included sequelae of arteriosclerotic ischemic leg, diabetes mellitus, and post-traumatic anesthetic lesions. The procedure was performed under pneumatic tourniquet control, maintaining a soft-tissue cuff around the pedicle in order to ensure adequate neurovascularity to the filleted toe flap.

Results—One filleted second-toe flap for a dorsal chronic diabetic foot ulcer developed a postoperative deep wound infection and subsequent flap necrosis. The remaining eight flaps survived intact and initially attained postreconstructive coverage. Two patients required below-knee and first ray amputations after developing postoperative infections 2 years and 7 months later, respectively.

Discussion—Etiologies of chronic forefoot wounds and trophic ulcers include repeated trauma with nerve dysfunction, repeated trauma with pathological deformity, and tissue ischemia due to vascular insufficiency. Neighboring skin may be damaged in trophic ulcers caused by structural abnormalities or diabetic neuropathy. Similarly, an ischemic limb can produce deleterious effects on same limb local flap microcirculation. Therefore, the use of several flap designs might not be possible. The prevention of ulcer recurrence may be achieved with treatment of the underlying etiology—bypass revascularization in ischemic cases, and bone remodeling in structural deformities. In addition, tight blood sugar control and regular foot care are of the utmost importance in ulcers secondary to diabetic neuropathy. The filleted toe flap is a simple and effective method for the coverage of forefoot defects.—*E. Zarutsky*

♦ The authors report their experience with filleted toe flaps for coverage of dorsal and plantar forefoot defects. The sacrifice of a digit in the form of a soft-tissue blanket yielded a sensate flap of between 4 and 5.5 cm in diameter. Nine patients were reported, with five requiring coverage for dorsal defects and four with plantar defects. Eight flaps survived with only one failure.

The sacrifice of a toe to provide a durable soft-tissue replacement, particularly on the plantar surface, is a relatively small price to pay. Often, plantar ulcers are associated with a dislocated or flail toe, so that there is no real functional loss. Additionally, filleted toe flaps can be converted to an island, which renders it a bipedicled flap with a greatly enhanced arc of rotation. The authors use a dorsal splitting technique, although either a dorsal or plantar approach may be used.—*G.P. Jolly, D.P.M.*

The Reversal Sural Artery Neurocutaneous Island Flap in Composite Lower Extremity Wound Reconstruction

Isenberg JS (University of Oklahoma Health Center and Midwest Regional Medical Center, Midwest City, OK)
J Foot Ankle Surg 39(1):44–48, 2000

Introduction—Reconstruction of complex wounds of the lower extremity is a challenging process. This retrospective study/case presentation reviews the use of the reversal sural artery neurocutaneous island flap (RSANIF) for lower extremity wound management. The study cohort was made up of 15 individuals of 65 years or older. All wounds, which were either ischemic or pressure related, were managed preoperatively with wet-to-dry saline dressing changes. All subjects received a RSANIF. All subjects healed without flap loss.

Case 1—A 72-year-old diabetic male with peripheral vascular disease (PVD) presents with an open, necrotic wound of the right ankle. The wound with underlying osteomyelitis was debrided and treated daily with whirlpool and silverdene dressing. Five days status-postdebridement, the wound was closed with a RSANIF. The patient healed uneventfully and went on to returned to ambulation.

Case 2—A 68-year-old diabetic female with PVD, cirrhosis, and chronic peripheral edema presents with a left lateral ankle pressure wound. The patient has had previous debridement of the wound site with skin grafting that had failed. The patient was treated with a RSANIF. The patient healed uneventfully and went on to return to ambulation.

Discussion/Conclusion—Wound reconstruction in the foot and ankle is a challenging process as there are limited units of muscle and soft tissue available for use. Microvascular transplants do provide the necessary coverage for the most part but are associated with higher morbidity and operative time. Fasciocutaneous flaps incorporating neural elements and associated arterial networks offer the advantages of microvascular transplants, but avoid the disadvantages of morbidity and operative time. The RSANIF additionally has no significant impact on lower extremity perfusion and, as a result, can safely and reliably be used in the elderly patient. The application of the RSANIF in the treatment of complex lower limb wounds is preferred over microvascular transplantation.—*D.D-Q. Tran, D.P.M.*

◆ Soft-tissue reconstruction of the lower leg and rearfoot has always been problematic for surgeons. By and large, significant defects in this area have been addressed by free muscle flaps and more recently free fasciocutaneous flaps. Although retrograde, pedicled flaps based on the anterior tibial, posterior tibial, and peroneal arteries have been described, they have not found much favor in the United States or Europe, due in large part to the sacrifice of a major vascular element of the lower extremity, as well as difficulties with venous congestion. The author reports his experience using a reverse sural artery flap. Although this flap was previously described by Hasegawa et al., Jeng and Wei, Yilmaz et al., and others, this paper reports on a cohort of 15 patients who were 65 years of age or older, all of whom had either diabetes, peripheral vascular disease, or both.

Reported outcomes were universally good with no major flap failures, and the fact that the operation could be done under local anesthesia is quite desirable in this older population with significant comorbidities. Since this flap makes use of the accompanying arteries to the lesser saphenous veins, the operation is technically simpler and avoids the need for venous anastomosis. The average duration of the procedure was less than 2 hours. It is important to note that no attempt was made to preserve the sural nerve, but the sensory loss in the lateral territory of the foot was not reported as problematic. This may well come to replace free muscle flaps for many indications in the lower extremity. This flap can also be modified as a adipofascial flap, used in conjunction with a skin graft for coverage of the Achilles tendon. — *G.P. Jolly, D.P.M.*

Soft-Tissue Reconstruction for Recalcitrant Diabetic Foot Wounds

Cohen BK, Zabel DD, Newton ED, Catanzariti AR (The Western Pennsylvania Hospital, Pittsburgh, PA; University of Pittsburgh Medical Center, Pittsburgh, PA)
J Foot Ankle Surg 38(6):388–393, 1999

Introduction—It is widely known that diabetes mellitus and plantar foot ulceration often are a difficult problem, and various soft-tissue reconstruction methods have been described as aids in the healing of these ulcerations. Medial plantar artery (MPA)-based fasciocutaneous flaps are one such method that has been described, but has not thoroughly been reviewed for efficacy.

Methods—In a retrospective study 33 consecutive patients with plantar soft-tissue defects managed by a single surgeon were reviewed. MPA reconstruction was performed on the heel, midfoot, and forefoot with the average tissue deficit of 13 ± 9 cm^2, most common being in the midfoot. Follow-up averaged 19 months with the etiology of the plantar ulcers consisting of neuropathic neuropathy causing bony deformities. Early (<30 days postop) and late (>30 days postop) complications as well as major (flap failure and amputation) and minor (marginal necrosis and infection resolving uneventfully) complications were identified and noted. All patients had failed previous conservative care (wound care and/or off-loading devices), and each patient had ankle-brachial indices >0.80.

Operative Procedure—After sharp debridement and resection of bony prominences and wound conversion to clean-contaminated wounds, a rotational flap with the intacted ligated medial plantar artery deep to the plantar fascia and tightly adherent to the harvested flap was placed into the area of the defect. Slightly different techniques were used to harvest the MPA flap for forefoot, midfoot, and rearfoot ulcers in order to obtain adequate coverage. All donor sites by flap rotation were covered with skin graft at the time of the surgery.

Results—There were four patients with minor complications, and six with major complications as described earlier. All the patients with major complications were on hemodialysis for renal failure. There were seven patients who underwent readvancement of a previously healed flap to cover recurrent ulcers. Twelve rerotations were performed in those seven patients with an average of 13 months from the initial flap dissection to rerotation.

Discussion—Due to high shear stresses on the weightbearing surfaces of the feet, reconstruction of recalcitrant ulcers with similar tissue is ideal. Medial plantar artery fasciocutaneous flaps not only provide the unique structural features of the plantar foot, but they also allow for continued readvancement of healthy tissue in the diabetic patient who has a increased susceptibility to reulcerate.—*S.B. Heninger*

♦ The authors report their experience with a flap based on the medial plantar artery. Thirty-three patients were reviewed, and all flaps were designed as rotation flaps, rather than islands. Rearfoot and heel defects were closed by rotation of medially based flaps and transection of the medial plantar artery distal to the flap, thereby preserving antegrade flow through cutaneous collaterals. Forefoot defects were closed by medially based flaps with retrograde flow.

Of the 33 flaps, 12 required rerotations to close recurrent ulcerations. Two flaps resulted in frank necrosis. What is difficult to understand is the fact that the 12 rerotations were not considered to be failures. Rerotations were required in approximately one out of every three patients. This is almost the same proportion of failures reported last year by the same authors in this journal. In their previously published report, the majority of their failures were associated with ulcers under the lateral column. Unfortunately, the specific location of the recurrent lesions in this series was not reported.

It is also difficult to assess whether the flaps which survived did so because of the presence of perforators from the medial plantar artery or from the collateral flow from the dorsalis pedis artery via the medial tarsal vessels.—*G.P. Jolly, D.P.M.*

Salvage of the Distal Foot Using the Distally Based Sural Island Flap

Jeng S-F, Wei F-C, Kuo Y-R (Chang Gung Memorial Hospital at Kaohsiung, Chang Gung University, Taiwan, ROC)
Ann Plast Surg 43(5):499–505, 1999

Introduction—Distal foot reconstruction has been difficult especially if there is a lack of local tissue. Current techniques allow for ankle and proximal heel reconstruction. This study presents a technical modification to allow for forefoot reconstruction.

Patients and Methods—Eight patients received distally based sural flap reconstruction to correct for a traumatic soft-tissue defect in seven patients and a chronic ulcer in the last patient. The flap size varied from 6 × 8 cm to 14 × 8 cm. The axis of the flap is marked along the lesser saphenous vein from the politeal fossa to the Achilles tendon. The pivot point is above the lateral malleolus, sparing the medial sural nerve. The skin flap is then moved with the lesser saphenous vein and its accompanied arteries. The skin flap is rotated 180° and passed through a subcutaneous tunnel to reach the defect. The flaps were innervated by coaptation between the lateral sural cutaneous nerves and either the medial or lateral plantar nerves. All flaps were resurfaced with a split-thickness skin graft.

Results—Seven flaps survived and one developed distal necrosis, which was managed successfully. All patients could ambulate well and weightbearing forefoot flaps were sensate and durable. No one developed an ulceration over the transferred flap.

Discussion—Reconstruction of a distal defect of the foot ideally uses sensate tissue from the same region. Many other techniques are possible, but only for small defects. An alternative to skin flaps is muscle flaps with skin grafts, but again these can only fill small defects. Reverse-flow flaps are used in current techniques, but they may cause serious vascular compromise. In other studies, the original skin flap was safe only if taken from the lower two thirds of the posterior leg along the course of the superficial sural artery. In this study, the skin flaps were designed on the lesser saphenous vein in the proximal third of the leg and could reach the forefoot and distal plantar heel. The coaptation of the lateral sural cutaneous nerve provided protective sensation, especially important in weightbearing areas. In summary, this technique is simple and rapid when performed, has a reliable blood supply, does not sacrifice any major blood vessels, and keeps the patient sensate at the flap site.—*F. Nejad*

♦ The authors present a series of eight patients who underwent soft-tissue reconstruction of the foot using a distally based skin island from the sural artery. All patients were operated on because of traumatic soft-tissue loss. All injuries involved the distal forefoot. The lateral sural nerve was coapted to either the medial or lateral plantar nerves, and according to the authors, the flaps retained sensibility, with static two-point discrimination between 17 and 30 mm. No subsequent ulcerations were reported.

The clinical use of this flap, based on its frequency in the literature, appears to be increasing. Despite the distance that the pedicle has to pass, venous congestion did not develop. Despite the distance and bend that the pedicle was forced to take, the flow through the lesser saphenous vein was unaffected. This is in contrast to smaller island flaps where the cross section of those veins is significantly smaller in relation to the diameter of the supplying arteries. — *G.P. Jolly, D.P.M.*

16 Interesting Cases/ Case Reports

Stuart Tessler, D.P.M.

Squamous Cell Carcinoma Arising from Lesions of Porokeratosis Palmaris et Plantaris Disseminata

Seishima M, Izumi T, Oyama Z, Maeda M (Ogaki Municipal Hospital, Minaminokawa-cho, Japan)
Eur J Dermatol 10:478–480, 2000

Introduction—An autosomal dominant condition termed porokeratosis palmaris et plantaris disseminata (PPPD) exists as a rare variant of porokaratosis. Lesions traditionally first appear on the palms and soles in the 2nd decade of life and progressively involve the entire trunk and extremities. PPPD lesions present an increased incidence of squamous cell carcinoma. Treatment consists of oral retenoids, which are purported to decrease the likelihood of malignant changes.

Case Report—At the age of 28, a Japanese man with a negative familial history of the disease was diagnosed with PPPD. The patient reported to the Ogaki Municipal Hospital in Japan at the age of 43. At that time, he was noted to have numerous papules ranging from 1 to 1.5 mm in diameter on both the dorsal and plantar surfaces of his hands and feet with no involvement of the face, scalp, or trunk. Histological examination of a biopsy revealed tightly packed columns of parakeratotic cells in the cornified layer, absence of a granular layer, and dyskeratotic keratinocytes in the lower epidermis. The patient was treated with etretinate (10–50 mg/day) and with 10% topical urea ointment for approximately 14 years. Due to the consistent size and location of the lesions, the patient decided to discontinue treatment. At age 63, this gentleman reported to Ogaki Hospital with bilateral posterior calcaneal erosions of which a 2-mm punch biopsy was taken. Histological findings were consistent with squamous cell carcinoma: atypical keratinocytes in the epidermis with mononulccear infiltration of the upper dermis. CT of the entire body was negative for any abnormal findings and a Gallium scan did not indicate any presence of metastasis. Subsequently the diagnosis of squamous cell carcinoma secondary to PPPD was made and five erosions were removed within 1 cm of the margins.

Discussion—With absent familial involvement, histological evidence of PPPD provided the criteria necessary for the diagnosis. The cessation of the retinoid treatment for 1.5 years did not exacerbate the extent of the disease in this patient. The research yields conflicting results: both absence and cessation of retinoid therapy show similar relapse rates. It has been shown that the lesions of PPPD evolve from hypertrophy of abnormal basal coronoid cells resulting in malignant changes. Lesional keratinocytes of PPPD tend to overexpression of the p53 oncogene in malignant transformation. In this case, the lesions noted by histological evaluation to be squamous cell carcinoma were noticed by the patient only 9 months after cessation of retinoid treatment. Although the mechanism is unknown, this suggests retinoids might have an inhibitory effect on malignant changes caused by PPPD.—*K.E. Van Voris*

♦ The condition that commonly is characterized by multiple hyperkeratotic lesions of the palms and soles may not be as benign as we often expect. As it is reasonable that individuals with the lesions of porokeratosis palmaris et plantaris disseminata (PPPD) and similar conditions may find themselves seeking treatment for the foot lesions, biopsy of characteristic lesions is indicated to assist in the diagnosis. There is a need for awareness of the potential for malignant change in the lesions. This case provides one experience that the retinoid, etretinate, may have protected against the development of squamous cell carcinoma in a man with PPPD. The author points out other reports of the use of oral retinoids being effectively used in PPPD and the protection from malignant changes in the lesions.—*S. Tessler, D.P.M.*

Treatment of Keratoderma Blennorrhagicum with Tazarotene Gel 0.1%

Lewis A, Nigro M, Rosen T (Baylor College of Medicine, Veteran's Affairs Medical Center, Houston, TX)
J Am Acad Dermatol 43(2):400–402, 2000

Background—Hereditary or acquired palmo-plantar keratodermas are a heterogeneous group of diseases characterized by hyperkeratosis of the palms and/or soles. In diseases such as Reiter's syndrome, therapy is traditionally determined by and directed toward arthropathy, not the cutaneous manifestations. As a result, current treatment of keratoderma has been inconsistent and transient, with little reported efforts to determine efficient and effective treatment.

A case of Reiter's syndrome is presented here, where the major cutaneous manifestation, keratoderma blennorrhagicum, is nearly completely obliterated after topical application of tazarotene gel 0.1%.

Case Report—A 64-year-old man with a 15-year history of Reiter's syndrome presents with keratoderma blennorrhagicum. His keratoderma had been consistently refractory to treatment with keratolytics (salicylic acid and urea) or topical corticosteroids.

On physical exam, the patient had erythematous thick and painful superficial erosions. The treatment consisted of daily application of tazarotene gel 0.1% to the soles. In 4 weeks, the patient had significant reduction in pain and hyperkeratosis. At 8 weeks, the keratoderma was completely resolved. The patient stopped using the gel and at 12 weeks follow-up, the patient remained free of the disease.

Discussion—The cutaneous keratodermas share a common characteristic of hyperkeratosis. Regardless of the origin or cause, current treatments are ineffective against these disorders.

Reiter's syndrome is similar to psoriasis/psoriatic arthropathy in presentation and feature. These features include radiologic, cutaneous, and histologic findings; nail abnormalities; sausage digits; oligoarthropathy; sacroiliitis; and heel pain. They both are rheumatoid factor and antinuclear antibody (ANA) seronegative and have increased incidence of HLA-B27 positivity. Keratoderma blennorrhagicum and the skin lesions of psoriasis are both hyperproliferative cutaneous diseases.

Due to the similarities between these two diseases, there has been increased interest in treating keratoderma blennorrhagicum with agents proven to be effective for psoriasis. One agent that has been effective in treating psoriasis is retinoids. Since clinical and histopathologic features of keratoderma blennorrhagicum are almost identical to pustular psoriasis, topical tazarotene was used to treat this recalcitrant case of keratoderma blennorrhagicum.

Retinoids have been found to form complexes with receptors that modulate transcription and thus hyperkeratosis. This mechanism is probably why topical tazarotene worked in this case of keratoderma blennorrhagicum. Tazarotene is receptor selective and allows for decreased side effects, compared to other retinoids. The limited systemic absorption of tazarotene makes it safer than oral retinoids and immunosuppressive drugs in the treatment of regional cutaneous disorders.—*O.T. Wang, D.P.M.*

♦ While not a commonly presenting disease, Reiter's syndrome patients may complain of foot-associated problems initially. The keratoderma blennorrhagicum may be the secondary symptom in the foot behind the arthralgia and heel pain. The thick keratotic plaques, often accompanied by fissures, had lent itself to regular debridement and the use of salicylic acid preparations for chemical debridement. These methods have not been particularly satisfactory, as the process does not lead to resolution of the lesions.

The report's use of tazarotene gel 0.01%, a retinoid, currently prescribed for the treatment of the keratotic plaques of psoriasis and for acne, apparently acts by suppressing the development of hyperkeratosis. Interest may develop to investigate the use of tazarotene gel in other situations with profound hyperkeratosis of the soles, which do not fall within the categories of psoriasis or Reiter's syndrome. — *S. Tessler, D.P.M.*

Methicillin-Resitant *Staphylococcus aureus* Infections in 2 Pediatric Outpatients

Feder HM Jr (Connecticut Children's Medical Center, Hartford, CT)
Arch Fam Med 9:560–562, 2000

Introduction—Community-acquired methicillin-resistant *Staphylococcus aureus* (MRSA) infections are unusual in children. The author presents two unrelated cases of unsuspected MRSA infections in children.

Case 1—A 19-month-old girl was seen and treated with oral cephalexin for cervical adenitis. After 3 days of outpatient therapy, the patient was hospitalized. On admission, her temperature was 104°F, peripheral leukocyte count was 24.5×10^9/L, erythrocyte sedimentation rate (ESR) was 45 mm/h, and a 3×4 cm tender cervical node was present. She was treated with intravenous cephazolin for 3 days, without resolution. She was then taken to the operating room where an incision and drainage were performed. Cultures were positive for MRSA and therapy was changed to vancomycin. Her symptoms resolved over the next 5 days. Careful history revealed no exposure to someone at risk for MRSA.

Case 2—A 10-year-old girl presented to her physician with a 1-week history of a tender, erythematous, swollen fourth toe. There was no history of trauma or prior problems with the toe. Physical examination was significant only for edema, erythema, calor, and pain to the distal portion of the toe. Radiographs were normal. The patient was treated with oral cephadroxil for 10 days, without resolution. Radiographs upon follow-up showed a lytic lesion of the middle phalanx of the digit, consistent with osteomyelitis. Complete blood cell count and ESR were normal. She was admitted for surgical debridement. Cultures were positive for a pure heavy growth of MRSA, susceptible to several antibiotics. The patient was treated with 4 weeks of intravenous clindamycin, with complete resolution. She had no exposure to someone at risk for MRSA.

Discussion—Reports of community-acquired MRSA infections have recently been reported in children. In some studies, up to 48% of pediatric patients hospitalized with MRSA infections had community-acquired MRSA without an identified exposure. In contrast to nosocomial MRSA, community-acquired MRSA is usually sensitive to a number of antibiotics, including clindamycin. — *T.C. Melillo, D.P.M.*

◆ There needs to be an increasing awareness that MRSA may not only be hospital-acquired. This troubling pathogen is increasingly found in community-acquired infections, and as presented in the reported cases, in children. Perhaps we should not assume that the superficial infection that has so readily responded to penicillin and cephalosporin in the past will continue to do so. There is need to monitor patients with infections and make a greater effort to obtain cultures when there is a failure of the infection to respond to the prescribed antibiotics. Fortunately, as reported, most MRSA are still sensitive to vancomycin and often other antibiotics including clindamycin, trimethoprim/sulfamethoxazole, and quinolones.—*S. Tessler, D.P.M.*

A New Ambulatory Foot Pressure Device for Patients with Sensory Impairment. A System for Continuous Measurement of Plantar Pressure and a Feed-back Alarm

Pataky Z, Faravel L, Da Silva J, Assal JP (University Hospital of Geneva, Geneva, Switzerland)
J Biomech 33:1135–1138, 2000

Background—The ability to sense pain is critical in the prevention of injury, and those with nerve damage are at risk of ulceration. Patients without protective pain sensation from metabolic disorders like diabetes mellitus, infectious diseases like leprosy, or from traumatic lesions leading to paraplegia are all in danger of ulcerating under areas of unusually high plantar pressure. Elsevier Science Ltd. has created a device which diagnostically records these areas of excessive plantar pressure and, more importantly, provides the patient with a signal, warning them to off-load the area. Such a device could reduce the morbidity of plantar ulceration and amputations, and ultimately reduce the mortality of this at-risk population.

Methods—It has been reported that 94% of diabetic ulcers occur under areas of increased pressure. Combining this plantar pressure with sensory neuropathy and peripheral vascular disease leads many diabetics down a complicated road of ulcers and difficulty in healing. Reducing excessive plantar pressure has been paramount to the treatment of neuropathic ulcers, and hence to the prevention of amputations. A device has been developed to measure peak pressure and to warn the patient when pressures get dangerously high; its description follows.

The ambulatory foot pressure device (AFPD) utilizes a Holter-type instrument of plantar pressure acquisition allowing for continuous in-shoe recordings for up to 8 hours of ambulation. The device works on Force Sensing Resistors 174 sensors coated with 1-mm-thick silicon and exhibits roughly 98% reproducibility. The AFPD can measure maximum pressure values, integrals of pressure over time, and the duration of plantar pressure. The sensors are applied to areas of risk such as metatarsal heads, the hallux, or the styloid process of the fifth metatarsal. The sensor is then connected to the AFPD—15.5 × 9.5 × 3.2 cm^3 in size—which is worn at the belt. The AFPD is rigged with an audible alarm activated by pressures exceeding a predetermined threshold. This Critical Risk Pressure (CRP) is adjusted by the physician, calculated at 20%, 40%, or 60% of peak pressure. The AFPD stores in its memory peak pressures, duration of plantar pressures over the CRP, the number of gait cycles, as well as the number of cycles over the CRP. After 8 days or 60,000 gait cycles, the data are downloaded into a computer.

Discussion—When a diabetic patient develops peripheral neuropathy, ulcers tend to form in areas of excessive pressure because of their reduced protective threshold. Off-loading these areas is key to ulcer healing. The AFPD offers not only a diagnostic tool for podiatric physicians to pinpoint areas at risk for ulceration, but provides neuropathic patients with a protective modality. With the acoustic signal, behavioral changes and alterations of gait can reduce plantar pressures to a safe level.—*C. Jacka*

♦ The success of this device in preventing or, as an adjunct, in closing plantar ulcers is solely dependent on the motivation of the patient. There is a subset of our patients with diabetes and neuropathy who are so motivated that when confronted with the logical course of the development of the plantar ulcer, they may be able to modify the weightbearing stresses to the forefoot. This is accomplished, in part, by reducing the stride length and speed of walking. Any device that is dependent on the user's voluntary participation is not likely going to be effective in the long term. These patients do not voluntarily modify their shoes and other behaviors, even when faced with the prospect of amputation, and likely will not respond to an acoustic alarm. The stride length shortening effect of the use of a rocker sole shoe which reduces the forces at toe-off will be much more effective in preventing and closing plantar ulcers.—*S. Tessler, D.P.M*

Chronic Ergot Toxicity: A Rare Cause of Lower Extremity Ischemia

Garcia GD, Goff JM Jr, Hadro NC, O'Donnell SD, Greatorex PS (Womack Army Medical Center, Ft. Bragg, NC; Walter Reed Army Medical Center, Washington, DC; Uniformed Services University of the Health Sciences, Bethesda, MD)
J Vasc Surg 31:1245–1247, 2000

Introduction—Chronic ergot toxicity, usually a result of long-term usage of ergot-containing medication, is a rare cause of lower extremity ischemia. Ergot toxicity, whether acute or chronic, is most often associated with women in their mid-30s who suffer from migraine headaches. Ergot alkaloids induce central sypatholytic activity and peripheral alpha-adrenergic blockade and directly stimulate smooth muscle. More importantly for migraine sufferers, ergotamine decreases the vasodilation of cranial arteries. However, three classes of side effects may occur with ergot toxicity: neurologic side effects, alimentary side effects, and vascular side effects. A case report of long-term ergot use for migraine headaches in a woman who developed severe chronic lower extremity claudication is presented here.

Case Report—A 34-year-old woman presented with a 4-year history of progressive, bilateral lower extremity claudication and consequently was able to ambulate 50–75 feet before the onset of bilateral calf pain. She had a history of migraine headaches, which were first diagnosed at age 13, and since then has taken ergot-containing medication (Cafergot and Migri Diaxadol) almost daily. Physical exam revealed absent pedal pulses bilateral, atrophic pedal skin, and superficial ulcers on the great toes of both feet. Vascular ergot toxicity was discovered through the use of an arteriogram. At this time, all ergotamine-containing medications were discontinued and aspirin was prescribed. Within 3 months, the patient had showed progressive improvement and palpable pedal pulses were found. The superficial ulcers healed and the patient reported that she could walk 100 yards before the onset of pain.

Discussion—Ergot toxicity treatment primarily consists of discontinuing the use of cigarettes, caffeine, and all ergot-containing medications. Although no specific treatment is used uniformly, conservative measures, such as observation and administration of antiplatelet agents, have been found to be effective if they are implemented after the discontinuance of ergot-containing medications. However, should the symptoms progress to rest pain or gangrene, surgical treatment is an option and therefore should be considered.

Conclusion—After a 34-year-old woman presented to the clinic with chronic arterial insufficiency, it was found that her 20-year history of ergot use was the cause. Caffeine use, cigarettes, and all ergot-containing medications were stopped and aspirin was given. The patient's condition improved remarkably after 3 months. —*A. Duckworth*

♦ This is one of those cases that may cause the light bulb over one's head to light, explaining the apparent vascular insufficiency in an otherwise healthy young female. Ergot intoxication is indeed uncommon. I have encountered this only once in 29 years of practice. In that case the woman was consuming vast quantities of the ergotamine over a long period, having become dependent on it and requiring increasing quantities for relief of the migraine headaches. She presented with superficial ulcers of the heels, fifth toes, and plantar fifth metatarsal heads. The publication of this case can increase our index of suspicion for ergot toxicity.—*S. Tessler, D.P.M.*

Fine Needle Aspiration of Tophi for Crystal Identification in Problematic Cases of Gout: A Report of Two Cases

Rege J, Shet T, Naik L (Bai Yamunabai Laxmanrao Nair Charitable Hospital and Topiwala National Medical College, Mumbai, India)
Acta Cytol 44(3):433–436, 2000

Introduction—Demonstration of monosodium urate crystals in the synovial fluid or biopsy provides a definitive diagnosis of gout. Similarly, gouty tophi are one of the important differential diagnoses of periarticular nodules. Yet, the recognition of the nodules as tophi is often missed due to the fact that the clinical diagnosis of gout is not straightforward. Consequently, the use of fine-needle aspiration cytology (FNAC) in such a setting could facilitate the clinical diagnosis and treatment of gout.

Case 1—A 36-year-old chronic alcoholic male presented with three swellings: one on each malleolus (the swelling on the lateral malleolus had ulcerated and was infected) and one on the base of the left fifth metatarsal. The patient's serum urate was normal and radiologic findings of the foot were normal. FNA was performed on the nonulcerated nodule of the base of the fifth metatarsal. The aspirating needle was flushed with absolute alcohol, which was then subjected to polarization microscopy.

Case 2—A 50-year-old diabetic male presented with multiple nodules on the middorsum of the foot, sole, and lateral malleolus. Bony erosions, suspicious for gout, were found at the second metatarsophalangeal joint on a foot roentgenogram, but joint aspiration failed. The patient's uric acid levels were normal. Similar to case I, FNA was performed on a nodule on the dorsum of the foot.

Results—In case 1, papanicolaou-stained smears produced easily recognizable crystals and acute and chronic inflammatory cells, which were scattered throughout. In case 2, blood in the background made crystal identification using stained smears difficult; however, at high power, delicate crystals trapped in blood could be seen. In both cases, long, thin, needle-shaped crystals were discovered using the wet mount preparations from the needle washings.

Discussion—FNAC can be utilized to confirm the diagnosis of gout. It provides an alternative to synovial biopsy and joint fluid analysis because it has the advantage of being simpler, less painful, and easily repeatable and not requiring an operating room or sterile setup. In addition, as the crystals are preserved in stained smears, they can be employed for polarization and confirmation of gout.—*A. Duckworth*

♦ Fine-needle aspiration of a periarticular nodule in the foot yielding a chalky white material is an effective and easy way to arrive at a diagnosis of gout. There should be a high index of suspicion for gouty tophi in the situation of a superficial nodule at, for instance, the DIPJ of a lesser toe. The skin is often slightly movable over the firm nodule that may or may not be tender. Attempted aspiration of the nodule with an 18- or 22-gauge needle reveals the characteristically appearing chalky white material. Often, the material can be more easily extruded through the opening created with the 18-gauge needle than can be aspirated. While it is most often assumed, cytology of the specimen with emphasis on observation for crystals should be performed on the aspirant or extruded material for confirmation of gouty tophus.—*S. Tessler, D.P.M.*

Diabetic Bullae: 12 Cases of a Purportedly Rare Cutaneous Disorder

Lipsky BA, Baker PD, Ahroni JH (University of Washington School of Medicine and General Internal Medicine Clinic, Veterans Affairs Puget Sound Health Care System, Seattle, WA)
Int J Dermatol 39:196–200, 2000

Background—About one in three patients with diabetes mellitus suffers from some cutaneous disorder. Defects in collagen production, vasculopathy, neuropathy, and immune deficits can often be the underlying cause. Skin disorders, some common like acanthosis nigricans and diabetic thick skin, others less so like necrobiosis lipoidica diabeticorum, pigmented purpuric dermatoses, acquired perforating dermatoses, and yellow skin, are all considered markers of the disease. Three cutaneous disturbances are essentially diagnostic of diabetes: syndrome of limited joint mobility and waxy skin, diabetic dermopathy, and diabetic bullae. These recurrent bullae that erupt mostly on acral surfaces have unknown etiology. The syndrome is purportedly rare, yet 12 cases were seen at VA Puget Sound Health Care System within an 8-year period, and are reported here.

Methods—The above site specializes in the care of diabetic foot problems and receives referrals from the university-affiliated hospital. Diagnoses of the diabetic bullae were established by clinical findings without any other tenable diagnosis. To be included, the lesions had to painless, free of primary infection, and filled with clear drainage; the history had to be free of trauma and hypersensitivity or any other cutaneous or systemic disorder. The lesions resolved with no specific treatment leaving no scar; bullae were aspirated, some of which were sent to pathology for culture.

Results—Within 8 years, 12 diabetic bullae were diagnosed, most commonly involving the toes. Two cases involved the heel and two others affected the anterior tibia. Recurrence without history of trauma appeared to be the trend, as eight of nine patients whose information was available related similar episodes in the past, although a diagnosis was never made. For most patients, the bullous lesions resolved with local care alone; five patients received oral antibiotics and one was given topical antibiotics for secondary infections incurred during the course of treatment, and all initially healed without scar. Two patients, however, required amputation of the affected limb secondary to complications at least partially related to the bullous pathology.

Discussion—A clinical presentation with sudden appearance of painless and tense blisters, usually but not confined to acral regions of the body, is indicative of this distinct skin disorder in patients with diabetes mellitus. Once termed "bullosis diabeticorum," this diabetic bulla shows correlation with peripheral neuropathy, yet previous reports indicate adequate lower extremity perfusion. Lesions most commonly present at the distal tips of the toes or the plantar surfaces of feet show no surrounding erythema or induration, and can be as large as several centimeters and as small as a few millimeters. Bullae arise as tense blisters containing clear fluid, unless secondary bleeding or infection creates sanguineous or cloudy drainage, and becomes more flaccid as they increase in size. Given 2–5 weeks, these lesions will spontaneously heal without a residual scar, consistent with a cleavage plane above the dermoepithelial junction. Proposed causes of impaired anchoring fibrils are microangiopathy, immune-mediated vasculitis, and disturbed calcium, magnesium, and carbohydrate metabolism. Treatment is directed at preventing infection and letting it heal on its own. Aspiration minimizes discomfort and prevents accidental rupture; the superficial skin provides good covering for the lesion and should be left intact, simply covering with a sterile dressing. The incidence of diabetic bullae appears to be more common than previously thought; therefore podiatrists and diabetologists alike should be aware.—*C. Jacka*

♦ The treating physician likely does not recognize bullae that present in people with diabetes as "diabetic bullae," often believing the lesions are the result of excessive shoe friction or resulting from a thermal injury. As these patients are insensate, and are not necessarily reliable in providing an accurate history, we too often do not believe the bullae arise without antecedent trauma. In communication with others who see large numbers of patients with diabetes, these lesions should not be considered rare, a conclusion reached by the authors. The treatment should focus on preventing infection and education of the patient to act appropriately if new lesions occur.—*S. Tessler, D.P.M.*

Correction of Scar Contracture Deformities of the Big Toe with a Multiplanar Distraction Device

Lin S-D, Tsai C-C, Lin T-M, Lee S-S (Chung-Ho Memorial Hospital, Kaohsiung Medical University, Kaohsiung, Taiwan)
Ann Plast Surg 44(3):320–323, 2000

Introduction—Gradual skeletal distraction/distraction osteogenesis techniques are derived from Ilizarov procedures, and are usually used on long bones for extremity reconstruction. The Multi-Guide is the next generation of these devices and has previously been used in mandibular reconstruction work. This device has many applications as it offers multiplane correction. The following is a case report in which the Multi-Guide device is used for correction of a multiplane digital deformity.

Case Report—A 65-year-old female presents with contracture deformities of her right hallux and second toe secondary to heavy scarring. The patient has been unable to wear shoes for 28 years secondary to the deformity of her digits. The patient also had a recent unhealed ulcer on the dorsum of her foot that had resolved after the application of a fillet flap harvested from the second toe. The Multi-Guide device was employed to position the hallux into a more functional position. Two pins were placed from dorsal to plantar in both the first metatarsal and proximal phalanx, respectively. The pins were placed perpendicular to the long axis of the respective bone. The patient was seen as an outpatient, and adjustment was performed on the device twice a week. The hallux deformity was corrected from 43° to 0° in the sagittal plane and from 22° to 0° in the transverse plane. This correction was achieved after 3 weeks, and the device was maintained in place for an additional 4 weeks. Kirschner wires were placed into the proximal phalanx to maintain the correction and were removed after 6 weeks. At 8 months follow-up, the hallux was noted to still be in good functional position.

Discussion—For multiplane deformities, conventional correction would involve complicated surgical procedures. These complicated endeavors are not without challenge and results may be unpredictable. Through the use of the Multi-Guide device, complicated surgical intervention was avoided.—*D.D-Q. Tran, D.P.M.*

♦ The ultimate uses of the multiplanar distraction devices for the correction of foot deformities have not been fully explored. It is interesting to see the device used for a strictly soft-tissue-maintained deformity. There is an acknowledged basic impatience on the part of many surgeons and also patients that often precludes the use of the distraction devices in foot surgery. There may be situations following extensive tissue loss with associated contractures and deformity where extensive surgical intervention may not be desirable. With the use of a distraction device to prepare the soft tissues for a separate surgical intervention to accomplish the structural correction, perhaps more secure results could be obtained with less soft-tissue trauma. The use of the devices to correct the common structural and positional deformities of the foot should be studied utilizing sound investigational procedures. — *S. Tessler, D.P.M.*

Dorsalis Pedis Artery Aneurysm: Case Report and Literature Review

McKee TI, Fisher JB (Easton Hospital, Easton, PA)
J Vasc Surg 31(3):589–591, 2000

Case Report—A 71-year-old noninsulin-dependent diabetes mellitus female patient presented to a general surgeon's office to evaluate a cyst on her right foot. The mass was noticed 2 months earlier and had been increasing in size. The patient experienced no pain and only related some pruritis. The lesion was palpated as a pulsatile mass over the dorsalis pedis artery. The patient underwent a duplex scan to confirm a diagnosis of dorsalis pedis artery aneurysm. The aneurysm was excised and measured 1.5 cm × 0.6 cm.

Background—Aneurysm of the dorsalis pedis artery is a rare finding; in fact only 14 cases have been reported to date. Some are true aneurysms, while others are traumatic/pseudoaneurysms. Four cases have been found to be true aneurysms, while the others are secondary to trauma or imaging modalities. With a true aneurysm of the dorsalis pedis artery, duplex scan of the abdominal aorta, iliac, femoral, and popliteal arteries should be performed to rule out multiple aneurysms.

Discussion—Of the four true aneurysms only two were described histopathologically. They were idiopathic or isolated lesions. In the 71-year-old female, the lesion was found to be an aneurysm associated with epithelioid hemangioma. Ligation with or without excision is performed in most cases, and some authors feel the two segments should be anastomosed. If the posterior tibial artery demonstrates adequate foot perfusion, ligation may be indicated. A dorsalis pedis artery aneurysm is truly a rare finding; however, if one is to ever see one, it is imperative that a duplex scan of the abdominal aorta, iliac, femoral, and popliteal arteries be performed. — *K. Carriero*

♦ This interesting report was made more so by the number of cases cited from the podiatric literature. The authors reported that in their 71-year-old patient, they elected to ligate the dorsalis pedis (DP) artery versus anastomosing the remaining normal artery after excision of the aneurysm. They evaluated the posterior tibial

(PT) artery on the arteriogram and determined it was patent. The presence of a palpable PT pulse may be sufficient information to proceed to ligating the DP in situations of inadvertent injury as can occur in the resection of a dorsal boss and associated bursa or midtarsal arthrodesis when subperiosteal dissection is not performed appropriately.—*S. Tessler, D.P.M.*

Vancomycin-Resistant *Enterococci* Infected Puncture Wound to the Foot

Hayes DW Jr, Mandracchia VJ, Buddecke DE, Rissman LJ (Broadlawns Medical Center and University of Osteopathic Medicine and Health Sciences, Des Moines, IA)
Clin Podiatr Med Surg 17(1):159–164, 2000

Introduction—*Enterococci* are common nosocomial pathogens implicated in bacterial infections, including the urinary tract, surgical wounds, and bacteremia. The prevalence of Vancomycin-resistant *enterococci* (VRE) infections is increasing in hospitals nationwide, typically affecting the sick and elderly. Difficult to eradicate, VRE appears to be transmitted person-to-person, with isolates recovered from many common surfaces. Infective risk factors include prior surgery, immunosuppression, antibiosis with broad-spectrum cephalosporins or aminoglycosides, and prolonged hospitalization. Vancomycin resistance is more frequent with *Enterococcus faecium*.

Case Report—A 26-year-old man presented to the emergency department with a superficial puncture wound to the right lateral rearfoot. He denied any trauma and there was no sign of infection. The wound was cleansed, dressed, and the patient was prescribed Darvocet N-100 and cephalexin 500 mg. One week later, the patient noted minor discomfort in the affected area; the wound appearance was unchanged with minimal clear drainage. Both medications were continued. On presentation to the podiatry service 3 weeks later, the patient could not ambulate and complained of severe pain unrelieved by medication. The wound demonstrated no visible improvement with completion of the cephalexin regimen; it was edematous and warm with purulent drainage. Cellulitis was localized to the lateral rearfoot and ankle. Right ankle range of motion was absent. Neurovascular status was intact, protective threshold and sharp-dull discrimination were present, and radiographs revealed no foreign body in the wound area.

Clinical evidence of severe infection mandated immediate incision and drainage. The wound demonstrated purulence but neither sinus tracts nor osteomyelitic changes to the lateral calcaneus. The wound was cleansed with pulse lavage and packed open with 0.25-inch nu-gauze. Deep cultures grew Vancomycin- and tetracycline-resistant *E. faecalis*, with corynebacterium, *S. aureus*, and *S. epidermidis*, but no anaerobes. The patient was prescribed levofloxacin 500 mg, Percocet, and discharged to home. He returned 3 days postoperatively reporting minor discomfort at the 4 × 2 cm wound.

Edema and erythema were slight without cellulitis or drainage. The packing was removed to allow healing by secondary intention. At 10 days follow-up, the wound demonstrated significant granulation with no clinical signs of infection. All health care workers were alerted to the presence of VRE infection to help prevent its transmission.

Discussion—This case is unique because VRE is rarely seen in a young healthy adult and the patient had none of the typical risk factors associated with such infections. This is the first reported incident of VRE secondary to a puncture wound of the foot. Since the patient's symptoms were not improved by cephalexin, and because corynebacterium is often a contaminant, it is likely that *E. faecalis* was a pathogen. The method of transmission was not determinable.

Conclusion—Laboratory susceptibility testing is crucial for antibiotic selection. Beyond levofloxacin, the combination of ceftriaxone plus Vancomycin and gentamicin can be effective against VRE. With the frequent empiric Vancomycin administration for various infections when methicillin-resistant staphylococci is suspected, resistant strains appear. The prudent assessment of Vancomycin use is imperative. A new class of antibiotics in development, the semisynthetic streptogramnins, offer promise for the treatment of multiresistant infections. Synercid, a bacterial protein synthesis inhibitor, is now available for severe cases of VRE.—*D. Collman*

♦ Until recently, most podiatrists did not encounter Vancomycin-resistant *enterococci* (VRE) in practice. The hospital-acquired infection with the organism requires scrupulous attention to detail and following the institution's policies and procedures to isolate the patient and prevent the spread of the organism. Hospitals maintain registries of their patients who have had positive cultures demonstrating VRE and consider the patient infected or a carrier until negative cultures from multiple sites are obtained. Even though the patient may be admitted for an unrelated problem months after a previous culture positive for VRE, expect the infection control procedures to take precedent. In outpatient surgery, the resulting changes in the time of the case, patient handling, and room preparation are all designed to prevent transmission of VRE.—*S. Tessler, D.P.M.*

Author Index

Subject Index

Note: Page numbers followed by letters *f* and *t* indicate figures and tables, respectively.